"The pivotal role of critical psychotherapy in the emancipation of disabled people has been largely ignored. This foundational reading drives an essential conversation surrounding the potential of depth-oriented, subversive and liberatory psychotherapy. It uncovers the links between ableist ideology, material barriers to participation, and the subjective worlds of disabled people, through interrogating the unconscious underpinnings of inequality."

Brian Watermeyer, Ph.D., *Associate Professor, Stellenbosch University, Division of Disability & Rehabilitation Studies*

"This extraordinary comprehensive handbook is the first to provide a relational and family-focused, systemic, contextual, and disability studies informed framework. This 'go-to' text will be an extremely valuable resource to seasoned clinicians, scholars, and graduate students across mental healthcare disciplines. Manasi and colleagues provide a wealth of evidence-based therapeutic interventions as well as training and programmatic guidelines to help meet the challenges for disabled individuals, couples, and families."

John Rolland, Ph.D., *Professor of Psychiatry, Northwestern University; Co-Founder, Chicago Center for Family Health*

THE HANDBOOK OF DISABILITY-AFFIRMATIVE SYSTEMIC THERAPY

This comprehensive handbook provides therapists, social workers, educators, and mental health professionals with effective clinical interventions for working affirmatively with disabled clients and their families.

Using an intersectional and strengths-based perspective, Manasi Shankar brings together interdisciplinary experts to outline the history of the disability community in the United States, their resultant experiences, and best practices in clinically affirmative care. Chapters are authored by disabled scholars, marriage and family therapists, disability activists, and researchers to amplify the voices of disabled experts. Topics include models of disability, ableism, disability in older populations, sexuality, disability, and persons of color, moving toward the critical role of marriage and family therapists and the ways they can integrate affirmative approaches into their work.

Filled with case vignettes, this handbook offers clinical applications of treatment strategies as well as pedagogical features for educators to supervise and instruct graduate students in working with disabled clients in therapy. This book aims to inspire therapists to incorporate disability dialogue into clinical practice, deconstructing the fragmentation of disability as outside the scope of marriage and family therapy (MFT).

This text is an essential reading for graduate and licensed marriage and family therapists, clinical social workers, counselors, and educators in MFT, counseling, and psychology.

Manasi Shankar, Ph.D., is a clinician, educator, and scholar who specializes in disability-affirmative systemic therapy. She is the founder of *Therapy at Bay* – a private practice based in the San Francisco Bay area and – provides national and international training on systemic therapy with disabled clients and families.

THE HANDBOOK OF DISABILITY-AFFIRMATIVE SYSTEMIC THERAPY

Effective Clinical Care with Disabled Clients and their Families

Edited by
Manasi Shankar

Routledge
Taylor & Francis Group
NEW YORK AND LONDON

Designed cover image: Mariam Paré. Portraits of Spinal Cord Injury: Oppo (2023)
Image Credit: "By courtesy of the Association of Mouth and Foot Painting Artists Worldwide."

First published 2026
by Routledge
605 Third Avenue, New York, NY 10158

and by Routledge
4 Park Square, Milton Park, Abingdon, Oxon, OX14 4RN

Routledge is an imprint of the Taylor & Francis Group, an informa business

ISBN: 978-1-032-42388-3 (hbk)
ISBN: 978-1-032-42386-9 (pbk)
ISBN: 978-1-003-36258-6 (ebk)

DOI: 10.4324/9781003362586

Typeset in Times New Roman
by codeMantra

To families around the world who live with, and resist disability and disablism; may this work stand as a reflection of humility, perseverance, and a commitment to creating accessible, safe, and healing mental health spaces that have long been overdue.

CONTENTS

ABOUT THE COVER ARTIST

Mariam Paré became a quadriplegic after surviving an act of gun violence at the age of 20. Determined to pursue her passion for art, she relearned how to paint by holding brushes with her mouth, evolving into a distinguished visual artist and mouth-painter. With over two decades of creative experience, Paré is known for her exceptional mouth-painting technique and compelling multimedia works that often explore the disability experience. She is a 3Arts Fellow and collaborates with the Disability Culture Leadership Initiative at the University of Illinois at Chicago. She is also a proud member of the Association of Mouth and Foot Painting Artists Worldwide. Today, Paré continues to create in her home studio in the western suburbs of Chicago, dividing her artistic output among still life, portraiture, and semi-abstract modes.

About the Cover Artwork

Portraits of Spinal Cord Injury: Oppo (2023)
Watercolor on paper
8″ × 8″
Painted by mouth

Image Credit

"By courtesy of the Association of Mouth and Foot Painting Artists Worldwide."

EDITOR BIO

Manasi Shankar, Ph.D., LPCC, NCC, is a licensed clinician, educator, supervisor, and scholar specializing in disability-affirmative mental health care. She is the founder of *Therapy at Bay*, a private practice in the San Francisco Bay Area, where she offers clinical services and consultation through a systemic, justice-oriented lens. Dr. Shankar holds a Ph.D. in Couple and Family Therapy from Virginia Polytechnic Institute and State University and a Master's degree from Syracuse University, home to one of the nation's first disability-specialization programs. A former clinical fellow at the Chicago Center for Family Health, Dr. Shankar brings over a decade of experience in providing clinical care to structurally marginalized populations. Her work centers on expanding access to inclusive, disability-affirmative therapy, with a particular focus on systemic and relational approaches. She has served as adjunct faculty at the University of San Francisco and currently offers national and international training for graduate programs, clinical organizations, and interdisciplinary teams working to integrate disability-affirmative frameworks into practice. Dr. Shankar also serves as Advisory Director of the *Tinkesh Ability Foundation* in India, where she contributes to cross-national efforts advancing accessibility, representation, and disability justice.

CONTRIBUTORS

Madeline Barger, MS, LMFT, BCBA, CST, is a Licensed Marriage and Family Therapist, Certified Sex Therapist through the American Association of Sex Educators, Counselors, and Therapists, and the Lead Behavior Analyst for UW Health and UW Madison, wherein she leads the teen and adult clinic. Barger has been a trainer, speaker, and panelist at international conferences, training and advocating for positive change for people on the autism spectrum. Barger's work advocates for the human right to a pleasurable and fulfilling sex life for people of all abilities.

Megan C. Carlos, Ph.D., is an Associate Professor with the California School of Professional Psychology (CSPP) at Alliant International University. She also has a private practice in Berkeley, California. Dr. Carlos has previously served on the American Psychological Association's committee on disability issues and is the Vice-Chair of the National Council of Schools and Programs in Professional Psychology's disability Committee.

Ellis Scout Cliff is a neurodivergent public interest lawyer in Washington, D.C. Ellis is an alumnus of the University of Cincinnati College of Law, and Earlham College.

Katy Evans is currently completing an M.Sc. in Mad Studies and working as a co-researcher across a number of projects that focus on the lived experiences of disabled people. Katy is also a trainer for Spokz People – a UK-based social enterprise. She was born disabled and the lack of access to safe and effective mental health care encouraged her to contribute to the development of accessible mental health care for disabled communities.

Gabrielle Ficchi, Ph.D., is a full-time faculty member at the University of Phoenix, where she teaches courses in counseling. She is also the Chief Operating Officer of *Care 4 the Caregivers*, working to build a community of support among caregivers, with disabled children, raise awareness, and better the lives of disabled people in her community. Her work at her therapy practice, New Perspectives LLC, focuses on providing mental health services to the disabled community and their families.

Lyndon Frommer is a Ph.D. candidate in the Science and Technology Studies department at Virginia Tech. He received his undergraduate degree in Science, Technology, and Society and his Master's in Integrative Social Sciences from Arizona State University. His research interests focus predominantly on trans medicine and health care. His current work with the DisCoTec research group is to get disabled consultants into different lab settings to get researchers into conversations with disabled people early on in projects.

Briana Gaines, Ph.D., LPC, CCTP, is an Assistant Teaching Professor in the Counselor Education Program at North Carolina State University. With a specialization in Marriage and Family Therapy, she has practiced as an outpatient therapist and clinical case manager at a non-profit organization where she worked with underserved and underrepresented populations.

Kami L. Gallus, Ph.D., LMFT, is a Professor of Human Development and Family Science and the Associate Director of the Center for Developmental Disabilities at Oklahoma State University. A Licensed Marriage and Family Therapist, Dr. Gallus' scholarship focuses on enhancing individual functioning, belonging, and relationship outcomes among vulnerable, often marginalized, and traditionally under-served populations, including female trauma survivors, at-risk youth, and disabled individuals.

Shakeela Gray, LGPC, NCC, is pursuing a Ph.D. in Counselor Education and Supervision at Bowie State University. She has over seven years of experience in case management and supervision, supporting Maryland's Developmental Disabilities Administration and Maryland's Autism Waiver program. In her newest pursuits, Ms. Gray founded Village Values LLC, a company that provides a variety of disability support to individuals and their families.

Angélica Guevara, Ph.D., J.D., is a neurodivergent Latina scholar whose work centers on disability rights law and non-apparent disabilities. She holds a J.D. from UC Berkeley Law and a Ph.D. in Education from UC Berkeley. She previously served in the U.S. Department of Labor and the American Bar Association. Dr. Guevara is currently an Assistant Professor at Indiana University's Kelley School of Business, where she integrates disability justice into her teaching of Business Law and Ethics.

Mel Halacre is a clinical therapist working since 2009 with disabled clients and families. She is the founder of Spokz People CIC, a UK-based non-profit social enterprise whose aim is to provide disability-affirmative therapy to disabled communities. The enterprise now runs a low-cost well-being platform with a psychoeducational program, videos, weekly live events, and a forum to train therapists to work affirmatively with disabled clients.

Caitlin Hernandez is a blind writer, writing nonfiction essays about total blindness, queerness, and the intersections thereof that appear in the disability studies textbook: *Barriers and Belonging: Personal Narratives of Disability* and *Firsts: Coming of Age Stories by People with Disabilities.* A two-time Lambda Literary fellow, her unpublished novel, *Even Touch Has a Tune*, which centers on a queer, blind girl who finds love and survives sexual assault, is represented by Emily Keyes of Keyes Agency.

Garrett M. Jones is a lived experience expert with the Center for Developmental Disabilities at Oklahoma State University. Mr. Jones utilizes his experience working and living in inclusive communities to advocate for building relationships between people with and without disabilities.

Jennifer L. Jones, Ph.D., is a Professor of Human Development and Family Science and the Director of the Center for Developmental Disabilities at Oklahoma State University. Her works in communities and in academia over the past 25 years have focused on improving the quality of life for individuals with intellectual and developmental disabilities and their families.

Rebecca Kammes, Ph.D., LMFT, is a Licensed Marriage and Family Therapist and a clinical specialist at the University of California, Los Angeles, where she leads clinical groups for individuals with developmental disabilities, specializing in working with parents and young adults interested in dating and romantic relationships. She also engages in private practice work through the Honeycomb Therapy Center where she specializes in working with disability and couples, individuals who have experienced sexual trauma, and gender or sexuality nonconforming individuals.

Catherine Kapphahn is an educator, writer, speaker, and storyteller. Her memoir *Immigrant Daughter: Stories You Never Told Me* received The Center for Fiction's Christopher Doheny Award and was published by Audible. She has received artist grants from the Queens Council on the Arts and City Artist Corps and her writing has appeared in Queensbound, *Motherwell Magazine*, *Croatia Week*, *Newtown Literary*, the Feminist Press Anthology, *This Is the Way We Say Goodbye*, as well as *CURE Magazine*. Catherine is an adjunct lecturer in Lehman College in the Bronx at the City University of New York where her students' stories inspire her.

Steven T. Licardi, LCSW, is an Autistic/neurodivergent social worker, spoken word poet, actor, science fiction writer, artist, and performance activist working at the intersections of art and social policy. He travels internationally using the power of storytelling to create empathic dialogue around, to confront the realities of, and to assist communities in dismantling historic narratives around mental health and madness. His work can be found at *thesvenbo.com/books* and *thesvenbo.substack.com.*

Alan Santinele Martino, Ph.D. (he/him), is an Assistant Professor in the Community Rehabilitation and Disability Studies program in the Department of Community Health Sciences at the University of Calgary. His work has been published in multiple journals, such as *Disability Studies Quarterly*, *Sexuality and Disability*, and *Culture, Health and Sexuality*, as well as edited volumes focused on disability and/or sexualities studies. He is the lead of the Disability and Sexuality Lab at the University of Calgary.

Onyinye F. Mbanefo is a graduate student on the Master's to Ph.D. track and a graduate research assistant at the Center for Gerontology at Virginia Tech. Her research focuses on elder abuse and neglect of vulnerable adults, particularly those living in underserved communities, and surrogate decision-making. She has been awarded scholarships such as an AARP Scholarship and the Mancini Research Award.

Debra L. Miller, PhD, LMSW, is a Licensed Clinical Social Worker who holds a clinical faculty appointment with Michigan State University, College of Medicine where she provides behavioral health education and research support to family practice residents at the University of Michigan Health System's Family Practice Center. She is the Associate Director of the Family Therapy Training Institute of Miami, supporting the implementation of Brief Strategic Family Therapy throughout the United States. She is the coauthor of *Deliberate Practice for Systemic Family Therapy*, a book designed to support practitioners' skill development in key systemic family therapy approaches.

Melissa Miller (she/her) holds a bachelor's degree in Community Rehabilitation and Disability Studies from the University of Calgary. Melissa has had an extensive career in the disability services field spanning 15 years and has presented at numerous conferences such as the Calgary Board of Education Support Staff Conference, the Greater Edmonton Teacher's Association Conference, and most recently the Canadian Sociological Association's annual conference.

Eleni Moumos (she/her) is a recent graduate from the University of Calgary with a Bachelor of Arts in Psychology. She is currently a research assistant in the Disability and Sexuality Lab where she works under the supervision of Dr. Alan Santinele Martino.

Rhoda Olkin, Ph.D., is a Distinguished Professor in the California School of Professional Psychology at Alliant International University and the Executive Director of the Institute on Disability and Health Psychology. A disabled trailblazer in the field of psychotherapy, she authored *What Psychotherapists Should Know About Disability* (1999) and has profoundly shaped the integration of disability-affirmative practice into the field of psychotherapy.

Jordan Parks (she/her) is an undergraduate student from the University of Calgary completing a combined degree in Psychology (BA) and Community Rehabilitation and Disability Studies (BCR). Jordan is currently a research assistant in the Disability and Sexuality Lab under Dr. Alan Santinele Martino's guidance.

Lydia Qualls, Ph.D., is a Licensed Clinical Psychologist at the Cook Counseling Center, Virginia Tech. Dr. Qualls attended Vanderbilt University for her bachelor's degree in Psychology, graduating in 2009, and spent two years after, obtaining her graduate degree working at the Vanderbilt Kennedy Center on various research projects with Autistic children and teens. In her tenure at Cook Counseling Center, she has served as the assessment coordinator and the liaison to the Services for Students with Disabilities Office at Virginia Tech. Dr. Lydia Qualls identifies as Autistic, queer, and hard-of-hearing.

Natalie M. Richardson, Ph.D., LMFT, is a Licensed Marriage and Family Therapist and the Assistant Academic Program Director for the Marriage and Family Therapy and Advanced Studies in Human Behavior graduate programs at Capella University, with a background in Medical Family Therapy.

Jody Russon, Ph.D. (she/her), is an Associate Professor in the Department of Human Development and Family Science (Marriage and Family Therapy Program Area) at Virginia Tech. Within her department, she is the principal investigator of the Alliance for Suicide Prevention and Intervention through Relationship Enrichment (APSIRE) research team. She is an AAMFT Approved Supervisor and an instructor of Dr. Harry Aponte's Person-of-the-Therapist (POTT) training model. Dr. Russon trained and co-taught master's students with Dr. Aponte for several years before developing a POTT capstone practicum course for doctoral students at Virginia Tech.

Toni Saia, Ph.D., is an Assistant Professor and the Director of the Rehabilitation Technology Certificate at San Diego State University within the Department of Administration, Rehabilitation, and Postsecondary Education. She is a disabled woman and is one of the originators of the American Rehabilitation Counseling Association's (ARCA) Disability-Related Counseling Competencies, informing the work of 55,000 counselors nationally.

Derek X. Seward, Ph.D., LMHC, NCC, is an Associate Professor in the Counseling and Human Services Program in the School of Education at Syracuse University. Dr. Seward's scholarly interests focus primarily on the multicultural and social justice development of mental health professionals. He is a Licensed Mental Health Counselor in New York State, National Certified Counselor, and an Approved Clinical Supervisor.

Manasi Shankar, Ph.D., LPCC, NCC (she/her), is a licensed clinician, supervisor, educator, and scholar specializing in disability-affirmative mental health care. Her work centers on advancing accessible, inclusive mental health care for disabled individuals and families, with a particular emphasis on systemic, relational approaches. Dr. Shankar frequently provides training and consultation at both national and international levels, supporting graduate programs, clinical organizations, and interdisciplinary teams in the integration of disability-affirmative frameworks into systemic therapy. She currently owns *Therapy at Bay*, a private practice in the San Francisco Bay Area.

Pramod Shankar is a published author, storyteller, and spoken-word-poet. A constant learner and a true creative, he has worn many hats throughout his career. He is currently working as a coach, communicator, performer, and creative consultant. He is also disabled, living with ALS for over 30 years.

Ashley Shew, Ph.D., is an Associate Professor of Science, Technology, and Society at Virginia Tech, and specializes in philosophy of technology at its intersection with disability studies, animal studies, and emerging technology. She is a co-founder of the Disability Caucus at Virginia Tech. She is a co-recipient of an Andrew W. Mellon grant called *Just Dis Tech*. She has authored two books and co-edited three books; her most recent book is *Against Technoableism: Rethinking Who Needs Improvement.*

Kahyen Shin (she/her) is a Ph.D. student in Counseling and Counselor Education at Syracuse University. Her research interests focus on low-income communities, cross-cultural experiences, and development of culturally tailored interventions for populations with mental health stigma.

Shalini Srinivasan, M.A. (she/her), is a doctoral student in the Marriage and Family Therapy program at Virginia Tech. Her research focuses on sexual socialization, sex education, and relationship well-being. Shalini is interested in the sexual and relational experiences of South Asians through a sociocultural framework. Shalini received her B.A. in Psychology, Sociology, and Economics and M.S. in Counseling Psychology from Christ University, Bangalore, India.

Pamela B. Teaster, Ph.D., M.A., M.S., NREMT, is a Professor and Director of the Center for Gerontology at Virginia Tech. She serves on the Editorial Boards of the *Journal of Elder Abuse and Neglect* and the *Journal of Trauma, Violence, and Abuse Review* and is in her second term as a Commissioner for the American Bar Association for Law and Aging. She became a nationally registered EMT, licensed in Virginia in 2023.

James Tillett, Ph.D. (he/him), received his doctorate in Marriage and Family Therapy at Virginia Tech and earned his M.A. in Marriage and Family Therapy from Appalachian State University. Broadly, Jim's research focuses on de-pathologizing neurodivergent, disabled, sexually minoritized, and gender minoritized ways of being in therapy. Jim is passionate about centering neurodivergent individuals and their relationships in the development of psychotherapies and challenging the idea that there is a "normal" or "right" way to be.

Brian Watermeyer, Ph.D., is a psychoanalytically oriented psychotherapist working with disabled clients, as well as a researcher and renowned scholar of disability studies. He also lives with disability himself, having been severely visually impaired since his early life. As a theorist, his work employs critical psychoanalysis as a lens with which to understand psychological and relational aspects of disability oppression, including both the unconscious dynamics implicated in prejudice and stigma, and the psychic impressions left on disabled people by othering, discrimination, and exclusion.

Brittany A. Williams, Ph.D., LCPC, NCC, is an Assistant Professor in the Counseling and Psychological Studies Department at Bowie State University. Dr. Williams is a Licensed Clinical Professional Counselor in Maryland, National Certified Counselor, and Approved Clinical Supervisor. With a focus on culturally sensitive practices, she aims to foster positive outcomes among marginalized populations, particularly within the Black community, through compassionate and individualized care.

Solomon Furious Worlds, J.D., is a Black, Muslim, disabled staff attorney with the ACLU of Pennsylvania, focusing on police misconduct, protesters' rights, free speech rights, and government transparency. Solomon earned two bachelor's degrees in Saxophone Performance and Social Psychology from the University of Iowa and a Juris Doctor from the University of Michigan Law School.

PREFACE

I was about ten years old when I first noticed my father's impairment. He was 16 when doctors misdiagnosed him with "Essential Tremors," a movement-related disorder. In his 20s, after numerous consultations, he received an accurate diagnosis of Amyotrophic Lateral Sclerosis (ALS). ALS is a (relatively rare) progressive neurodegenerative disease that affects nerve cells in the brain and spinal cord, leading to muscle weakness, paralysis, and eventually, possible respiratory failure. It is also the condition that renowned physicist Stephen Hawking lived with in the 60s. Unlike Hawking, my father's disability was not visually observable when you first met him. If you met him in the 90s, it would be his humor, creativity, and distinct artistic sensibilities that you would have noticed right away. What Hawking and my father shared, however, was their unprecedented longevity; each, in his own way, lived far beyond the number of years those around them had anticipated.

As I progressed through life's stages, so did my father's disability. Growing up, we lived in a home with a shared bathroom. I vividly recall the night that I heard my father cry, presumably from the pain in his fingertips. I use the word "presumption" intentionally. Like many families living with disability, conversations about impairment characteristics, the unpredictability and instability of symptoms, emotional vulnerabilities, and psychological impacts were not openly discussed. As I grew older, I became more aware of the relational, emotional, and systemic impacts of the disability on my family. In 2012, when my mother was diagnosed with cancer was when we recognized our capabilities as a family unit. Almost instantly, each of us took on roles that would eventually (and gradually) not only help us overcome the adversity of living with illness and disability, among other severe stressors, but also leave us feeling closer to one another in immeasurable ways. As a unit, we became stronger, and as individuals, and in our own rights, we became magnificently resilient. Today, as a woman in my 30s and an immigrant with thousands of miles between my family and me, I wouldn't describe growing up with a disabled parent as simply "good" or "bad." The experience was far more complex than any binary or mechanistic framing could ever capture.

In 2014, I moved from India to the United States to deepen my training and growth as a mental healthcare provider. I soon recognized that the relational, systemic way of thinking about the world that is characteristic of the discipline of Marriage and Family Therapy was deeply aligned with my own collectivistic tendencies. I had found my home within the field of psychotherapy. Another important quality of our discipline lies in its recognition of the need to understand individuals and experiences from an Intersectional perspective. As a collective, we are at the forefront of conversations and actions surrounding social justice, minoritized and oppressed identities, liberation, advocacy, and equal rights. I recall feeling hopeful for the state of our worlds during these conversations, as I waited patiently to hear about disability.

I never did.

The absence of disability-focused discourse was reflective of gaps in the broader field, the overmedicalization of disability, and the deeply hierarchical priorities of the world. During my doctoral program, I got to work with Dr. Ashley Shew, an incredible disabled scholar serving as an Associate Professor of Science, Technology, and Society at Virginia Tech. During one of our coffee shop conversations about disability and mental health, she shared "I am glad you are doing this work. Disabled people have a secret list of safe therapists that we pass around. A 'golden list' of sorts. Typically, therapy doors are closed to us."

This conversation with Dr. Shew, my ongoing professional development, and my personal experiences of living with a disabled family member all culminated in two profound realizations: the invaluable benefits that an effective family therapist would have had on my own family's functioning and well-being, and that marriage and family therapists are in an incredibly powerful position to serve the disabled community. With our skills, training, and competence related to mental health, our social justice orientation, interdisciplinary collaborations, and the genuine compassion in our hearts, we hold the power to work with disabled individuals to create a change that is long overdue. Through these enriching experiences, my thoughts and feelings began to crystallize into a tangible goal; to contribute to narrowing the frightening gap between disabled communities and effective, safe, systemic therapy.

You will read this statement in different forms and at different junctures throughout this handbook; we are underserving of labeling ourselves a diversity-focused field, if we are overlooking the largest minority group in the world. I hope instead dear reader that we can work to *earn* that title. Thank you for picking this book up. As therapists, we know that insight, awareness, and the motivation to learn are often the most critical steps to creating transformational change.

ACKNOWLEDGMENTS

This handbook is dedicated to the innumerable individuals, families, and communities who are and have been impacted by disability and disablement. For far too long, their experiences have been silenced, deprioritized, overmedicalized, and excluded from broader conversations on inclusion and diversity. Disabled communities have had limited access to safe, effective, affordable mental health care, and have often faced these barriers in isolation. Reflections shared by disabled clients, friends, and colleagues, in moments of vulnerability, have inspired this work in deeply meaningful ways.

This text owes so much to the ever-evolving discipline of Marriage and Family Therapy, and to the scholars who continue to shape it. The field's deep commitment to social justice, advocacy, and holistic care makes it the ideal home for work that seeks to challenge inaccessibility and promote safe, evidence-based care for minoritized communities. Systemic thinkers such as Dr. Rhoda Olkin, Kimberlé Crenshaw, and Salvador Minuchin have paved the way for many of the ideas held within these pages. The compassion at the heart of our discipline is precisely what is needed, and long overdue for disabled communities.

I am deeply grateful to the educators and mentors who have shaped my professional journey. Since immigrating to the United States, I have grown in immeasurable ways, and much of that growth is owed to the guidance and generosity of my mentors. The faculty and staff at Syracuse University's Clinical Mental Health Counseling program laid the essential foundations of my career. During my doctoral studies at Virginia Tech, colleagues and mentors such as Dr. Megan Dolbin-MacNab and Dr. Ashley Shew were instrumental in the initial conceptualization of this work. I am eternally thankful to, and for, Dr. Pamela Teaster, whose advisory role extended far beyond my dissertation. Dr. Teaster, while working on this book, I realized how much stronger a writer I had become under your mentorship. Thank you. I value and cherish you.

I am so deeply grateful to the faculty at the Chicago Center for Family Health – Drs. John Rolland, Froma Walsh, and Steven Zuckerman, whose training and collaboration helped crystallize the urgent need to think relationally about disability and chronic illness. John, your advice and guidance at multiple stages of this handbook have been truly invaluable.

To the Taylor & Francis, Routledge team – thank you for recognizing the importance of this work, embracing its urgency, and offering the opportunity to collaborate on something meaningful and impactful. A heartfelt thank you to Julia Giordano, editor at Routledge, for your unwavering support and thoughtful guidance through every stage of bringing this book to life. You were a treat to work with.

To every contributor of this handbook, thank you. The conversations we shared during the early stages, the passion with which you live, your resilience, your expertise, and your commitment to this community have blown my mind. It has been both humbling and inspiring to witness. Thank you also to our artists, who brought richness, depth, and vibrancy to this text in ways only they could. You are all truly incredible.

Any immigrant living far away from family will tell you just how invaluable friendships away from home can be. I am fortunate to have the most wonderful friends who have supported me through this journey – in the form of accountability, patience, encouragement, and love. I think especially of Dr. Léa Barber, Dr. Allie King, Tasha, Sriram, Vijaya, Goutham, Ashwin, Divya, Irene, Anand, Amma, and Appa, among many others. Thank you for your steadfast love and support.

I owe so much of this handbook's very existence to my husband, Arun. His empathetic ways of thinking about complex constructs helped me engage in key insights around content, structure, and language. His patience and unwavering support over the past few years made it possible for this work to come to fruition. I am in constant awe of his intuitive kindness and the way he continues to extend compassion to the world – even when it is difficult to do so.

The acknowledgment of my family, Amma, Acha, and Appu, makes me pause. No expression of gratitude could fully capture the depth of what they have given me. Through their own experiences of disablement, financial hardship, and so much more, they supported me every step of the way, to where I am today. But what I feel most grateful for is the kind of people they are – deeply caring, kind, and inclusive. These values have profoundly inspired both who I am and the foundations of this handbook.

INTRODUCTION

Manasi Shankar

Objectives, Scope, and Limitations

Three key objectives guide the structure of this handbook. First, we aim to deepen systemic therapists' understanding of the historical experiences of disabled individuals, families, and communities, as well as the evolving discourse surrounding disability, specifically in the United States. The hope is that this knowledge will actively draw marriage and family therapists (MFTs) into claiming a seat at the table of disability advocacy and systemic change. Second, we seek to raise awareness about the urgent need to address the mental health and relational needs of the disabled community – a population that has long been overmedicalized and whose psychological well-being has too often been neglected. Third, we hope to offer an accessible introduction to tangible theories and concrete clinical applications for working with disabled clients and their families within the therapy space.

However, given the vast diversity of identities and experiences within the community, it would be both unrealistic and potentially harmful to assume these interventions can be universally applied to every therapeutic context. All our contributors acknowledge that impairments (and the experiences that accompany them) vary widely. Our goal is to offer an overview of affirmative practice, rather than to make claims about its universality or applicability. Therefore, therapists must rely on their clinical intuitions, training, supervision, and personal work to discern what experiences are relatively common among many disabled people (such as feelings of isolation and disablement) and what experiences are unique to a specific client (such as developmental history and the model of disability to which they adhere).

Similarly, the perspectives and strategies presented in this handbook are based on a particular cultural, social, and clinical context. While we strive to offer

 DOI: 10.4324/9781003362586-1

inclusive, affirmative approaches, these ideas may not fully account for the diverse cultural, socio-economic, or geographic factors that influence the experiences of disabled individuals and families around the world. For example, the disability discourse in India is vastly different; with cultural, religious, and social underpinnings that would make some chapters feel inapplicable, or even irrelevant to readers there. As such, the recommendations made in this text are not universally applicable, and adaptations may be necessary, depending on the specific circumstances and social location of each client or family.

Language and Terminology

"Language, regardless of intent, is very powerful. It can be used to uplift or degrade someone depending on how it is used" (Stuntzner, 2012, p. 40). This statement is particularly true for historically marginalized populations where language directly impacts treatment, which, in turn, can influence the formation of laws and policies that affect disabled lives directly. Outdated or inaccurate terminology can encourage and promote, even if unintentional, poor and negative perceptions and feelings about disabled people; some of which include the words "*invalid, suffering, afflicted, victim, handicapped, crippled,* and *wheelchair-bound*" (Titchkosky, 2001, p. 127). In the context of therapy, language and repeated use of negative and disempowering words can influence the ways clients view themselves, particularly when such experiences are internalized. This, in turn, can have detrimental effects on the therapeutic alliance and client's feelings of safety.

Another dominant debate that has polarized the community is related to "person-first" (person with Autism) versus "identity-first" (Autistic person) language. For the purposes of this handbook, identity-first language is utilized whenever appropriate. This practice was carried out intentionally for a few important reasons. First, at the time of the development of this text, identity-first language has been acknowledged as the preferred terminology by many communities and organizations such as the American Psychological Association (2021). This is in line with the social model of disability that emphasizes the role of society on the experience of "disablement", rather than a focus on an impairment. The term "disabled" places the onus on societies, rather than individuals, to dismantle inaccessible structures. To demonstrate the role of disablement, Olkin (1999, p. 27.) says "if the whole world signed, deafness would not be much of a disability".

Second, when considering important, minoritized identities, we often use identity-first language. For instance, rather than saying "man who is Black" or "man who is gay," we say, "Black man" or "Gay man" to emphasize the pride inherent in these identities. However, person-first language is utilized in chapters where that is the preference of the writer living with disability. Person-first language is also utilized in contexts where it is more appropriate to the specific disability culture to do so (e.g., many self-advocates and organizations that support individuals with Down syndrome prefer person-first language). Ultimately, while this text uses identity-first language, the most accurate language is the one chosen by the disabled individual.

Artists and Authors

During the initial phases of conceptualizing this handbook, I began to recognize how important it was to challenge the archaic ways in which we tend to think of textbooks and handbooks. Art has played a pivotal role in disability history, providing a means of expression for a community that has been silenced for centuries. The theme of this book revolves around disabled voices and lived experiences – stories of grief, anger, and injustice, but also of triumph, beauty, and healing, which have, in turn, informed rigorous scholarship. To reflect this quality within the community, every section is introduced by a disabled artist, alongside the book cover created by incredible visual artist and mouth-painter, Mariam Paré.

The majority of our authors also self-identify as disabled and/or a person with a disability. This was important to me in my effort to contribute towards dismantling decades of academic writing entrenched in ableist tendencies and practices. The iconic motto of several disability communities-"Nothing about us Without us", rings throughout the pages of this text.

Structure

This handbook is organized into four broad sections – each with a specific objective that is addressed through the multiple chapters within it. As noted earlier, every section of the handbook is introduced by a disabled artist- an expert of their own craft.

Section I: History, Law, and the Sociopolitical Context of Disability

Introduced by Steven T. Licardi, author, spoken word poet, actor, and licensed clinician, this section orients readers to the socio-cultural landscape of disability in the United States. Dr. Megan Carlos provides an accessible, yet thorough historical overview of the disability community, offering therapists a contextual foundation for understanding the evolution of disability rights and advocacy in the U.S. Building on this, Solomon Furious Worlds and Ellis S. Cliff, drawing from their expertise in disability law, present a foundational examination of the legal system and disability rights, emphasizing the relevance of legal frameworks to therapeutic practice. Dr. Angélica Guevara then explores the predominant models of disability, including the medical and social models, which have critically shaped public and clinical discourse around disability. The section concludes with a compelling chapter by renowned psychotherapist and author Dr. Rhoda Olkin, who interrogates the historical role of ableism within academia, and calls for systemic transformation toward greater inclusivity and equity.

Section II: Contextualizing Disability through an Intersectional Lens

Introduced by the incredible Caitlin Hernandez-a blind, queer, woman of color, this vital section highlights key intersections that therapists must consider when working with disabled clients. While not exhaustive, the chapters in this section aim to address some of the most pressing and underexamined intersectional dynamics shaping disabled lives. A significant section of the disabled population includes older adults. In their chapter, Dr. Pamela Teaster and Onyinye F Mbanefo, examine the unique challenges faced by disabled older adults, and offer practical strategies to enhance their quality of life. Recognizing that communities of color are disproportionately affected by disability due to systemic inequities and limited access to resources, Dr. Angélica Guevara explores the intersection of race and disability, illuminating how racial injustice compounds disablement. Alan Santinele Martino and colleagues draw from Intersectionality and Crip theory to investigate the lived experiences of 2SLGBTQ+ individuals, another community often marginalized through intersecting systems of ableism, heteronormativity, and cisnormativity. Together, these chapters highlight the essential role of critical intersectional frameworks in disability-affirmative therapy.

Section III: Foundations of Disability-Affirmative Systemic Therapy

Catherine Kapphahn – published author, speaker, and storyteller – introduces this foundational section on disability-affirmative therapy. The section opens with a deeply reflective chapter by Dr. Brian Watermeyer- a leading scholar in disability studies, educator, and clinical psychologist. Drawing from Psychoanalytic traditions, Dr. Watermeyer invites clinicians to critically examine their own intuition, countertransference, and unconscious responses when engaging with disability in therapeutic contexts. This powerful contribution is followed by a chapter from Katy Evans and Mel Halacre, who illuminate the often-overlooked harm of subtle microaggressions within the therapy space and offer concrete strategies for cultivating more inclusive therapeutic practices.

Shifting the focus to systemic frameworks, Dr. Kami Gallus and colleagues underscore the essential role of systemic therapists-particularly MFTs, in supporting the overall well-being and relational health of disabled individuals and their families. Building on this, Dr. Rebecca Kammes and colleagues offer couples therapy interventions, when disability is present within the couple system. Dr. Manasi Shankar then presents a two-part series on working affirmatively with families that include one or more disabled members. The first chapter articulates foundational, philosophical assumptions grounded in the field of family therapy, while the second chapter offers a practical and adaptable framework for clinical application with disabled families.

The section concludes with an incisive chapter by Dr. Toni Saia and Dr. Gabrielle Ficchi, who challenge traditional understandings of accessibility in therapy. Through a disability justice lens, the authors unpack the deeper meaning of accessibility and offer thoughtful guidance on how clinicians can construct truly accessible therapeutic environments and processes.

Section IV: Disability-Affirmative Education: Transforming the Future of Therapist Training

This final section is introduced by Pramod Shankar – a storyteller, published author, and poet, inviting readers to reflect on the transformative power of education, supervision, and research in shaping a more inclusive clinical future. The section opens with a chapter by Dr. Brittany Williams and colleagues, who address the persistent absence of disability content in therapy graduate programs. They offer concrete strategies for integrating disability into existing counseling curricula, aiming to shift disability from a "checklist item" to the center of clinical training. Following this, Dr. Lydia Qualls and colleagues explore the ethics and practices of inclusive, collaborative research. Emphasizing fairness and equity, their chapter highlights how research grounded in disability justice can inform more accessible and responsive therapeutic approaches.

Building on the theme of training, Shakeela Gray and colleagues underscore the importance of disability-affirmative supervision. They provide guidance on how clinical supervisors can support trainees in developing competence and confidence in working with disabled clients. To extend this conversation, Dr. James Tillett and colleagues apply the Person-of-the-Therapist model (Aponte & Kissil, 2016) to supervision in disability-centered cases. Through case examples, they illustrate how supervisors can engage trainees in reflective, identity-conscious work that deepens their clinical effectiveness with disabled populations.

Accessibility Statement

This handbook was created with a deep awareness that accessibility is not simply a technical requirement-it is an act of care. In the words of disability activist, Mia Mingus, "access is love". We believe that accessible scholarship is essential to disability justice, and we recognize that many disabled readers have historically been excluded from engaging fully with academic texts due to inaccessible formats and design.

This book, like the field it serves, is part of an evolving journey toward greater access. While it is far from being accessible in all formats, both the publisher and I have taken important steps toward that goal with the resources currently available. Taylor & Francis now aims to meet the WCAG 2.2 AA level of accessibility across all new titles and has discontinued its "fixed layout only" model, committing instead to publishing EPUB (version 3.3) formats for all books, including this one. Our title is also scheduled for a manual accessibility review prior to publication, to help ensure a more reader-friendly experience for digital users. While more specialized formats such as braille and large print remain dependent on manufacturing logistics and third-party services, the publisher has expressed openness to supporting remediation where possible. Additionally, the rights team is actively exploring possibilities for an audiobook or translation version, though these formats also depend on third-party partnerships. We believe that accessibility is an ongoing commitment – not a box to check. We acknowledge that this work is still in progress, and that this book has accessibility-related limitations.

Positionality Statement

As a temporarily non-disabled person, I write and edit this handbook from an outsider-perspective, recognizing that I do not experience disability in my own bodymind, and that my current experience of being non-disabled is neither fixed nor permanent. Ability is socially constructed, shaped by cultural, structural, and environmental contexts, and can shift across time and space. I acknowledge the impermanence of my own embodied status, and the numerous privileges that come with it.

At the same time, my proximity to disability is deeply personal. I was raised by a disabled parent, and my early life was shaped by witnessing and navigating the systemic, cultural, and familial dynamics that disability brings into focus. Though I do not hold the lived experience of disability directly, I carry a relational understanding of what it means to exist in a world that often marginalizes disabled people and their families. This proximity has deeply informed my clinical values, my professional commitments, and my orientation toward disability justice.

I (and other contributors of this work) understand disability as a minority experience and an oppressed identity, rather than a medical issue that demands a "fix". In fact, it is for this reason that disability has been categorized as an experience, rather than being tied to one type of impairment, example: "physical disability" or "mental disability". Our work as clinicians, centers around the experience of "disablement", while acknowledging any challenges that come with living with an impairment. I also acknowledge the existence of the bodymind unity. Bodymind represents alignment with a disability-justice perspective that resists Cartesian dualism (the separation of body and mind) and affirms the integrated nature of lived experience (Price, 2015). We also see, recognize, and honor the experiences of congenital, acquired, apparent, non-apparent, and all other variations of disablement.

I also write as an Indian immigrant, shaped by cultural frameworks and systemic dynamics that differ from those of the United States. My immigrant experience offers a critical lens through which I engage with U.S.-centric models of therapy and disability. It allows me to question dominant narratives, while also recognizing that certain cultural rules, norms, and nuances within U.S.

disability discourse may be less familiar to me. As an international author among others in this handbook, I view these perspectives as a strength. The work of disability-affirmative therapy is not confined to one cultural or geographic context-it must be informed by global, plural, and decolonial ways of learning.

In conclusion, I write and edit this work not to speak for disabled people, but to contribute to the field of systemic therapy, that urgently needs more reflexive, systemic, and disability-affirmative perspectives. My position calls for ongoing self-reflection, humility, and accountability to disabled communities, whose lived expertise must remain central in both theory and practice.

References

American Psychological Association. (2021). *Inclusive language guidelines*. https://www.apa.org/about/apa/equity-diversity-inclusion/language-guidelines

Aponte, H. J. & Kissil, K. (Eds.). (2016). *The person of the therapist training model: Mastering the use of self.*

Olkin, R. (1999). *What psychotherapists should know about disability*. The Guilford Press.

Price, M. (2015). The bodymind problem and the possibilities of pain. *Hypatia*, 30(1), 268–284. https://doi.org/10.1111/hypa.12127

Stuntzner, S. (2012). *Living with a disability: Finding peace amidst the storm*. WestBow Press.

Titchkosky, T. (2001). *Disability, self, and society*. University of Toronto Press.

Bibliography

Charlton, J. I. (1998). *Nothing about us without us: Disability oppression and empowerment*. University of California Press

SECTION I

History, Law and the Sociopolitical Context of Disability

PART I

*he printed his name with his right hand**

Steven T. Licardi

Our task is to imagine the futures we want with the histories we have.

in 1999, my mother feeds me vanilla ice cream at 6 AM with jagged bits of depakote in it. my madness is mediated by mellaril, the bureaucracy of buspar, & a rhapsody of risperdal. i'm ten years old. the years do not matter.

/ he has a mixture of several psychiatric disorders /

i exist in multiple realities at once. a life awash with half-lives. the interplay between what is & what could have been. an ever-present unknowing. the pharmacokinetics of entropy—spooky action potentials at a distance that suggest there is something wrong with me.

/ because of disruptive behavior /

The task at hand is to subvert historic narratives that claim to constitute normalcy; to overthrow the ways such narratives persist in our lived experiences; to push back against praxis, against policy, to continuously hold them accountable.

i wake up on a couch in a language lab. the lamps bask the room in jaundice yellow. for a moment, i don't know where i am. there's a two-way mirror in front of me. the room on the other side is dark. its 2012, but the years do not matter.

/ he has a long standing history /

memory is a fickle thing. its 1995. the room is off-white. the linoleum floor, the walls, the ceiling tiles—all a different shade. i know they watch me from behind the mirror. i'm six years old. i play.

/ banging his head / throws himself on the floor /

Our task is to push the world toward new realities, new ways of being; not merely inclusive, but expansive; to terraform the human conscience, with terror and love, into a cosmic consciousness; beyond even what is conceivable and comprehensible.

DOI: 10.4324/9781003362586-3

the smell of saline gel. 2011. i'm an electroencephalogram technician, studying psychopaths. my story is a toed line between the incarceration of ableism & a chasm of infinite other ways of being. i am the fulfilled dream of mainstreamed suburban rematriculation. a capitalism- contributing (functional) member of society. i work three jobs. i'm a full-time student. i'm masking all the time.

/ recently he pulled the fire alarm during lunch /

my head is tethered to the wall by an electroencephalograph. my mother sleeps on the floor beside my hospital bed. its 1997, but the years do not matter. the nurse brings me two breakfasts. the bacon tastes like acetone.

/ he had shown habits of throwing his pencil /

The task at hand is to supplant the systems we are entrenched in; to re-contextualize our positions within legacy; to un-erase the lives set before us.

it's 2008. the years do not matter. i'm enrolled in a course the community college calls "Abnormal Psychology." i'm an artist, flirting with archeology, thanatology, & elevator mechanic. i just learned that i'm autistic; metagnosis. my own psychology is abnormal.

/ a long history /

in 2018, i stand on the banks of a lake with unmarked graves at my back. the final resting place of patients from the local insane asylum. demolished now, aside from a few luxury condos & a boutique hotel. i wonder—what does it mean that i can come & go as i please? what does it mean to the dead? who will speak for them? for whom do they speak?

/ crawling in the closet /

Our task is to create the world we want from the one we have.

/ white male / learning / the history / blames himself
he strives for perfection /

Note

* *Italicized words have been lifted verbatim from the author's own health record.*

1

AN OVERVIEW OF THE HISTORY OF DISABILITY IN THE UNITED STATES

Megan C. Carlos

Introduction

Throughout history, societies have held a wide range of beliefs about diversity in body types, sensory differences, cognitive ability, emotionality, and neurodiversity. Certain types of diversity in physical, cognitive, neurological, and socioemotional functioning have been marginalized because they are not like "normal" bodies or minds within a specific cultural context. As historian Douglas Baynton (2013) insightfully observed, "Disability is everywhere in history once you begin looking for it, but conspicuously absent in the histories we write" (p. 52). This absence is not coincidental – it reflects the cultural tendency to ignore or erase disability as a meaningful category of analysis. Marginalization due to bodily diversity is typically not emphasized within history courses taught in elementary school, high school, or college. It is not unusual for students to be exposed to very little information about the history of disability within the United States. Moreover, it is not uncommon for therapists in training to have limited awareness of how American culture has historically responded to bodies with physical, cognitive, or socioemotional differences. Understanding disability history in the United States is critical for therapists working with disabled individuals because it sheds light on the systemic oppression, marginalization, and stigma the community has endured over time.

This knowledge helps therapists grasp the roots of collective and intergenerational trauma, recognize the broader social and historical contexts that shape their clients' experiences, and approach their work with greater cultural humility, empathy, and awareness of the structural barriers that continue to impact the lives of disabled people. In light of this, the purpose of this chapter is to provide an overview of how disability has been viewed across the history of the United States, offering

DOI: 10.4324/9781003362586-4

context for understanding more about the experiences of the disability community and its subsequent marginalization. Therapists must learn about disability community history to provide client-focused mental health care, as understanding the historical oppression faced by disabled clients enables therapists to recognize the lasting effects of stigma, discrimination, and marginalization, and to approach clients with greater sensitivity to how these experiences shape their identities, mental health, and sense of agency. This knowledge allows therapists to offer more effective, compassionate care by addressing not only the symptoms but also the broader socio-cultural forces that impact their clients' lives.

Themes across the History of Disability

While this chapter focuses on the history of disability within the United States, it is essential to acknowledge that the history of disability across societies and nations spans thousands of years. Diversity in body types and abilities has been present since the beginning of the human race, which has triggered a multitude of cultural reactions to these bodily differences. Fear, disgust, ambivalence, and acceptance have each, at different points in time and in different cultural contexts, characterized how disabled individuals are viewed. Across time, one very common conceptualization of disability has been the pathologizing of body types and bodily differences (Rembis, Kudlick, & Nielsen, 2018). This perspective is consistent with the medical model of disability, which has served as a core foundational principle for the practice of psychotherapy. Therapists need to be mindful that practicing psychotherapy within a medical model framework may inadvertently echo injustices committed against the disability community across history and need to become more aware of how such a framework has harmed the community over time. Possessing such understanding is necessary for cultural competence, developing rapport, and understanding patterns of transference and countertransference among temporarily able-bodied therapists and disabled clients.

An alternative conceptualization to the medical model has been the framing of disability as a form of human diversity and a means of focusing attention on the marginalization of disabled individuals (Rembis, Kudlick, & Nielsen, 2018). This model, typically termed the social model of disability, is reflected in both pre-colonial and more modern views of disability. The social model, and the historical movements supporting it, is important for psychotherapists to understand. There is growing literature that suggests that disabled individuals who adopt a social model of disability are more likely to develop a positive experience of disability, which is associated with higher levels of self-esteem and life satisfaction, and lower levels of distress (Bogart & Dunn, 2019; Zapata, 2020, 2022).

As this chapter unfolds, you will notice how different bodies and body types created a myriad of responses across different cultural contexts. Following colonization within the United States, patterns of keeping disabled individuals sequestered, institutionalized, or hidden away in their homes were prevalent. However, with the onset of the medical model, American culture came to focus on rehabilitating those with disabilities and ambivalently tolerating their presence in communities. Eventually, however, as disabled individuals created community with one another, disability slowly began to be defined as a marginalized identity status that was a reaction to the lived history and generational trauma of disabled individuals within the United States.

Disability in Pre-Colonial North America

It is important to distinguish between pre-colonization and post-colonization experiences of disability in the United States, for disabled individuals were treated in notably different ways during these two periods of history. Pre-colonial, or indigenous, perspectives on disability were characterized by inclusivity, such that disabled individuals were valued for what they brought to their community and the roles they played within these communities (Weaver, 2018). According to Native-American worldviews, each individual had a skill or a purpose that they were meant to utilize in their life (Nielsen, 2012), and these abilities were valued within community, regardless of the disability, cognitive, or health status of an individual. Because the focus within Indigenous communities was on individuals' skills and traits, as opposed to what they lacked, there was no word or concept for disability (Nielsen, 2012). Indigenous communities focused on fostering those skills or abilities that individuals were able to accomplish, while utilizing those skills for the good of the community. For example, Nielsen (2012) described how a boy with an intellectual impairment might serve as a strong water carrier and emphasized how the community benefited from that ability. As Nielsen (2012) described, "As long as an individual could sustain meaningful relationships that involved emotional or labor reciprocity-regardless of cognitive, physical, or emotional capacities… they were not considered disabled" (p. 3).

Indigenous beliefs about mental health were similar. Just as there was no word or concept for disability in indigenous cultures, there was no recognition of the notion of mental illness either (Nielsen, 2012). Instead, indigenous communities focused on the idea that an individual's spirit, mind, and body needed to be in harmony with one another (Nielsen, 2012). Experiences such as hearing voices, seeing visions, or being unable to sit still were often interpreted as a psychological gift, a sign of wisdom, or an indicator that an individual's spirit, mind, and body were out of balance or harmony (Nielsen, 2012).

Within indigenous communities, because of the physical toll of nomadic life on bodies, it was not unusual for individuals' bodies to be scarred, be missing fingers or toes, or possess other signs of physical variability (Nielsen, 2012). Because of the commonplace nature of the impact of lifestyle on human bodies, less cultural attention was paid to variability among bodies and abilities (Nielsen, 2012).

European Colonizers' Views of Disability

Colonizers brought very different value systems with them to North America about disability than was seen in indigenous cultures. In the 15th and 16th century, Europeans came from cultures where disability was viewed in a much more negative manner. From the time of the Middle Ages, the general view of disabled people in Europe was characterized by indifference, fear, and neglect (Minnesota Governor's Council on Developmental Disabilities (MGCDD), 2024). Disabled individuals were often confined to asylums or prisons (MGCDD, 2024). Beginning in the late 1700s in Britain, concerns developed that population growth was not sustainable with the current food resources. This marked the beginning of the harmful eugenic mindset within Europe. Thomas Malthus, a British clergyman and economist, was credited with developing the first social plan for the management of disabled individuals (MGCDD, 2024). He proposed controlling the population size with birth control and sexual restraint. Further, he argued that individuals who did not appear, behave, or function like the majority of the population (i.e., disabled individuals) should be eliminated. Thus, the eugenics movement developed in Britain and was brought to North America by colonizers. Principles of capitalism and the notion of 'return on investment' play a central role in understanding eugenic perspectives (MGCDD, 2024). Return on investment, a concept still seen in modern American society, is the notion that an individual's worth is not based on their unique individuality or contribution, but on the ability to be productive to society and repay the community for resources that have been put into that individual (MGCDD, 2024).

Disability in Colonial America

Ideas about disability and body-type influenced the identities of European settlers in Colonial America. It determined who was sent on voyages across the Atlantic to North America; individuals with body variability seen as undesirable or unlikely to make the long trip were not allowed to travel (Nielsen, 2012). Further, individuals who became sick or passed away on the voyage were thrown overboard. As such, the colonizers who arrived in North America represented mostly able-bodied individuals who were able to provide labor to create settlements. As the colonies grew, body diversity due to birth trauma, disease, genetics, or accidents became relatively typical (Nielsen, 2012). As long as individuals were able to engage in labor and be economically profitable, there was somewhat less focus on body differences. However, attention was placed on individuals with cognitive disabilities in early legal frameworks within these colonies. Laws reflected that colonies provided more oversight of cognitively disabled individuals than other disabled individuals. For example, in Massachusetts, the law mandated that cognitively disabled individuals could not be made to perform public service if they were unable to and protected cognitively disabled individuals who were considered to be incapable of making sound financial decisions (Nielsen, 2012). Additionally, colonial laws prevented disabled individuals from punishment if they could not understand a law that they had broken (Nielsen, 2012).

During the mid-1700s, institutions to care for disabled individuals began to emerge across the American colonies (Nielsen, 2012). It is important to acknowledge that the care provided in these early institutions was very poor, and often residents of these institutions were punished with whippings or chained to walls. However, it does show that the American colonies were grappling as a society with how to better support and provide treatment for disabled individuals, as misguided as the attempts were (Nielsen, 2012).

Finally, it is pertinent to recognize that the practice of enslavement, which began in the 1500s and continued through and beyond the founding of the United States, was based in deep-rooted ableism (and racism) (Nielsen, 2012). Individuals who practiced enslavement did so on the ableist and racist assumptions that Africans were mentally and physically inferior and abnormal compared to those of European descent (Nielsen, 2012). Further, abhorrent physical and emotional treatment of African and African American individuals created physical disability, social marginalization, educational marginalization, and generational trauma among this community (Hicks, 2015).

Eugenics

The Eugenics Movement strongly shaped beliefs about disability held by European colonizers and the growing colonies in North America. As described earlier, eugenic practices were created in Britain as a strategy for population control across Europe and to lands being colonized by Europeans. While it is widely known that eugenics principles played a significant role in promoting the extermination of millions of Jewish people under Hitler in World War II, what is less known and less explicitly acknowledged is that many prominent European and American psychologists, including Frances Galton, Karl Pearson, Lewis Terman, Henry Goddard, and Edward Thorndike, identified as eugenicists and that eugenic beliefs significantly shaped the practice of psychology in the United States.

Eugenics and the History of Psychological Assessment

Psychological assessment practiced by American psychologists in the early 1900s was deeply influenced by eugenic beliefs. Terman, Goddard, and Thorndike played instrumental roles in creating standardized tests for intellectual ability in the United States (Stoskopf, 2002), and specifically sought to use these tests to advance their eugenic agenda. Using the normal curve and other basic statistical principles, psychologists had tools to classify individuals as "normal" or "abnormal" (Emanuel, 2022). Intelligence was conceptualized as a "given inherited feature" (Pilgrim, 2008, p. 278), and clinical psychologists utilized testing to separate children and adults into groupings based on cognitive functioning. Terman (1916), who later became the president of the American Psychological Association in 1922, wrote:

> Thus far intelligence tests have found their chief application in the identification and grading of the feeble-minded. It is safe to predict that in the near future, intelligence tests will bring tens of thousands of these high-grade defectives under the surveillance and protection of society. This will ultimately result in curtailing the reproduction of feeble-mindedness and in the elimination of an enormous amount of crime, pauperism, and industrial inefficiency.
>
> (Terman, 1916, pp. 5–7)

Throughout the 20th century, mental health professionals continued to utilize assessment and standardized testing to determine the placement of disabled individuals into special education classes, certain types of employment, and institutional care, based on ability (Stoskopf, 2002; Winzer, 1993). These assessments, which were guided by a medical model perspective, focused on identifying impairments in disabled individuals and impinged upon personal or family autonomy to make decisions. Further, allegations that testing methods promoted racial and ethnic discrimination became endemic to the use of psychological testing (Byrd et al., 2021). A disproportionate number of children from minority backgrounds and immigrant families were funneled into special education classes, particularly in urban school districts, because of their scores on standardized tests (Stoskopf, 2002). Given that assessment procedures were shaped by the eugenics movement that was then utilized to limit personal autonomy and justify societal oppression (Coble-Temple et al., in press), it is crucial that therapists understand how the disability community may experience contemporary mental health assessment in a negative manner based on its misuse for generations.

Eugenics and Forced Sterilization

Another result of the eugenics movement in the United States was the utilization of forced sterilization. By 1924, approximately 20 states had instituted forced sterilization laws, which primarily targeted disabled, Black, and Brown individuals. It is estimated that the United States sterilized 60,000 individuals between 1900 and 1960 (Andrews, 2019), and women of color are overrepresented in those who have been sterilized. It is notable that sterilization practices in the United States pre-dated similar practices in Nazi Germany (Andrews, 2019). In fact, several practices that were criticized by American judges in the Nuremberg trials following World War II were modeled from the work of American physicians practicing eugenics, deemed as acceptable by the US Supreme Court on multiple occasions (Andrews, 2019). While sterilizations decreased over time, as of 2022, 31 states and territories still had laws or court precedents that allow for forced sterilization (National Women's Law Center and Autistic Women and Nonbinary Network, 2022). Further, federally forced sterilization remains legal within the United States. It is important for therapists who work with disabled individuals to understand that forced sterilization is not necessarily a relic of the distant past, but may be part of a client's lived history.

Disability and the Industrial Revolution

The transition from an agricultural-based economy to an industrial-based one had critical implications for disabled people in the capitalist-driven United States economy. As described earlier in this chapter, the ability to labor and produce economically has been valued since the colonization of North America. As long as disabled individuals could provide labor and economic value, disability was generally downplayed. When the foundation of the US economy shifted in the Industrial Revolution, this had a cascading impact on those with disabilities. As individuals shifted from working in the home in an agricultural-based economy to engaging in factory-work, less accommodation was available for disabled individuals and typical working hours were standardized based on non-disabled workers (Newman & Turner, 2024). Disabled workers and aging workers were slowly displaced from the workforce, which contributed to higher rates of institutionalization (Newman & Turner, 2024). Andrews (2019) explained that "industrial capitalism tended to marginalize people with disabilities, who were forced to compete against non-disabled workers" (p. 7). Further, industrialization and factory work also began to rely on standardized tests as a tool for businesses to match workers with specific jobs (Katz, 2022). As described by Nair et al. (2023), standardized testing "evolved as a tool for exclusion and oppression of disabled identities [and served] as a tool for pathologizing Black and Brown children with cognitive, language, communication, and behavior impairments because of their embodied differences" (p. 2).

Ugly Laws

Between the end of the Civil War and the beginning of World War I, increasingly negative social beliefs about disability and disabled people were reflected in a series of municipal statutes across the country that made it illegal for disabled individuals to appear in public (Schweik, 2009). These municipal statues were aptly referred to as the "Ugly Laws", and sought to prevent individuals who were "diseased, maimed, mutilated, or in any way deformed, so as to be an unsightly or disgusting object" (Chicago City Code, 1881), from appearing in public. Versions of the Ugly Laws stayed in effect in several cities within the United States until 1974 (Schweik, 2009).

The Ugly Laws reflected general fear and distastefulness of disabled individuals within the United States. Nielsen (2012) explains that these laws reflected a broader societal unease – despite the Progressive Era's efforts from the 1890s to the early 1920s to study, regulate, and improve society, bodily difference persisted, and misfortune remained prevalent. In fact, industrialization itself became a significant source of disability (p. 89). During the same time, in the late 19th century, laws were passed to restrict voting and property ownership among those with disabilities (Nielsen, 2012). These laws further reflected society's unease with and ambivalence toward those with disabilities.

Institutionalism as a Means of Disability Management

The 19th century also marked the rise of institutionalism within the United States. Institutions to care for disabled individuals initially came about to support injured veterans returning from the Civil War (Nielsen, 2012). At the time, this was the government's plan for ways to manage individuals who were unable to care for themselves, and who did not have family members available to provide care (Noll, 2018). While preliminary institutions were created within the framework of the medical model, geared toward rehabilitating injured veterans, they were influenced by the eugenics movement and were gradually transitioned into environments that protected disabled people from society and protected society from disabled people (Noll, 2018). Families were encouraged to place disabled children in institutions and were told that it would be better for their non-disabled children to have disabled siblings placed outside of the home (Nielsen, 2012).

As institutions grew in the United States, so did their struggles to run successfully. To be financially solvent, many institutions took on more patients than they could realistically manage. Further, institutions led family members to believe they could cure disabled individuals in a certain time frame (Noll, 2018). Not surprisingly, institutions could not deliver on this promise of a cure, and, as a result, lost funding to run smoothly. Soon, institutions became chronically underfunded and short staffed. As a result, they often relied on their own patients for labor. Many stories of abysmal treatment in institutions surfaced, including patients being beaten, chained to walls or furniture, and used for medical experimentation (Noll, 2018). Moreover, because institutions were an opportunity for socialization for disabled folks, over time institutions became environments that unintentionally facilitated reproduction. Again, as a result of the eugenics movement, sterilization was introduced as a strategy for birth control in institutions, the constitutionality of which was held up by the Supreme Court in 1927 (Noll, 2018).

War Veterans and Early Disability Movements in the United States

The Civil War, World War I, and World War II are important to examine as a part of understanding the history of disability, since many veterans returned from war with significant disabilities. The Civil War resulted in extensive injuries and resultant disabilities, especially amputations, among soldiers (Andrews, 2019). The influx of disabled veterans forced the United States to face the question of how to "rebuild war cripples into economically viable citizens" (Linker, 2006, p. 1). The Civil War was the first war within the United States in which decisions needed to be made about supports and plans for disabled veterans. Following the Civil War, the government offered injured veterans medical care and pay. While these resources allowed veterans to not return to the labor market, this pattern created long-term concerns from the government that the pension system would be overburdened by veterans (Linker, 2006).

Therefore, when the United States reached the end of World War I, the government considered the position of veterans in a notably different way (Linker, 2006). An economic agenda and the capitalistic values of the United States were reflected in the political campaigns related to veterans post-World War I, given the strong political support for transforming disabled veterans into wage earners (Linker, 2006). Federal programs for physical and vocational rehabilitation services were developed in 1920 and continued to be offered via the Veteran's Administration. As Linker (2006) articulates, "with proper physical and vocational reconstruction, blind men, deaf men, and dismembered men could all produce wealth and contribute to society" (pp. 1–2). She further explains that the initial rehabilitation programs moved away from a eugenic approach to disability toward a medical model approach. Notably, this change was driven by strong financial incentives. Linker (2006) explains that the government,

> Sought instead to educate the nation to accept disabled soldiers while also providing the injured with the tools to reintegrate back into "normal" life as seamlessly as possible. Such ambitions formed the foundation of federal rehabilitation programs that began during the Great War; those ambitions also continued to shape America's healthcare policies and veteran welfare programs well into the 1960s.
>
> (p. 4)

World War II

Similar to the aftermath of World War I, there was a large emphasis on physical rehabilitation of injured and disabled veterans following World War II. Howard Rusk was an army physician who took a new approach to the rehabilitation of World War II veterans. He viewed rehabilitation in a more holistic manner, advocating that rehabilitation centers should feel more home-like than the traditional military-style rehabilitation centers (Andrews, 2019). Following these changes in how rehabilitation was viewed, Veterans Administration medical centers developed programs for rehabilitation that included medical care, vocational rehabilitation, occupational therapy, physical therapy, psychotherapy, and recreational activities (Andrews, 2019). As such, the care of veterans helped to shape the quality of rehabilitation services available to individuals following accidents and other major medical issues. Further, as an increasing number of disabled veterans sought to use the Servicemen's Readjustment Act of 1944 (which became known as the GI bill) to pay for their return to school, this placed pressure on university campuses to make their facilities and programs accessible to disabled individuals. While universities began to develop programs for disabled students to meet the needs of veterans returning to school, the influx of disabled students into higher education increasingly highlighted the inaccessibility of many colleges and universities (Madaus, Miller, & Vance, 2009). This is just one example of how disabled veterans advocating for greater accessibility helped to initiate the long path of increasing physical accessibility within the United States.

Civil Rights Bill

The 1960s brought strong arguments for racial and gender equity within the United States. The Civil Rights Act of 1964 prohibited discrimination on the basis of race, national origin, religion, and sex (Civil Rights Act, 1964). However, the Civil Rights Act remained silent on the identities of disabled individuals. A major reason that disability was not included in the Civil Rights Act was the complications involved in mandating greater accessibility in buildings and city infrastructure (e.g., transportation systems) (Andrews, 2019). The National Commission on the Rehabilitation of the Handicapped was formed in 1965 to begin to address lack of physical accessibility in federal buildings. The work of this commission laid the groundwork for the passage of the Architectural Barriers Act of 1968 that set initial accessibility standards within the United States (Andrews, 2019).

The Independent Living Movement

In the late 1960s and the 1970s, the San Francisco Bay Area served as the center of many types of civil rights activism; especially true for disability rights (Andrews, 2019). Disabled writers and activists credit the San Francisco Bay Area as the birthplace of the disability community (Shapiro, 1994). One activist whose work is often cited, and who is considered the father of the independent living movement, is Ed Roberts. Roberts, a young man who had polio, enrolled at the University of California (UC) at Berkeley, in 1962. He was the first student at UC Berkeley who was a wheelchair user. Roberts, who utilized an iron lung, could not be accommodated in the dormitories at Berkeley. As such, he negotiated the opportunity to live in the student health center on campus. As the word spread among families of disabled students that UC Berkeley had accommodated Roberts' needs, more disabled individuals applied to the campus and came to live with Roberts in the student health center (Andrews, 2019).

After graduating from Berkeley, Roberts is credited with beginning the Independent Living Movement. This movement was based on two core ideas: first, that disabled people should not be institutionalized; and second, that disabled individuals should be full participants within their communities (Andrews, 2019). Advocates argued that quality of life and living conditions are poor in state hospitals and nursing homes, and that community-based living was far less expensive in human and financial cost (Andrews, 2019). The first Center for Independent Living (CIL) opened in Berkeley, California, in 1979, and focused on providing disabled individuals with skill-building, advocacy, and peer support (Andrews, 2019). This center became a model for other CILs around the country.

Rehabilitation Act 504

Beginning in the 1970s, more federal legislation was passed to secure the rights of disabled individuals. The most significant legislation that was passed during this time was the Rehabilitation Act of 1973, which stated that disabled individuals could not be discriminated against by institutions that received federal funding. This represented a significant step forward in reducing discrimination and securing accessibility in public institutions for people with disabilities. However, after the passage of this act, the Secretary of Health and Human Services, Joseph Califano, refused to sign Section 504 of the newly passed act. Further, a taskforce was created by Health and Human Services to revise the language of Section 504 and to weaken the reinforcement of the act. As a result, in April 1977, over 100 disabled individuals began a sit-in protest at the Health and Human Services offices in the San Francisco Federal Building (Andrews, 2019). The sit-in lasted for 25 days and was the longest-ever occupation to occur in a federal building. Disabled individuals, personal care attendants, and disability community allies lived in the building during the sit-in and were supported by a network of supporters outside of the building who provided food, portable showers, mattresses, and other necessities to make the lengthy protest possible. It resulted in Joseph Califano signing Section 504 of the Rehabilitation Act as originally written (Andrews, 2019).

When Califano signed Section 504, he was also signing the Education for All Handicapped Children Act, which mandated that public schools provide education to disabled students in the least restrictive environment (Education for All Handicapped Children Act, 1975). While this was a significant event in disability rights history in the United States, it is important to point out that the primary leaders of this occupation, including disability rights activist, Judy Heumann, were White. Many of the key activists in US disability history who argued for increased civil rights for people with disability were in fact primarily White individuals with mobility impairments (Frederick & Shifrer, 2019).

Fighting for Transportation Accessibility in the 1980s

Following the passage of the Rehabilitation Act, disabled individuals had increased access to education and employment. However, disabled individuals often did not have access to public transportation. In Denver, Colorado, following new city busses not being equipped with wheelchair lifts, a group of disability activists surrounded and blocked the front and back of a city bus so that it couldn't move. The activists blocked traffic and refused to disband for two days. As a result, the city of Denver agreed to be the first city in the US to provide accessible bus transit for disabled individuals (Andrews, 2019).

The activists who secured accessible busses in Denver came to be known as the American Disabled for Accessible Public Transit (ADAPT). They were considered a radical activist group, and frequently utilized nonviolent civil disobedience to call attention to their cause (Andrews, 2019). The types of protests carried out by ADAPT included disabled activists chaining themselves to the White House fence, utilizing sledgehammers to destroy curbs to convince local legislators to create curb cuts, and blocking entrances at a transportation conference for legislators (Andrews, 2019).

Americans with Disabilities Act

The strides that were made in the 1970s and 1980s in increasing rights and accessibility of those with disabilities led to momentum to pass a civil rights bill for disabled individuals. President George H.W. Bush signed the Americans with Disabilities Act (ADA) which came into effect on July 26, 1990. The ADA has been described as the most monumental legislation to be passed in support of disability rights in the United States (Andrews, 2019). The ADA transformed the way that individuals with disabilities are educated, granted rights as consumers and citizens, and altered the way disabled people are treated at the workplace. Similar to earlier civil rights legislation that protected disparate minority groups, the ADA made it illegal to discriminate on the basis of disability and granted sweeping access to public accommodations and services for the disabled (Karger & Rose, 2010).

Life in the Post-ADA World

While the ADA brought important changes to life for individuals with disabilities in the United States, this legislation has not brought about change regarding beliefs about disability. As such, attitudes toward disability and disabled individuals remain quite negative (Scope, 2022; Olkin, 2001). Despite it being 34 years past the passage of the ADA, disabled individuals report experiencing regular discrimination (Keller & Galday, 2010) and there are ongoing legal and political attempts to roll back the strides made by the ADA (Wylonis, Wylonis, & Sadoff, 2017). As Peace (2015) describes, "In the post-ADA era, discrimination is far more insidious and polite" (p. 104). Emanuel (2022) further argues that post-ADA systemic ableism in the United States is routinely unacknowledged, that the disability experienced is often sensationalized through inspiration pornography (Young, 2014), and that there is ever-present pressure for those individuals with disabilities to conform to ableist notions of normality. Emanuel (2022) also contends that ability discrimination may be far more aggressive by arguing, "In our contemporary culture, people with disabilities-particularly those with intellectual, developmental, and psychiatric disabilities, are regularly hated and perceived to be threatening. For example, people with intellectual and developmental disabilities are often accused of violence and even white supremacy" (p. 187).

Conclusion

Throughout this chapter, we recognize how the view of disability and disabled individuals has been in constant flux, from pre-colonial times to the present. The response to disabled individuals in the United States has ranged from fear and rejection to uneasy tolerance. While initial responses to disability reflected sequestering of those with disability, a growing number of disabled veterans and an increasingly medicalized view of disability gave rise to focusing on treatment and minimization of disability. History has demonstrated that attitudes towards disability are widely impacted by the capitalist values in the United States, and that the ability to labor has been crucial in distinguishing whether individuals have been viewed as worthy. These capitalist values also allowed for disability and ableism to be utilized to justify enslavement of Africans and African Americas; there was a very significant economic payoff for the United States to utilize ableism to pathologize and vilify Black bodies. In more recent history, as members of the disability community have come together to fight for accessibility, a shared sense of marginalization has given rise to the social model of disability and promoted pride within the disability community.

There are several key takeaways from the history described in this chapter that can provide useful guidance to therapists working within the disability community. First, the health care that is offered to those with disabilities – including the practice of mental health assessment and psychotherapy – is steeped in a medical model framework, which is focused on pathologizing disability. Relatedly, this medical model framework has served as a backdrop of mistreatment of disabled individuals by physicians and medical institutions. As such, it should not come as a surprise if a disabled client does not trust their mental health provider. Finally, research has demonstrated the significance of adopting a social model of disability and utilizing the disability community's expertise for learning about their mental health needs. Mental health professionals may wish to convey this information to their clients with disabilities to support the development of resiliency and positive mental health.

References

Andrews, E. E. (2019). *Disability as diversity: Developing cultural competence*. Oxford University Press.

Baynton, D. C. (2013). Disability and the justification of inequality in American history. *The Disability Studies Reader*, *17*(33), 33–57.

Bogart, K. R., & Dunn, D. S. (2019). Ableism special issue introduction. *Social Issues*, *75*(3), 650–664. https://doi.org/10.1111/josi.12354

Byrd et al., 2021. Byrd, D. A., Rivera Mindt, M., Clark, U. S., Clarke, Y., Thames, A. D., Gammada, E. Z., & Manly, J. J. (2021). Creating an antiracist psychology by addressing professional complicity in psychological assessment. *Psychological Assessment, 33*(3), 279–285. https://doi.org/10.1037/pas0000993

Civil Rights Act of 1964, Pub. L. No. 88–352, 78 Stat. 241 (1964).

Coble-Temple, A., Carlos, M., Caprio, E., Zhang, B., & Chen, J. (2024). Psychological assessment with clients with physical and medical disabilities. In A. J. Wright (Ed.), Essentials of culture in psychological assessment (pp. 467–486). John Wiley & Sons.

Education for All Handicapped Children Act, Pub. L. No. 94–142 (1975).

Karger, H., & Rose, S. R. (2010). Revisiting the Americans with Disabilities Act after two decades. *Journal of Social Work in Disability & Rehabilitation, 9*(2–3), 73–86. https://doi.org/10.1080/1536710X.2010.493468

Keller, R. M., & Galgay, C. E. (2010). Microaggressive experiences of people with disabilities. In D. W. Sue (Ed.), *Microaggressions and marginality: Manifestation, dynamics, and impact* (pp. 241–268). John Wiley & Sons.

Emanuel, C. (2022). A white and nondisabled psychoanalyst: Owning racism and ableism in the clinical process. *Psychoanalysis, Self, and Context, 17*(2), 181–195.

Frederick, A., & Shifrer, D. (2019). Race and disability: From analogy to intersectionality. *Sociology of Race and Ethnicity, 5*(2), 200–214. https://doi.org/10.1177/2332649218783480

Hicks, S. R. (2015). *A critical analysis of post traumatic slave syndrome: A multigenerational legacy of slavery*. California Institute of Integral Studies.

Katz, Y. (2022). Intelligence under racial capitalism. *Monthly Review, 74*(4), 32–52. https://doi.org/10.14452/MR-074-04-2022-08_4

Linker, B. (2006). *For life and limb: The reconstruction of a nation and its disabled soldiers in World War I America*. Yale University.

Madaus, J. W., Miller, W. K., & Vance, M. L. (2009). Veterans with disabilities in postsecondary education. *Journal of Postsecondary Education and Disability, 22*(1), 10–17.

Minnesota Governer's Council on Developmental Disabilities. (2024). *A history of developmental disability.* Retrieved from: https://mn.gov/mnddc/parallels/5e.html

Nair, V. K., Farah, W., & Cushing, I. (2023). A critical analysis of standardized testing in speech and language therapy. *Language, Speech, and Hearing Services in Schools, 54*(3), 1–13. https://doi.org/10.1044/2023_LSHSS-22-00141

National Women's Law Center, and Autistic Women, & Nonbinary Network. (2022). *Forced sterilization of disabled people in the United States.*

Newman, S. L., & Turner, D. M. (2024). Disability, gender and old age in the Industrial Revolution: Cultural historical and osteoarchaeological perspectives. In *The material body* (pp. 205–235). Manchester University Press.

Nielsen, K. E. (2012). *A disability history of the United States* (Vol. 2). Beacon Press.

Noll, S. (2018). Institutions for people with disabilities in North America. In M. Rembis, C. Kudlick, & K. E. Nielsen (Eds.), *The Oxford handbook of disability history* (pp. 307–326). Oxford Academic.

Olkin, R. (2001). *What psychotherapists should know about disability.* New York, NY: Guilford Press.

Peace, W. J. (2015). Parenting and disability: The final frontier. *Houston Law Review, 5,* 101–109.

Pilgrim, D. (2008). The eugenic legacy in psychology and psychiatry. *The International Journal of Social Psychiatry, 54*(3), 272–284. https://doi.org/10.1177/0020764008090282

Rembis, M., Kudlick, C. J., & Nielsen, K. (Eds.). (2018). *The Oxford handbook of disability history*. Oxford University Press.

Schweik, S. M. (2009). *The ugly laws: Disability in public*. New York University.

Shapiro, J. P. (1994). *No pity: People with disabilities forging a new civil rights movement.* Crown.

Stoskopf, A. (2002). Echoes of a forgotten past: Eugenics, testing, and education reform. *The Educational Forum, 66*, 126–133. https://doi.org/10.1080/00131720208984814

Terman, L. M. (1916). The uses of intelligence tests. In *The measurement of intelligence* (pp. 3–21). Houghton, Mifflin and Company. https://doi.org/10.1037/10014-001

Weaver, H. N. (2018). Disability through a Native American lens: Examining influences of culture and colonization. In *All my relations: Understanding the experiences of Native Americans with disabilities* (pp. 18–32). Routledge.

Winzer, M. A. (1993). *The history of special education: From isolation to integration.* Gallaudet University Press.

Wylonis, L., Wylonis, N. T., & Sadoff, R. (2017). Navigating the rolling hills of justice: Mental disabilities, employment and the evolving jurisprudence of the Americans with Disabilities Act. *Behavioral Sciences & the Law*, *35*(2), 178–185.

Young, S. (2014). *I'm not your inspiration, thank you very much* [Video file]. Retrieved from: https://www.ted.com/talks/stella_young_i_m_not_your_inspiration_thank_you_very_much?subtitle=en

Zapata, M. A. (2020). Disability affirmation and acceptance predict hope among adults with physical disabilities. *Rehabilitation Psychology*, *65*(3), 291–298. https://doi.org/10.1037/rep0000364

Zapata, M. A. (2022). Disability self-worth and positive personal meaning in disability: Correlates of hope among U.S. residents with physical disabilities. *Rehabilitation Counseling Bulletin*, *65*(2), 150–160.

Bibliography

Hutcheon, E. J., & Lashewicz, B. (2020). Tracing and troubling continuities between ableism and colonialism in Canada. *Disability & Society*, *35*(5), 695–714.

Leong, F. T. L., & Park, Y. S. (2016). *Testing and assessment with persons and communities of color.* Council of the National Psychological Associations for the Advancement of Ethnic Minority Interests.

Lieffers, C. A. L. (2020). *Imperial Ableism: Disability and American Expansion, c. 1850–1930* (Doctoral dissertation, Yale University).

Tuck, E., & Yang, K. W. (2012). Decolonization is not a metaphor. *Decolonization: Indigeneity, Education & Society, 1*(1), 1–40.

2

DISABILITY AND THE LAW

Challenges and Opportunities in the U.S. Legal System

Solomon Furious Worlds and Ellis Scout Cliff

Introduction

A foundational understanding of disability rights and the legal system is invaluable for therapists, as it equips them to better support and advocate for their clients. While therapists are not expected to be legal experts, familiarity with broad legal principles and key legislation would enhance their ability to recognize systemic barriers and provide informed, affirming care. Legal protections significantly impact mental health and well-being since they shape clients' access to employment, education, health care, education accommodations, and more. By integrating a basic knowledge of disability law into their practice, therapists can foster a more inclusive therapeutic environment, empower clients to navigate institutional challenges, and ensure they are upholding ethical and equitable standards of care.

What we call "the law" is greatly influenced and informed by politics and natural observations, so all matters of opinions-positive, negative, or otherwise about the spectrum of disabled people have been or presently are part of "the law." The U.S. legal system is a descendant of the British legal system, which revolved largely around the idea that property rights (meaning both real estate and personal property, like money and livestock) take precedence over all else, and those with property and wealth have more rights and more favorable societal standing. Those who were not born into wealthy families must be "functioning" members of the labor force to have any moniker of worth. And so, a disabled person who could not work, learn, or engage in public life in the ways non-disabled society was accustomed to recognizing, were (and are) less protected and were (and still are) even criminalized (Dowd, 2020; Greiwe, 2019). The concept of "functioning" has evolved over time with the increasing inclusion of disabled people in everyday life. This shift can be attributed to figures like President Franklin D. Roosevelt and

DOI: 10.4324/9781003362586-5

the nearly one million disabled veterans following World War I and II (Reft, 2017), as well as advancements in adaptive technologies such as Braille and hearing aids (Assistive Devices for Disability, 2020).

The natural sequel to disability representation and technological advancements has been the increased understanding of disabled people as rich and complex with an untold number of valid variations, like any other people. Indeed, in 2006, the United Nations adopted the Convention of the Rights of Persons with Disabilities which called upon all governments of the world to "recognize the inherent dignity and worth and the equal and inalienable rights" of disabled people. The word "disability" is "an evolving concept," in part, because one's disability "results from the interaction between [oneself] with impairments and attitudinal and environmental barriers that hinders their full and effective participation in society on an equal basis with others" (United Nations Convention on the Rights of Persons with Disabilities, 2006; Stein, 2007).

Unfortunately, as this chapter later notes, federal statutes meant to address disability discrimination did so in such a way to perpetuate arcane and belittling notions of what it means to be a disabled person (Americans with Disabilities Act, 1990; Fair Housing Amendments Act, 1988; Rehabilitation Act, 1973). However, in 2009, the U.S. Congress passed a law that replaced the outdated phrase "mental retardation" with "intellectual disability" in all its present statutes, a clear recognition of the inherent dignity of disabled people and the societal harm disabled individuals often endure (Rosa's Law, 2010). Indeed, various social, economic, and technological advancements have even brought the social model of disability into the law (Powell, 2022; Bagenstos, 2000) to replace, albeit slowly, its outdated and disgusting medical model counterpart (Hogan, 2019).

This chapter focuses on those aspects of law that were created to explicitly affect disabled people. It explains the U.S. legal system's structure, examines several impactful federal court cases that advanced legal protections for disabled people, and reviews the major statutes that further afforded disabled people legal protections. The law is far from a perfect vehicle to enact social change, or to fully protect the inherent rights that all disabled people, or any other peoples, deserve and are entitled by virtue of being human. Still, in serving as an accurate introduction to "the law" that affects disabled people, this chapter hopes to offer more good news than bad.

Branches and Levels of Government in the American Legal System

The American legal system is a series of different legal systems stacked on, and within, one another, forming a tapestry of bureaucracy meant to govern its inhabitants. There are three main branches of government—judicial, legislative, and executive—that exist on three separate levels—federal, state, and local.

The judicial branch (i.e., federal, state, and local courts) adjudicates statutes, regulations, challenges to government actions, and disputes among private parties by determining whether parties violated the Constitution or some other law (e.g., federal or state statutes, regulations, and past judicial orders); then, the judicial branch creates law by issuing judicial orders called opinions. The legislative branch (e.g., Congress, state general assembly, and local school board) creates laws, known as statutes, that allow for or criminalize any number of activities. The executive branch (e.g., the president, governor, mayor, secretary of state, and secretary of education) carries out and regulates statutes, and creates law by executive orders or directives through its own power and by regulations through government agencies. Each state has the same three-branch structure of government within it, and most local governments (e.g., cities, towns, school districts) have legislative and executive branches.

The U.S. Constitution states that federal law takes precedence over most state laws in what is commonly referred to as "the Supremacy Clause," and most states' constitutions have a similar provision giving state law precedence over most local laws (U.S. Const. art. 6, para. 2). This means that any federal disability protections – including constitutional provisions, Supreme Court opinions, or Congressional statutes – collectively represent the *minimum* protections that must be afforded to all disabled people in the United States. Therefore, states are constitutionally prohibited from taking actions that limit the rights of disabled people in ways that conflict with federal law, and cities and school districts are prohibited from doing the same in ways that conflict with state law. This means that the protections afforded to disabled people can vary from state to state, and sometimes city to city, with some governmental entities creating more protections, and others choosing to make very few additions.

While some areas of law are entirely created, changed, or managed by one branch or at one level of government, all three branches at all three levels work together to form what is comprehensively known as disability law. Below are some of the most impactful and foundational court cases and statutes that define and shape disability law. However, this chapter does not provide an overview of regulations that directly affect disabled people because they tend to address specific aspects of the statute to which they are connected and can change often. Likewise, this chapter does not explore state and local disability law because there are so many state and local variations that an entire encyclopedia set would be needed to do so properly. However, it is important to note that state and local law often offers more protections than federal law.

Constitutional Law and Influential Court Cases Effecting Disabled Persons' Rights

The Fourteenth and Fifth Amendments' (U.S. Const. amend. XIX; U.S. Const. amend. V) equal protection and due process clauses are the driving force for every U.S. civil rights movement after the Civil War. Both guarantee equal treatment under the law by forbidding any government agency or actor from arbitrarily treating one class of persons better or worse than another (Schneider v. Rusk, 1964;

Bolling v. Sharpe, 1954). The Fourteenth Amendment applies to state and local governments, and the Fifth Amendment applies to the federal government (*Schneider v. Rusk,* 1964*; Bolling v. Sharpe,* 1954*).*

Their due process clauses, by their plain texts, guarantee notice and hearing by forbidding any government agency or actor from taking away a person's liberty interests without first giving them notice and an opportunity to defend their liberty interests (U.S. Const. amend. XIX; U.S. Const. amend. V). The due process clause is also thought to protect substantive liberty rights-like the rights for parents to raise their children (*Santosky v. Kramer,* 1982), privacy (*Griswold v. Connecticut,* 1965), and same-sex marriage (*Obergefell v. Hodges,* 2015), from unnecessary, unreasonable, or arbitrary government action. When invoked in the manner first described, the law refers to it as procedural due process; likewise, when invoked in the manner described second, the law refers to it as substantive due process (Chemerinsky, 1999). However, U.S. Supreme Court Justice Clarence Thomas disagrees with decisions wherein the due process clause is employed in a substantive manner and recently suggested that the high court "should reconsider all of this Court's substantive due process precedents" in future cases because, in his view, they are "demonstrably erroneous" – which includes the aforementioned cases where the U.S. Constitution was found to protect the rights for parents to raise their children, privacy, and same-sex marriage (*Dobbs v. Jackson Women's Health Organization,* 2022). Though this radical departure from decades of jurisprudence has been proposed, at the time this chapter was written, the "fundamental" rights protected by the substantive use of the due process clause remain intact.

Since the Fourteenth Amendment was passed in the immediate aftermath of the Civil War as a way to address the nation's long history of racialized slavery, it was immediately understood to apply across racial lines using the equal protections clause (*Slaughter-House Cases*, 1872) and, soon after, fundamental rights (e.g., voting, religious expression, freedom of speech, and marriage) using the due process clause (*United States v. Carolene Products Company,* 1938). Because of this, Courts analyze government actions that implicate race, ethnicity, national origin, or a fundamental right under strict scrutiny, meaning the action must be narrowly tailored to further a compelling government interest (*Miller v. Johnson,* 1995). For example, in the 1967, U.S. Supreme Court case *Loving v. Virgina*, the Court held that statutes forbidding interracial marriages violated the Fourteenth Amendment's equal protection and due process clauses because such statutes implicated a protected class (i.e., race) and a fundamental right (i.e., marriage) without there being a compelling enough government reason to do so (*Loving v. Virginia,* 1967). Courts apply intermediate scrutiny when analyzing government actions that implicate a quasi-suspect class (e.g., sex and gender) (*Mississippi University for Women v. Hogan,* 1982), and rational basis when reviewing government action that does not implicate a suspect or quasi-suspect class (*Romer v. Evans,* 1996). However, in 1985, the U.S. Supreme Court eventually recognized that the Fourteenth Amendment's equal protection clause applied to disabled people.

In *City of Cleburne, TX v. Cleburne Living Center*, a proposed operator of a group home for disabled people challenged a city's zoning ordinance that made it illegal for such homes to exist in a particular zoning district. A lower court held in favor of the proposed group home operator by calling disabled people a quasi-suspect class and thus subjecting the zoning ordinance to intermediate scrutiny (*City of Cleburne, TX v. Cleburne Living Center*, 1985). The Court held that disability status is different from one's sex in that "the sex characteristic frequently bears no relation to ability to perform or contribute to society," implying that being disabled diminishes one's ability to contribute to society (*City of Cleburne, TX v. Cleburne Living Center*, 1985; *Frontiero v. Richardson*, 1973). Though ableist, the Court continued stating that though it refused to recognize disabled people as a quasi-suspect class, its opinion "does not leave [disabled people] entirely unprotected from invidious discrimination" because disabled people "have and retain their substantive constitutional rights in addition to the right to be treated equally by the law" (*City of Cleburne, TX v. Cleburne Living Center*, 1985). The Court held that the zoning ordinance failed under rational basis review because its treatment toward disabled people was, in fact, irrational and thus not related to any legitimate government interest (*City of Cleburne, TX v. Cleburne Living Center*, 1985).

Though the Court did not decide to apply the same strict level of scrutiny towards government actions and regulations that specifically implicate disabled people, and claimed to use rational basis review, it did decide to apply a heightened standard of review above what is normally used. Typically, a government only needs a rational reason for its action or regulation and the means by which they act just need to be related to the reason. Though the Court claimed to apply the same rational basis review standard in *Cleburne*, its reasoning has led the legal community to understand that there exists a certain "bite" to this application rational basis review. Thus, when government action that directly affects disabled people is challenged, Courts tend to apply a level of review that is above rational basis but below intermediate and strict scrutiny-called *rational basis with teeth or rational basis plus* by many (Pettinga, 1987).

Other Cases Regarding Legal Protections for Disabled People

Before and after the articulation of this heightened rational basis and the implicit recognition of disabled people as a *pseudo*-protected class under the U.S. Constitution, judicial opinions grapple with legal protections for disabled people

1 *Plessy v. Ferguson*, 163 U.S. 537 (1896) – The implications of this case's holding (i.e., the law it created) are no longer valid.

   a Held that segregation of people based on race, and implicitly permitting segregation based on any identity that was "thought to be inferior and unfit," when compared to white, land-owning, able-bodied, cis-males-did not violate the Fourteenth Amendment's equal protection clause where separate but "equal" accommodations were available (Cook, 1991).

2 *Buck v. Bell*, 274 U.S. 200 (1927) – The implications of this case's holding (i.e., the law it created) are no longer valid.

   a Held that compulsory sterilization of disabled people did not violate the Equal Protection Clause, while offering a full-throated defense of the eugenics movement of the 1920s and publishing one of the vilest sentences in 20th-century American law: "Three generations of imbeciles are enough."

3 *Pennsylvania Association for Retarded Citizens v. Commonwealth of Pennsylvania*, 334 F. Supp. 1257 (E.D. Pa. 1972)

   a In the first right-to-education lawsuit in the country, a non-profit organization that sought to advance the rights of disabled children and several disabled children who were "excused" or otherwise expelled from school represented a class of over 50,000 school-aged children. They brought this class action suit against the Commonwealth of Pennsylvania and claimed numerous state laws that allowed public schools to exclude children who had not reached the "mental age of five years" when they enrolled in first grade were unconstitutional under the due process clause of the Fourteenth Amendment.
   b The Commonwealth settled the case and entered into a consent decree wherein all Pennsylvania and its school districts were prohibited from using state law to deny disabled children education, and the settlement agreement was monitored by the court (The Public Interest Law Center, n.d.).

4 *O'Connor v. Donaldson*, 422 U.S. 563 (1975)

   a Held that the government violates the due process clause if it unnecessarily confines an individual to a mental hospital when the individual is not dangerous and is capable of surviving safely in freedom by themselves or with the help of willing and responsible family members or friends.

5 *City of Cleburne, TX, et al. v. Cleburne Living Center et al.*, 473 U.S. 432 (1985)

   a Held that claims alleging discriminatory action, in violation of the Fourteenth Amendment's equal protection clause, towards disabled people should be reviewed using the rational basis standard, but most recognize that the standard has "teeth"—meaning it is a higher standard than the typical rational basis standard. The court also held that government entities or government actors violate the Fourteenth Amendment's equal protection clause when they discriminate against disabled people simply because they are disabled, since doing so is irrational.

Anti-Disability Discrimination Statutes and Related Court Cases

While unchallenged Supreme Court decisions protect the fundamental rights of disabled people, federal statutes and state laws create the legal landscape that attempts to level the playing field. These laws shape where disabled people live and work, how they receive health care, how they are educated, how they are accommodated, and how they are integrated into their communities. There are multiple legal definitions of "disability," which establish who is protected by federal disability laws in various contexts. For the purposes of nondiscrimination laws, such as the Rehabilitation Act of 1973, the Americans with Disabilities Act (ADA), the Individuals with Disabilities Education Act, and the Fair Housing Amendments Act (FHAA), a person with a disability is defined as anyone who has:

a physical or mental impairment that substantially limits one or more major life activities
b a record of such impairment, or
c is regarded as having such an impairment (Definition of Disability, 2008).

This legal definition of disability broadly frames disability by its impact on the disabled individual, rather than limiting it to an enumerated list of symptoms or diagnoses. Notably, the legal definition features the word "impairment" three times. This pathologizing language mirrors the medical model of disability, which views disability as impairments to be corrected (Fisher & Goodley, 2007), rather than the social model of disability, which frames disability as social oppression that should be eliminated (Thomas, Gradwell, & Markham, 1997).

Although this legal definition of disability is intentionally broad, several statues carve out exceptions for whom it protects. For example, many people with Opioid Use Disorder ("OUD") are considered to have a disability under federal law (Opioid use disorder, 2024). This is because OUD is an addiction that can substantially limit major life activities, such as the ability to take care of oneself, work, communicate, think, or learn. However, federal law also creates an exception, and does not protect individuals who are currently using illegal substances.

The Rehabilitation Act

In 1973, the United States signed into law the Rehabilitation Act, one of the first federal laws that prohibits discrimination on the basis of disability in programs run by federal agencies, in programs receiving federal funding, and for federal employers and contractors (Rehabilitation Act of 1973, § 701, 1973). Examples of entities the Rehabilitation Act applies to include, public schools and universities, libraries, hospitals, fire departments, public transportation systems, public housing programs, fire departments, childcare centers, Head Start programs, federal courthouses, and museums (Rehabilitation Act of 1973, § 701, 1973).

Sections 501 and 503 prohibit discrimination in the employment practices of Federal agencies. Under Section 501, executive branch agencies are required to take affirmative action in hiring, assigning, and promoting disabled people (Rehabilitation Act of 1973, § 701, 1973). These requirements are extended to federal contractors through Section 503. Together, these sections additionally establish an Interagency Committee on Employees to ensure federal agencies comply with the mandates of the Rehabilitation Act (Rehabilitation Act of 1973, § 791(a), 1973).

Mirroring the language of civil rights laws protecting people from discrimination based on race and sex, Section 504 states that "no qualified individual with a disability in the United States shall be excluded from, denied the benefits of, or be subjected to discrimination." (Rehabilitation Act of 1973, § 794, 1973). Each federal agency has its own rules for complying with this tenant of Section 504 (U.S. Department of Justice, 2024). There are two ways these rules most commonly address discrimination based on disability. One way that agencies attempt to level the playing field is by creating accessibility standards, like requiring effective communication channels for people who have hearing or vision disabilities (U.S. Department of Justice, 2024). Another common rule federal agencies have created under Section 504 is the requirement to provide *reasonable accommodations* for disabled people (U.S. Department of Justice, 2024). A reasonable accommodation is a modification to a policy, program, service, or workplace that gives a disabled person access to full participation.

Before determining whether an accommodation is reasonable, a person with a disability must first demonstrate that the accommodation is necessary (U.S. Department of Housing and Urban Development, n.d.). They can prove this by showing there is a relationship between their disability and the requested accommodation (U.S. Department of Housing and Urban Development, n.d.). If an accommodation is necessary, several factors determine whether an accommodation is reasonable. These factors attempt to balance the rights of disabled people with practical considerations and resources of the service providers. First, an accommodation is not considered reasonable if it imposes an undue hardship on the operation of the program or activity (U.S. Department of Housing and Urban Development, n.d.). An accommodation imposes an undue hardship if it requires significant difficulty or expense when taking into consideration factors such as the nature and cost of the accommodation, the financial resources of the federally funded facility, and the impact the accommodation will have on the operation of the facility (U.S. Department of Housing and Urban Development, n.d.).

In 1998, the Rehabilitation Act was amended to include Section 508, which creates accessibility requirements for electronic information and technology utilized by the Federal government (Rehabilitation Act of 1973, § 794(d), 1973). Below are a few of the most impactful Rehabilitation Act cases:

1 *School Board of Nassau County v. Arline*, 481 U.S. 273 (1987).

  a In this case, the Court held that an individual with a long-term recurring illness (here, tuberculosis) was protected under Section 504 of the Rehabilitation Act.
  b The Court also recognized that disabled people have historically been subjected to "discrimination stemming not only from simple prejudice but also from 'archaic attitudes and laws' and from 'the fact that the American people are simply unfamiliar with and insensitive to the difficulties confront[ing]'" disabled people.

2 *Traynor v. Turnage*, 485 U.S. 535 (1988)

  a In this case, the Court held that Rehabilitation Act does not require benefits extended to one category of disabled people to be extended to all categories of disabled people. For example, just because low vision and/or blind individuals can have guide dogs as a reasonable accommodation does not mean that someone with ADHD could have the same.
  b More specifically, the Court held that a Veterans' Administration regulation defining alcoholism as "willful misconduct," and thus not as a disability, did not violate Section 504.

The Americans with Disabilities Act

For much of American history, people with disabilities have been denied the right to exist in public spaces, let alone access public accommodations due to inaccessible architecture, and discriminatory practices. Up until 1974, "Ugly Laws" even existed in communities across the country to keep poor and disabled people out of public spaces.[1] For example, a disturbing San Francisco law from 1867 prohibited "any person, who [was] diseased, maimed, mutilated or deformed in any way, so as to be an unsightly or disgusting object, [from exposing themselves] to public view" (Schweik, 2009).

Like the Rehabilitation Act, the Americans with Disabilities Act (ADA) prohibits discrimination based on disability but expands the reach of these protections to the everyday lives of disabled people in areas including employment, the activities of state and local governments, businesses that are open to the public, commercial facilities, transportation, and telecommunications (Americans with Disabilities Act of 1990, § 12101, 1990).

Title I of the ADA prohibits discrimination based on the disability in the employment arena (Americans with Disabilities Act of 1990, § 1201, 1990). It requires private employers with at least 15 employees to provide qualified people with disabilities equal access to employment-related opportunities in hiring, promotions, training, pay, social activities, and termination (Americans with Disabilities Act of 1990, §§ 12111, 12112(a), 1990). Religious entities are not exempt from the ADA (Americans with Disabilities Act of 1990, § 12113(d), 1990). Employers are prohibited from asking about an applicant's disability before making a job offer (Americans with Disabilities Act of 1990, §12112, 1990). Employers are also required to make reasonable accommodations for employees who have disclosed their disability status and have requested an accommodation unless there is an undue hardship (Americans with Disabilities Act of 1990, § 12112(b)(5)(A), 1990).

Title II of the Act applies to the actions of public entities, regardless of size or Federal funding (Americans with Disabilities Act of 1990, § 12131, 1990). Public entities include state and local governments, departments, agencies, special purpose districts, and commuter authorities (Americans with Disabilities Act of 1990, § 12131, 1990). This section requires public entities to provide each "qualified individual with a disability" equal access to their services, including public education, employment, transportation, recreation, health care, social services, courts, voting, and public meetings. Public entities are required to adhere to specific accessibility standards when constructing or remodeling their buildings (Americans with Disabilities Act of 1990, § 12146, 12147, 12148, 1990). Public entities are also required to make reasonable modifications to make policies, practices, and procedures accessible to avoid discrimination (Americans with Disabilities Act of 1990, § 12182(b)(2)(A)(ii), 1990). Notably, the Title II definition of disability more closely aligns with the social model of disability, rather than with the pathologizing definition that centers on the word "impairment" referenced earlier. It does this by defining a qualified individual as someone

> with a disability who, with or without reasonable modifications to rules, policies, or practices, the removal of architectural, communication, or transportation barriers, or the provision of auxiliary aids and services, meets the essential eligibility requirements for the receipt of services or the participation in programs or activities provided by a public entity.
>
> (Americans with Disabilities Act of 1990, § 12131, 1990)

Title III of the ADA applies to public accommodations and prohibits public-facing businesses, accommodations, and service providers from discriminating against disabled people (Americans with Disabilities Act of 1990, § 12182, 1990). Examples of public-facing entities include restaurants, movie theaters, private schools, concert venues, zoos, stadiums, hotels, and privately owned transportation services. Three primary practices are prohibited under Title III to prevent discrimination based on disability:

1 Denial of participation: The exclusion of individuals, on the basis of disability, from the opportunity to participate in or benefit from the goods, services,

facilities, privileges, advantages, or accommodations of an entity (Americans with Disabilities Act of 1990, § 12182(b)(1)(A)(i), 1990).

2 Participation in unequal benefit: To deny individuals, on the basis of disability, the opportunity to participate in or benefit from a good, service, facility, privilege, advantage, or accommodation that is not equal to that afforded to others (Americans with Disabilities Act of 1990, § 12182(b)(1)(A)(ii), 1990).
3 Separate Benefit: To provide individuals, based on disability, with a good, service, facility, privilege, advantage, or accommodation that is different or separate from that provided to other individuals, unless such action is necessary to provide the individual an opportunity that is as effective as that provided to others (Americans with Disabilities Act of 1990, § 12182(b)(1)(A)(iii), 1990).

Finally, Title IV of the ADA requires that telephone and television technology be made accessible for people with disabilities that impact their speech and hearing. Below are a few of the most impactful ADA cases:

1 *Olmstead v. L.C.*, 527 U.S. 581 (1999)[2]

   a The Court reinforced the right of disabled people to live in the community by holding that states unnecessarily institutionalizing disabled people constitutes discrimination in violation of the integration mandate of the ADA, and thus are required to provide services in the most integrated settings.
   b This case is often called the most important civil rights decision for disabled people in U.S. history.

2 *Board of Trustees of the University of Alabama v. Garrett*, 531 U.S. 356 (2001)

   a Weaken the effectiveness of the ADA by holding that state employees filing claims under the employment provisions of the ADA against state government agencies cannot obtain monetary damages as a part of the disposition of their suits because of the state sovereign immunity doctrine of the Eleventh Amendment to the U.S. Constitution.
   b The Eleventh Amendment usually prohibits claims for monetary damages by state employees and private individuals against states, unless the state explicitly consents to being sued for monetary damages.

3 *Johnson v. Gambrinus Co./Spoetzl Brewery*, 116 F.3d 1052 (5th Cir. 1997)

   a The Court held that the ADA and Texas state law protected a blind man's right to bring his guide dog on a Brewery tour, and that doing so did not violate applicable Food and Drug Administration regulations.

The Individuals with Disabilities Education Act

Both Section 504 Rehabilitation Act of 1973, and the ADA create protections for disabled students from discrimination. However, ensuring that disabled students are allowed to attend school does not inherently remove the many barriers that prevent students from accessing their curricula. To close this gap, the Individuals with Disabilities Education Act (IDEA)[3] provides the legal basis for children with disabilities to receive a free *appropriate* public education (Individuals with Disabilities Education Act, §1412, 2004).

The school district where a child lives is responsible for administering education services to any child with a disability who is evaluated and found eligible for an Individualized Education Program (IEP) (Individuals with Disabilities Education Act, 2004.) Before the passing of the IDEA, disabled students were either educated alongside their peers without the appropriate modifications or support to access the curriculum or were excluded from the classroom altogether. The IDEA was developed on the principle that students with disabilities should be educated alongside their nondisabled peers to the greatest extent possible because research has consistently shown the benefits of inclusion (NCLD, 2020).

Despite the intentions outlined by IDEA, the reality for many children with disabilities often falls short of the inclusive environment it advocates for. For example, Black, Indigenous, and Latine students with disabilities are disproportionately placed in these segregated settings compared to their white peers (NCLD, 2020). These disparities extend to disciplinary practices as well. Although IDEA provides extra legal protections for students who are facing suspension or expulsion, students with disabilities are still disproportionately disciplined (NCLD, 2020). Federal law offers limited protections against using restraint or seclusion as disciplinary practices in the education setting (Cho, 2021). Below are a few of the most impactful IDEA cases:

1 *Honig v. Doe*, 484 U.S. 305 (1988)

   a The Court held that the IDEA's "stay put" provision prohibited school districts from excluding or expelling a disabled student from the classroom setting for dangerous or destructive conduct that is a result of their disabilities.
   b Now, schools can only suspend disabled students for a limited amount of time without parental or court intervention.

2 *Jacob Winkelman v. Parma City School District*, 500 U.S. 516 (2007)

   a The Court held that parents may sue under the IDEA independent of their children because their statutory rights under the Act are separate from their child's rights.

3 *Timothy W. v. Rochester, N.H., School Dist*, 875 F.2d 954 (1st Cir. 1989)

   a The Court held that the IDEA guaranteed all disabled school-age children the opportunity to receive free appropriate public school that "emphasizes special education and related services designed to meet their unique needs."

The Fair Housing Amendments Act

The Fair Housing Amendments Act (FHAA) was enacted in 1988 to extend the protections of the Fair Housing Act of 1968 to disabled people. Through the FHAA, Congress recognized that "the right to be free of housing discrimination is essential to the goal of independent living" (H.R. Rep. No. 100-711, 1988; *Alliance for the Mentally Ill v. City of Naperville,* 1996). Just as *Olmstead* attempts to correct the harms of keeping disabled people cut off from their communities in institutional settings, the FHAA seeks to protect their right to choose to live where they want, by prohibiting practices that "discourage or obstruct [those] choices in a community, neighborhood or development" (The Fair Housing Amendments Act, 1988).

Under the FHA, it is illegal to discriminate against disabled people in the sale, rental, or financing of housing. It prohibits housing providers from refusing to rent or sell to people due to their disability status and requires that housing providers make reasonable accommodations for individuals with disabilities to ensure they have equal access to housing opportunities. This includes modifications to existing buildings or policies to accommodate the needs of individuals with disabilities. Section 504 of the Rehabilitation Act of 1973[4] reinforces the FHA by requiring federally funded housing providers to ensure that their programs are nondiscriminatory and accessible to disabled people. Most notably, it requires that federally funded housing that is newly constructed or altered meet accessibility standards outlined in the ADA. Below are a few of the most impactful FHAA cases:

1 *Regional Economic Community Action Program, Inc. v. City of Middletown,* 294 F.3d 35, 49 (2d Cir.), cert. denied, 537 U.S. 813 (2002)

   a The Court held that claimants do not need to prove that disability discriminatory animus was the only factor as to why the government did what it did, but that it was a significant factor under the FHA.
   b Courts in other appellate circuits have held the same (*Community Services, Inc. v. Wind Gap Municipal Authority,* 2005).

2 *Support Ministries for Persons with AIDS, Inc. v. Village of Waterford,* 808 F. Supp. 120 (N.D.N.Y. 1992);

   a The Court held that a change in a zoning ordinance in response to the effort to create group homes for persons who are HIV-positive, which generated intense community opposition, was the result of unlawful discriminatory intent and thus in violation of the FHA

3 Hamm v. City of Gahanna, 109 Fed. Appx. 744, 747-49 (6th Cir. 2004)

   a The Court held that a city did not violate the FHA by refusing to grant a variance to allow the plaintiffs to construct group homes for people who are elderly and have disabilities on their property because the decision was based on the city's desire to protect "property values" and the community opposition was based on concerns about property values rather than the disabilities of the residents.

Conclusion

Many of the cases, statutes, and other innovations discussed in this chapter start with the assumption that disability discrimination is like discrimination of any other kind; however, while aspects are identical, there are unique characteristics to discrimination along any single identity class. Too often, judges' and legislators' disability discrimination analyses and debates, respectively, are too "simplistic" and "reductive" such that they serve to "reinforce the white disability narrative" – wherein mostly (if not only) white, disabled cismen's opinions are solicited and listened to, and their narratives are the only ones retold (Chin, 2021). The legal world has long discussed the limits of the civil rights litigation model of obtaining rights and of the anti-discrimination paradigm endorsed through federal legislation (Bagenstos, 2004; Raj, 2021; Harris, 2020), especially since its framework "emphasizes individualism and self-sufficiency with the goal of assimilation" (Chin, 2021). These limits stifle the possibilities and usefulness of disability rights law such that it can only do so much to aid and assist disabled people, especially the most marginalized and under-resourced.

Disability Justice, as a socio-legal lens, offers today's legal advocates a set of principles to guide them (or rather, us) into the future. Those principles include recognizing the complexity and nuance of intersectional identity in challenging systems of oppression, pushing back against capitalist notions of productivity as a means to value one's worth, engaging in cross-disability movement building and cross-movement solidarity, and envisioning a "collective liberation where all bodyminds are valued" (Chin, 2021). As many attorneys seek and employ frameworks like Disability Justice in their everyday work advocating for disabled folks, they (as do we) also recognize that the law is an incomplete, slow, and often an ineffective tool to address harms and *today's* needs. That is why more attorneys refer their clients to, or partner with, other care workers, such as therapists, who are better equipped to address more immediate psychosocial needs.

Notes

1 *See* Schweik (2009), pp. 1–7, 291, for further discussion of ugly laws.
2 *See also* Cerreto (2001).
3 The Act was originally passed as the Education of Handicapped Children Act in 1975, and amended in 1990.
4 This statute was passed after tremendous struggle, pressure, advocacy, and efforts from an untold number of people and organizations. *See* Cone (2013).

References

Alliance for the Mentally Ill v. City of Naperville, 923 F. Supp. 1057, 1069 (N.D. Ill. 1996). https://casetext.com/case/alliance-mentally-ill-v-naperville

Americans with Disabilities Act of 1990, 42 U.S.C. §§ 12101, 12111, 12112, 12113,12116, 12131, 12146, 12147, 12148, 12182 (1990).

Assistive devices for disability: Past, present, and future (2020, March 31). *Disability Experts of Florida*, https://www.disabilityexpertsfl.com/blog/assistive-devices-for-disability-past-present-and-future

Bagenstos, S. R. (2000). Subordination, stigma, and "disability". *Virgina Law Review*, *86*(3), 428. https://www.jstor.org/stable/1073960

Bagenstos, S. R. (2004). The future of disability law. *Yale Law Journal*, *114*(1), 1–23. https://www.yalelawjournal.org/article/the-future-of-disability-law

Board of Trustees of the University of Alabama v. Garrett, 531 U.S. 356 (2001). https://casetext.com/case/board-of-trustees-of-univ-of-alabama-v-garrett

Bolling v. Sharpe, 347 U. S. 497, 499 (1954). https://www.loc.gov/item/usrep347497

Buck v. Bell, 274 U.S. 200 (1927). https://www.loc.gov/item/usrep274200

Cerreto, M. C. (2001). Olmstead: The Brown v. Board of Education for disability rights promises, limits, and issues. *Loyola Journal of Public Interest Law*, *3*, 47. https://heinonline.org/HOL/LandingPage?handle=hein.journals/loyjpubil3&div=7&id=&page=

Chemerinsky, E. (1999). Substantive due process. *Touro Law Review*, *15*(4), 15. https://digitalcommons.tourolaw.edu/lawreview/vol15/iss4/15

Chin, N. M. (2021). Centering disability justice. *Syracuse Law Review*, *71*(3), 683–691. https://lawreview.syr.edu/wp-content/uploads/2022/01/683-749-Chin.pdf

Cho, V. (2021). Significant disproportionality in special education: Current trends and actions for impact. *Connecticut Public Interest Law Journal*, *20*(1), 1. https://ncld.org/wp-content/uploads/2023/07/2020-NCLD-Disproportionality_Trends-and-Actions-for-Impact_FINAL-1.pdf

City of Cleburne, TX v. Cleburne Living Center, 473 U.S. 432 (1985). https://www.loc.gov/item/usrep473432

Community Services, Inc. v. Wind Gap Municipal Authority, 421 F.3d 170 (3d Cir. 2005). https://law.justia.com/cases/federal/appellate-courts/F3/421/170/

Cone, K. (2013). Short history of the 504 sit-in. *Disability Rights Education & Defense Fund (DREDF)*. Retrieved February 11, 2024, from https://dredf.org/504-sit-in-20th-anniversary/short-history-of-the-504-sit-in

Cook, T. M. (1991). The Americans with disabilities act: The move to integration. *Temple Law Review*, *64*(393), 404. https://www.templelawreview.org/lawreview/assets/uploads/2011/07/Cook_19911.pdf

Definition of Disability, 42 U.S. Code § 12102 (2008).

Dobbs v. Jackson Women's Health Organization, 142 S. Ct. 2228, 2300–01 (U.S. 2022) Thomas concurring. https://www.supremecourt.gov/opinions/21pdf/19-1392_6j37.pdf

Dowd, K. (2020, March 2). San Francisco once pioneered America's cruelest legislation: Ugly laws. *SF Gate*. https://www.sfgate.com/sfhistory/article/San-Francisco-once-pioneered-ugly-laws-15098902.php

The Fair Housing Amendments Act, 42 U.S.C. § 3601 (1988).

Fisher, P., & Goodley, D. (2007). The linear medical model of disability: Mothers of disabled babies resist with counter-narratives. *Sociology of Health & Illness*, *29*(1), 67–81. https://doi.org/10.1111/j.1467-9566.2007.00518.x

Frontiero v. Richardson, 411 U.S. 677, 686 (1973). https://www.loc.gov/item/usrep411677

Greiwe, E. (2019, May 11). How an 'ugly law' stayed on Chicago's books for 93 years. *Chicago Tribune*. https://www.chicagotribune.com/2016/06/23/how-an-ugly-law-stayed-on-chicagos-books-for-93-years/

Griswold v. Connecticut, 381 U.S. 479 (1965). https://casetext.com/case/griswold-v-state-of-connecticut

Harris, J. E. (2020). The frailty of disability rights. *University of Pennsylvania Law Review Online*, *169*, 29–38. https://scholarship.law.upenn.edu/penn_law_review_online/vol169/iss1/3/

Hogan, A. J. (2019). Social and medical models of disability and mental health: Evolution and renewal. *Canadian Medical Association Journal*, *191*(1), E16–E18. https://www.ncbi.nlm.nih.gov/pmc/articles/PMC6312522/

Individuals with Disabilities Education Act, 20 U.S.C. § 1400 et seq. (2004).

Loving v. Virginia, 388 U.S. 1 (1967). https://www.loc.gov/item/usrep388001

Miller v. Johnson, 515 U.S. 900 (1995). https://tile.loc.gov/storage-services/service/ll/usrep/usrep515/usrep515900/usrep515900.pdf

Mississippi University for Women v. Hogan, 458 U.S. 718 (1982). https://casetext.com/case/mississippi-university-for-women-v-hogan

National Center for Learning Disabilities (NCLD). (2020). Significant disproportionality in special education: Current trends and actions for impact. https://ncld.org/wp-content/uploads/2023/07/2020-NCLD-Disproportionality_Trends-and-Actions-for-Impact_FI

O'Connor v. Donaldson, 422 U.S. 563 (1975). https://www.loc.gov/item/usrep422563

Obergefell v. Hodges, 576 U.S. 644 (2015). https://www.loc.gov/item/usrep527581

Olmstead v. L.C., 527 U.S. 581 (1999). https://www.loc.gov/item/usrep527581

Opioid use disorder. (2024, June 11). *ADA.gov*. https://www.ada.gov/topics/opioid-use-disorder/

PARC v. Commonwealth of Pennsylvania, Complaint (1971). *Public Interest Law Center*. https://pubintlaw.org/wp-content/uploads/2012/04/1971-01-07-Complaint.pdf

Pennsylvania Association for Retarded Citizens v. Commonwealth of Pennsylvania, 334 F. Supp. 1257 (E.D. Pa. 1972). https://law.justia.com/cases/federal/district-courts/FSupp/334/1257/

Pettinga, G. L. (1987). Rational basis with bite: Intermediate scrutiny by any other name. *Indiana Law Journal 62*(3), Article 10. https://www.repository.law.indiana.edu/ilj/vol62/iss3/10.

Plessy v. Ferguson, 163 U.S. 537 (1896). https://casetext.com/case/plessy-v-ferguson.

Powell, R. M. (2022). Beyond disability rights: A way forward after the 2020 election. *St. Louis University Journal of Health Law & Policy*, *15*(2), 400. https://scholarship.law.slu.edu/jhlp/vol15/iss2/8/

The Public Interest Law Center. (n.d.). *Pennsylvania Association for Retarded Citizens (PARC) v. Commonwealth of Pennsylvania*. https://pubintlaw.org/cases-and-projects/pennsylvania-association-for-retarded-citizens-parc-v-commonwealth-of-pennsylvania-case-documents/

Raj, C. (2021). The lost promise of disability rights. *Michigan Law Review*, *119*(5), 933–976. https://repository.law.umich.edu/mlr/vol119/iss5/3/

Rehabilitation Act of 1973, 25 U.S.C. § 701 (1973).

Romer v. Evans, 517 U.S. 620, 631 (1996). https://www.loc.gov/item/usrep517620

Rosa's Law, Pub. L. No. 111-256, S. 2781, 111th Cong. (2010).

Ryan Reft, R. (2017, December 21). World War I: Injured veterans and the disability rights movement. *Library of Congress Blog*. https://blogs.loc.gov/loc/2017/12/world-war-i-injured-veterans-and-the-disability-rights-movement/

Santosky v. Kramer, 455 U.S. 745 (1982). https://www.loc.gov/item/usrep455745

Schneider v. Rusk, 377 U. S. 163, 214 (1964). https://www.loc.gov/item/usrep377163

School Board of Nassau County v. Arline, 481 U.S. 273 (1987). https://www.loc.gov/item/usrep480273

Schweik, S. M. (2009). *The ugly laws* (pp. 1–7, 291). NYU Press.

Slaughter-House Cases, 83 U.S. 36, 81 (1872). https://www.loc.gov/item/usrep083036

Stein, M. A. (2007). Disability human rights. *California Law Review, 95*(1), 75. https://lawcat.berkeley.edu/record/1121123?ln=en&v=pdf

Thomas, P., Gradwell, L., & Markham, N. (1997, July). Defining impairment within the social model of disability. *Greater Manchester Coalition of Disabled People Magazine*. https://disability-studies.leeds.ac.uk/wp-content/uploads/sites/40/library/thomas-pam-Defining-Impairment-within-the-Social-Model-of-Disability.pdf

Traynor v. Turnage, 485 U.S. 535 (1988). https://tile.loc.gov/storage-services/service/ll/usrep/usrep485/usrep485535/usrep485535.pdf

United Nations Convention on the Rights of Persons with Disabilities, December 13, 2006, https://www.ohchr.org/en/hrbodies/crpd/pages/conventionrightspersonswithdisabilities.aspx

United States v. Carolene Products Company, 304 U.S. 144, 152 n.4 (1938). https://www.loc.gov/item/usrep304144

U.S. Const. amend. XIX.

U.S. Const. amend. V.

U.S. Const. art. 6, cl. 2.

U.S. Department of Housing and Urban Development. (n.d.). Section 504. *HUD.gov*. https://www.hud.gov/program_offices/fair_housing_equal_opp/disabilities/sect504

U.S. Department of Justice. (2024, June 11). Guide to disability rights laws. *ADA.gov*. https://www.ada.gov/resources/disability-rights-guide/#rehabilitation-act

U.S. House of Representatives. (1988). *H.R. Rep. No. 100-711* (p. 13).

Bibliography

Disabled American Veterans. (2005). Wars & scars: A history of the disabled American veterans. *IPR Group American Printing*. https://www.dav.org/about-dav/history/

3

HUMAN VARIATION

Disability Models Explained

Angélica Guevara

Introduction

Disabled people do not inherently need to be empowered by others; they already hold within themselves the strength, resources, and capacity to thrive. Instead, what can be beneficial is for healthcare providers, especially mental health providers, to meet disabled individuals with nonjudgmental presence, recognizing and honoring all aspects of their identity and experience.

This process begins with how disabled clients are perceived, which greatly depends on the disability model adopted by the clinician. The more a healthcare provider is informed on how disability models can oppress, the more effective their services will be in therapeutic settings since they will be mindful of avoiding common trappings that have oppressed the community for centuries. Being aware of how to approach disabled clients and what not to say can impact future relationships not just with clients, but with their family members.

Every disabled person has a unique disability identity. Disabled individuals are often at different stages of acceptance and consciousness of their disability, all of which should be honored and respected within the clinical space. Embracing the disability identity adopted by the client, no matter the place in their journey, is crucial. It is important to not further burden the client with an already laborious reality of living in a world that does not readily accept them and their disability. One disability model specifically, the medical model, places the onus of the disability on the individual, while the other, the social model, places the onus on society. To combat the oppressive nature of the medical model readily adopted by society, the disability community has adopted the term "Disability" with a capitalized "D." This practice distinguishes the difference between illness and the social treatment that continues to disable individuals in our societies (Bagenstos, 2009; Jenks, 2019; Linton, 1998).

DOI: 10.4324/9781003362586-6

Embracing human variation is essential to avoid causing harm to disabled individuals (Linton, 1998). Disabled people already receive the social message that they are not the right way of being because they do not fit into a socially constructed able-body standard. Thus, taking human variation into account means acknowledging that there is no such concept as a standard way of being and that "the presence or absence of a disability [does not] predict [the] quality of life" of any individual (Hevesi, 2008; Johnson, 2003; Johnson, 2006; Kanter, 2010). By adopting a human variation ideology, the therapist's focus shifts to reconstructing the systems to become accessible instead of "fixing" the individual, so that they can better fit into existing systems (Kanter, 2010). Had individuals historically valued the utility of human variation, then perhaps the so-called able-body would not be the standard today (Ariotti, 1999; Gotto, 2009). As a result, disabled people are othered (Goffman, 2009), stigmatizing them even further. This stigma prevents some disabled people from openly disclosing or talking about their disabilities for fear of further marginalization. Others develop internalized ableism because of the innumerous times they may have been excluded within societal and familial settings, constantly being reminded that they are different from the able-body standard, which has erroneously been emphasized as the right way of being. Therapists can reduce the impact of the othering effect that disabled clients face in society and, at times, within their own families (Goffman, 2009), by understanding the medical model of disability, which perpetuates oppression, and the social model, which fosters greater inclusion for many disabled individuals.

Historically, the challenges faced by disabled individuals have been attributed to divine punishment, karma, or moral failing, and, following the "Enlightenment," to biological deficits (Shakespeare, 2006). As a result, therapists often may not know that they are using one model or the other, depending on how they have been socially conditioned to think about disability. Like others in society, therapists may be unaware of alternative realities due to a lack of personal experience with such circumstances. In addition, there is a tendency to compartmentalize the mind from the body when discussing disability issues. This compartmentalization occurs despite the understanding the unity of the mind and body. Thus, when considering the following disability models, it is important to view clients holistically, taking into consideration the mind and body as a single entity.

Disability models help explain the ideology that an individual currently adopts regarding disability, which then informs how they treat people with apparent and non-apparent disabilities. By learning how the disability models operate, an informed clinician can begin to dismantle the social conditioning that continues to oppress disabled people. Working toward embracing human variation is the goal, but in the meantime, knowing the dichotomy that exists, and the language currently used by disability scholars helps to not perpetuate oppression.

To start, let us differentiate between impairment and disability. An impairment is viewed as a personal condition, while a disability is structural and public (Shakespeare, 2006). Next, disabled people are distinguished from non-disabled people because the former is an oppressed group while the latter may contribute to the oppression (Shakespeare, 2006). Learning the difference between an apparent and a non-apparent disability is also valuable. A non-apparent disability is not visibly apparent but may become apparent through observation after a period of time (Price, 2011; Guevara, 2024). Some non-apparent disabilities become "intermittently apparent" (Price, 2015). For instance, stimming is an example of a moment when a non-apparent disability becomes intermittently apparent (Price, 2015). The term "non-apparent" is particularly used to supersede the notion of "visible" or "invisible" disabilities, as these terms are inherently ableist in assuming an objective standard of perception defined by only sight, othering people who are blind (Guevara, 2024).

For the scope of this chapter, I will define the medical model and explain how it's use is damaging when adopted by healthcare providers, but particularly harmful for therapists to utilize in case conceptualization. The social model of disability will then be defined, and examples will be provided to demonstrate how empowering and profound such a perspective is for both, disabled clients and future generations of therapists. Multiple contemporary disability models exist alongside the medial and social model, including, but not limited to, the biopsychosocial model, the human rights model, the minority group model, the capability approach model, and the affirmative model, all discussed toward the end of this chapter. These contemporary models are briefly described to make the reader aware of other frameworks that attempt to dismantle ableist views of disabled people. The time spent learning these models stands to have a significant social impact as more people become conscious of their subtle and not-so-subtle use. Focusing on the two traditional models will most effectively assist healthcare providers in immediately, directly, and effectively implementing the necessary ideological change. Despite the focus of this chapter on these two models, the author recognizes and acknowledges the value of the various other, contemporary models that are also becoming more popular in today's landscape of global disability discourse.

Medical Model

The medical model is cemented in the medical field, as doctors determine whether an individual has an impairment or loss of function (Bagenstos, 2009; Stone, 1986). The medical model is also known or referred to as the individual model. For those working in healthcare, it seems at times automatic to perceive people through the lens of this model. However, while this view temporarily assists healthcare providers in determining what medication to use to treat an illness, what type of prosthetic to design if the individual desires a prosthetic, or what treatment plan to implement, it becomes detrimental to use this view in general for all forms of treatment. This is especially true in therapeutic settings where an individual may already feel as though they are receiving therapy because they are not the "right" way of being.

Regrettably, the medical model has seeped into individuals' general psyches, to which therapists are not immune. This results in the view that disabled people are damaged or in need of "fixing." It is critical to remember that an illness is a condition that needs treatment (Ursano, 2011), which is separate from disability. Disability refers to how an individual is socially and legally treated. This is particularly important for those with chronic illnesses who are often viewed as sick and may have different experiences than those who are disabled by social and legal structures. Today, disability scholars are embracing the complex idea of the "healthy disabled versus the unhealthy disabled to better understand the problematic relationship between illness and disability" (Wendell, 2016). In other words, people sometimes navigate illness and disability simultaneously. Thus, moving away from the medical model when working with clients in therapy helps normalize the human variation within those with any type of disability. This is especially true for the experiences of chronically disabled people, who must often fight to be seen as being Disabled by societal structures, rather than someone who is always sick, and this illness being tied to their entire identity.

Despite many medical professionals adopting the viewpoint that "impairment is a purely medical phenomenon, while disability is a medical-administrative-legal phenomenon" (Stone, 1986), the larger society does not know to differentiate. Even medical professionals who often adopt this model, understand the difference but, at times, become obfuscated and forget not to utilize it outside of treating the illness. The American Medical Association understands this phenomenon and has stated that the "medical judgment of impairment is separate from the more subjective and value-laden judgment of disability" (Stone, 1986). Sadly, therapists and the general public remain unaware of the difference between impairment and disability, which further perpetuates the stigma against the community (Hahn, 1988). This chapter underscores the critical need for clinicians to move away from conceptualizing cases through the medical model of disability, as doing so risks further harming clients and reinforcing stigmatizing beliefs about disabled people.

The medical model is harmful because it lends itself to considering disability as a "'personal tragedy…,' which suggests that a disability is some terrible chance event that occurs at random to unfortunate individuals" (Guevara, 2021; Kanter, 2010).

This model places the "problem" of disability solely within the individual, effectively absolving society from the responsibility of addressing or considering disability further. It also perpetuates stereotypes of disabled people as incomplete or damaged and who need fixing to accomplish daily tasks (Oliver, 1990). As a result, it views the individual with pity, as defective, or as having an impairment that must be eliminated, treated, or cured (Goodley, 2014; Oliver, 1990; Stone, 1986). One scholar accurately wrote:

> Society, in agreeing to assign medical meaning to *disability*, colludes to keep the issue within the purview of the medical establishment, to keep it a

> personal matter and "treat" the condition and the person with the condition rather than "treating" the social processes and policies that constrict disabled people's lives.
>
> (Linton, 1998)

While this model has a detrimental impact on all disabled people, its harm reveals itself differently for people with non-apparent disabilities because when they disclose their disabilities, or the disability becomes apparent, the message received is that the disability is their personal problem to fix, and they are then encouraged to continue hiding it. As a result, those with non-apparent disabilities are often not believed. To be clear, while fabricating a disability can occur, it is extremely rare (Dorfman, 2021; Mittenberg et al., 2002; PsychDB, n.d.; Guevara, 2024). While rare, concerns about malingering should be approached with caution and cultural humility, as overemphasizing the possibility of symptom-fabrication can contribute to the ongoing stigmatization and dismissal of disabled individuals' lived experiences.

Currently, laws and policies are also based on the medical model of disability, forcing people into an ability/disability binary. According to the medical model, for the law to be accommodative of disabled people, a person is categorized as either disabled or not disabled and does not hold regard to fluctuating symptoms in disabilities that may render a body able one day and disabled the next. Laws, policies, and programs tailor assistance and solutions to fit the able-bodied world rather than normalizing human variation. It is important not to make that mistake as a therapist. One strategy is to incorporate Universal Design (UD) practices (Bayer, 1987; Mace, 1998) that serve most individuals in therapy sessions and as well as within the therapeutic alliance. More information about the principle and practice of UD is described in a different section of this chapter.

In summary, the medical model is harmful to most disabled people, but it particularly affects people with chronic disabilities in the following ways. First, under the gaze of the medical model, it inherently seems to imply a solution or a cure for the person being treated. Thus, those who encounter chronic illnesses feel as though they are automatically excluded from a sense of belonging. For example, when people are grateful for their good health, often met with the phrase, "health is wealth," it becomes challenging for those who encounter chronic disabilities to feel a sense of pride in their disability (Wendell, 2016). Thus, under this popular perspective, people with chronic disabilities and fluctuating symptoms struggle to normalize their existence. Instead, they must deal both with the impairment itself and the othering effect that then can lead to internalized ableism, which is yet another psychological barrier to overcome. When perpetuated in the therapy space, the client is left with having to manage the impacts of multiple layers of oppression, even after the therapy session has concluded.

Social Model of Disability

Unlike the medical model, the social model suggests that society disables individuals (Linton, 1998). In other words, our society's structures create disabilities when there is nothing deficient or wrong with an individual (Chappell, 1998; Linton, 1998; Shakespeare, 2013). The social model embraces the idea that there are many ways of existing in the world (Chappell, 1998; Shakespeare, 2013; Shakespeare, 1996). Michael Oliver developed the social theory of disability in *The Politics of Disablement*, in which he brings to academia, the perspective that society causes disability, an idea that is currently deeply rooted in the ideologies of the disability community (Oliver, 1990; Shakespeare, 2016).

The social model of disability embodies the idea that the society into which individuals are born into makes all the difference in how people experience and view their disability. The social model maximizes an individual's potential since it challenges traditional views of normalcy and forces an individual to examine any subconscious bias and assumptions about disability, thereby embracing universalism (Bickenbach et al., 1999). In doing so, decisions regarding and attitudes toward disabled people would be more inclusive. For example, instead of having a ramp to bypass stairs, a building would not have stairs from the inception of its construction. If elevators stopped working in a building, anyone could use a ramp. In other words, society's designs would be more accessible to all if we were to practice the social model of disability. Living under the social model of disability means the law would not rely on the medical model. The social construction of disability would be well understood. For example, for years, being gay was considered a psychiatric disability (Bayer, 1987), and women who deviated from gender norms were diagnosed with hysteria (Tasca et al., 2012). Today, it is well understood that these two "diagnoses" were more of a reflection of the times, indicating how these experiences and ways of being are socially constructed. These "able-body standards" of gender norms and behavioral expectations of women were established and embraced by the larger society. Similarly, if the social model of disability were embraced instead, society would have normalized human variation, and the categorization of disability itself would have ceased to be as harmful as it is today. Therapists now have the opportunity to use the social model of disability in their conceptualizations, to provide the necessary adjustments for clients to maximize their human potential, prioritizing client dignity.

Universal Design

The social model of disability prompts an individual to think inclusively about disabled people, a philosophical concept and practice known as UD (Dolmage, 2017; Mace, 1998). For instance, the dropped curb assists people in wheelchairs, people with strollers, and bicycle users (Dolmage, 2017; Price, 2011). UD's inclusive practices allow social participation for all, providing for unforeseen beneficiaries whether they have a disability or not. For example, many non-disabled individuals benefit from the handicap push-button that automatically opens doors, which was increasingly used in buildings during the coronavirus outbreak-it has a universal benefit (Dolmage, 2017; Price, 2011). In therapy, this may mean being conscious that some clients may need breaks during a therapy session, and offering this option to all, thereby normalizing the accommodation. It also emphasizes that such adjustments are offered to all clients, whether they have a disability or not. More broadly, UD represents a worldview where environments are not tailored to marginal groups but rather to a "form of hope; a manner of trying" (Dolmage, 2017). Therefore, a disabled person is "limited more by social attitudes and environmental barriers than any inherent 'defect' or 'deficiency' within the person, that must be remedied" (Kanter, 2010). A society that viewed the world through the social model of disability would embrace human variation and construct a system that benefits all, adjusting for individual needs to maximize all human potential.

Overall, categories should not exist, because human variation – a universal experience – defies neat categorization. The law requires categorizing individuals because categories are necessary to create legal, individual coverage. It is best to move away from the legal fix into an ideological fix, which would ultimately render a legal fix irrelevant. Moving in this direction also means employers would more readily provide accommodations for employees because there would not be accommodations that require legal enforcement, only adjustments to maximize human potential. This chapter is not arguing that we should not see disabilities; doing so would be a similar mistake to taking a color-blind view on racism. Under the ideological fix scenario, it would not matter how "severe" or "mild" the ability or disability is, because the dominant ideology would no longer be based on scarcity and instead, it would adjust for more inclusion. The universality of disability does not mean everyone's experiences are the same; it would mean the existence of a society where it would not matter what disability an individual has, because all will be accommodated. Maximizing human potential in all human variations would be the norm.

The ideology of capitalist production also contributes extensively to the oppressive nature that views disabled people as not whole or in need of fixing. Much of what perpetuates the current marginalization of disabled people stems from an ideology based on the assumption that disabled individuals cannot produce, reducing their worth to their production value (Althusser, 2006; Brewster & Althusser, 2001). Thus, when talking about maximizing human potential, it means truly embracing human variation by valuing what every individual can contribute through their mere existence.

The dominant ideology underpinning disability laws and policies is often ableist, as it continues to treat disabled people as incomplete, or in need of fixing to become productive members of society, thereby adhering to the medical model. The very act of having to define someone as disabled or not disabled creates the ability/disability binary that perpetuates ableist ideology, further marginalizing disabled people by embracing the idea of a right way of being.

Some normative solutions for long-term change would entail using schools, churches, and the family to teach and implement the social model of disability, shifting the dominant ideology in these formative systems. For example, in the context of schools, if students are taught the social model of disability before they enter the workforce, they will create, design, lead, and teach with a non-othering mentality and construct spaces of belonging for disabled people-maximizing human potential and capitalizing on human dignity. For now, therapists are on the frontlines assisting disabled clients to understand that they are not any 'less' than an able-bodied person, even though societal messaging may tell them otherwise. Pointing out to the client that there are other societies that treat disabled people differently can create a feeling of validation, hope, and belonging. Current examples of societies that prioritize feelings of belongingness for those deemed disabled in the Western world are the Anangu people in Australia and the Mixe people in southern Mexico, who embrace human variation because they value what any member of their community contributes (Ariotti, 1999; Gotto, 2009). A similar ideology that maximizes human potential in the Western world must be enforced within family systems and religious structures.

Furthermore, the very concept of disability *severity* would be irrelevant as human variation is embraced. Some providers view people with severe disabilities as needing dire investment of resources that may feel like a "waste" of these resources. They believe it is better to maximize the use of their resources. People with this ideology view disabled people as defective and unworthy of investment. Others who do not see disabled people as defective embrace the idea of just dividing the resources in an equitable manner (Bagenstos, 2003; Bagenstos, 2009). All disabled people are equally valuable, and severity is relative, depending on an individual's ideology. To say that only those closest to an able body are worth investing resources in, dehumanizes those on the other end of the ability/disability dichotomy. Therapists should understand how this belief system can affect disabled people depending on how society has categorized their disability under severity. In therapy, it is important to understand and address client differences as strengths worth investing in, similar to the ways of the Anangu and the Mixe peoples. These goals in therapy may seem ambitious for some, considering therapists are heavily influenced by the medical model throughout their education, but they are essential to creating a truly healing therapy experience for disabled clients.

Critiques of the Social Model

It is also valuable to understand the critiques of the social model of disability, should related issues arise in practice. The simplicity of the term, *the social model of disability*, and the idea itself have created some concerns among the community. Some believe it is because the social model of disability has been erroneously confused with social theory. Other scholars believe its weakness lies in its origin, where people with spinal injuries or other physical impairments headed a part of the original conversation defining the social model of disability without having people with non-apparent disabilities at the table (Shakespeare, 2016). When the model was first proposed, it did not include people with mental impairments (Shakespeare, 2016). For this reason, it was imperative to ensure that non-apparent disabilities were included in this chapter.

Arguably, perhaps the model would have been strengthened if it encompassed a broader view of disability, and it included people with non-apparent disabilities more explicitly. It may also have benefitted from acknowledging the very real, often painful characteristics of impairments; an important component of many disabled people's lives (Shakespeare, 2016). For instance, some clients may have Lyme disease with acute symptoms that may last for years, with the pain being an important part of their disability experience. HIV or AIDS could be deadly in poor communities, but in wealthier communities, there are ways to slow down its progress, resulting in a chronic condition.

Given its simplistic approach, the social model at times invalidates the inherent effects of the impairment, such as chronic pain. For many who have symptoms of pain, the "treatment" approach inherent in the medical model is relevant to their experience. To clarify, a chronic illness is typically seen as an illness that does not go away naturally within six months, cannot be reliably cured, and does not lead to death (Wendell, 2016). It is here that a distinction is drawn between the healthy disabled and the non-healthy disabled, as described in an earlier section of this chapter. For instance, people experiencing chronic conditions would like to be seen as disabled rather than ill to experience belonging. For instance, someone with lupus may deteriorate quickly, resulting in a sudden demise, while others may have diabetes, where symptom-formation may be more gradual (Wendell, 2016). Therefore, it is important to prioritize the client's definition of their own identity and journey.

> As individuals, most of us simply cannot pretend with any conviction that our impairments are irrelevant because they influence every aspect of our lives. We must find a way to integrate them into our whole experience and identity for the sake of our physical and emotional well-being, and, subsequently, for our capacity to work against Disability.
>
> (Shakespeare, 2016)

Christine Overall is a wonderful example. She was initially diagnosed with rheumatoid arthritis and later was re-diagnosed with viral arthritis. A part of her diagnosis was embraced by the disability community while simultaneously experiencing pressure to pass as "normal" (Wendell, 2016). This pressure could be diminished by minimizing the usage of the medical model which uses an able-body as the standard way of being. Therapists could embrace the social model of disability instead, which states that it is the structures in our society that are in fact disabling the client. Therapists can support clients in understanding the human variation that exists among us all, creating a safe and inclusive environment as a result. However, it is imperative that the client dictate to what extent the "treatment" of the pain is relevant to their progress. This allows clients to define their own identification with the healthy disabled vs the non-healthy disabled and prioritizes agency and autonomy.

Contemporary Models of Disability

The contemporary models of disability, in one form or another, derived and evolved from the traditional models of disability: the medical model and the social model. The traditional models of disability inspired a necessary ideological shift by first naming and defining disability. Moving away from a deficit model of disability inspired a few important contemporary frameworks. For example, the biopsychosocial model considers psychological, social, and biological factors impacting a client (Bolton & Gillett, 2019). The human rights model acknowledges the inherent human dignity and equal rights in all humans, thus viewing disability as a natural part of human diversity that must be supported in all forms (Baharna, 2013; United Nations, 2006). The minority group model affirms disability as a minority group status that demands recognition and representation (Hahn, 1996). The human development approach, also known as the capability approach model, focuses on an individual's capabilities rather than their perceived limitations (Nussbaum, 2011). The affirmative model promotes a positive representation of people with disabilities by emphasizing their strengths and contributions (Cameron, 2014). The development of these contemporary models is a source of encouragement and proof that an ideological shift is possible and ongoing. All of these models have unique contributions and objectives that can clearly be incorporated in a therapeutic setting, depending on the client's unique identities, experiences, and presenting issues. The following are examples of how some important contemporary models operate.

Human Rights Model of Disability

The Human Rights Model of disability emphasizes the rights and dignity of individuals with disabilities, framing disability as a matter of human rights rather than merely a medical or social issue that needs resolution (United Nations, 2006). The Disability Advocacy Resource Unit (DARU) highlights the key principles that the Human Rights Model of Disability recognizes. This includes the position that disability is a natural part of human diversity that must be respected and supported in all its forms, the awareness that disabled people have the same rights as everyone else in society, and the understanding that an impairment can never be used as reason to deny or restrict an individual's civil rights (DARU, 2019).

The model is grounded in the belief that disabled individuals should be offered the same resources, advantages, and access to policies, as their able-bodied counterparts. The Australian Human Rights Commission describes the model as "including a set of principles concerned with equity and fairness, where disabled individuals are living a life free from fear, harassment, or discrimination" (HRC, n.d.).

The Minority Group Model of Disability

Similar to the social justice component of the Human Rights model, the Minority Group model also encompasses socio-political elements. It is often referred to as the Sociopolitical model since it is an expansion of the Social Model that views disabled people as a minority group that is discriminated against and actively excluded from society (Nielsen, 2012). The Minority Group model emerged from the disability rights movements in the United States in the 1970s as the distrust of the medical model grew (Drum et al., 2010).

A driving force for the development of this model was to transfer the "burden of disability" from people with impairments to society at large, by creating a sense of community (Hahn, 1988). Similar to other minority groups (such as those based on race, gender, and sexual orientation), disabled people are also frequently experiencing oppression, marginalization, and discrimination. Drum et al. (2010) acknowledged that the Minority Group model is particularly important in the history of disability since it was instrumental in the passage and enactment of disability activism in the United States.

Biopsychosocial Disability Model

The Biopsychosocial Disability model also has its roots in the medical and social models. It attempts to recognize and account for the biological, psychological, and social elements of disability experiences. First proposed by Engel (1977), the model illuminates the importance of recognizing the interplay between biological, psychological, and social elements in the conceptualization of disability. Broadly, these elements include any physiological pathology; psychological experiences related to thoughts, emotions, distress, belief systems, coping methods, and/or attribution; and the socio-economic, cultural factors related to employment, benefits, and economies (Gatchel et al., 2007).

The conceptualization of disability through a Biopsychosocial framework also offers the opportunity for effective interdisciplinary collaboration- a critical factor that determines quality of care for many disabled individuals and their families. The benefit of this model lies in its recognition of economic and employment-related influences on a disabled person's life. This makes it the model of choice for the World Health Organization (World Health Organization, 2001). However, due to the inclusion of a medical component in the framework of the model, there has been some pushback from scholars who view the construct of disablement as a purely social phenomenon.

The Human Development Approach Model

The Human Development Approach to disability reframes disability as a developmental experience, focusing on expanding individuals' capabilities and freedoms rather than merely addressing impairments or barriers. Rooted in the broader capabilities approach developed by Amartya Sen and Martha Nussbaum, this model emphasizes the importance of enabling individuals to lead lives they value and have reason to value, regardless of their physical or cognitive differences (Nussbaum, 2011). It highlights the role of societal structures, education, and economic opportunities in fostering or constraining the capabilities of disabled people. The approach underscores that disability is not merely a lack of ability but also a reflection of inequitable societal arrangements that limit participation and inclusion. By prioritizing equity, dignity, and the removal of systemic barriers, the model advocates for policies and practices that empower disabled individuals to achieve their full potential while actively contributing to their communities (Mitra, 2018). This holistic perspective challenges traditional deficit-oriented models, aligning with current disability discourse.

Affirmative Model

The Affirmative model was developed to challenge the tragic viewpoint of disability that has historically plagued the world. The model is often described as a "non-tragic view" of disability and impairment, encompassing positive individual and collective social identities for disabled people (Swain & French, 2000). In this way, not only are disabled people viewed in a non-tragic manner but can also be celebrated for their unique strengths and contributions to society. Occupational therapists utilize this model frequently to recognize that differences can not only be acknowledged but also benefitted from, socially. This view significantly shifts traditional, and age-old narratives regarding ability in the workforce, and reductionistic ways of thinking about workplace and broader societal productivity.

Disability Justice Model

The Disability Justice model is a framework that extends beyond the limitations of traditional approaches, such as the medical or social models, by centering intersectionality and collective liberation. Originating from the activism of disabled queer, trans, Black, Indigenous, and people of color (BIPOC) communities, this model recognizes that disability cannot be understood in isolation from other systems of oppression, including racism, sexism, and capitalism (Piepzna-Samarasinha, 2018; Sins Invalid, 2019). Unlike models that focus solely on accessibility or rights, the Disability Justice model emphasizes community care, interdependence, and the dismantling of ableism at structural and cultural levels. It advocates for an understanding of disability as a natural and valuable part of human diversity, challenging societal norms that prioritize productivity and independence. This framework not only addresses physical and systemic barriers but also affirms the lived experiences and leadership of those most marginalized within disability communities (Sins Invalid, 2019).

Sins Invalid is another disability justice-based framework that celebrates the lives and experiences of disabled people, centering and led by disabled Black, Indigenous, and people of the global majority, queer, trans, and non-binary disabled people. It was founded by Berne and Moore Jr. in 2005 (Sins Invalid, 2019) and is gaining vast momentum within disability communities worldwide.

Conclusion

Disabled people are intrinsically made to feel less than or not whole in who they are. Often, friends and family members tend to make them feel an innate sense of deficiency and defectiveness since they also tend to succumb to dominant discourses surrounding defectiveness and/or pity. Despite their best intentions, they are not immune to social conditioning. However, clinicians providing psycho-social assistance through mental health treatment must be mindful of not perpetuating harm in this way. It is critical to recognize that it is further damaging when the professional who is assigned to assist a client, also perpetuates the general ideology that the client is trying to battle outside of therapy. It is critical that the therapist not view the client under the medical model of disability, which views them as broken or ill. Instead, their human variation should be embraced using the social model that states society disables them, or through more contemporary, rights-based models, depending on the client's personal narratives of their own disability experiences.

Therapists must help clients understand that there is nothing "wrong" with them as a whole being, while acknowledging and validating the role of impairments in their lives. The new normal should be consistently embraced and normalized, helping to diminish the heightened sense of difference clients experience outside of therapy. Clients can also benefit from therapists engaging in consistent, professional development to stay updated on related developments that can better serve their clients. In the simplest of terms, Michael Oliver said it best, "models are ways of translating ideas into practice and the idea underpinning the individual model was that of personal tragedy, while the idea underpinning the social model was that of externally imposed restrictions" (Shakespeare, 2016). Therapists are encouraged to self-examine and reflect from time to time which of these disability models is present in their therapy practices, to prevent future harm to disabled clients that seek care. Reading this handbook is already an important step in the right direction.

References

Althusser, L. (2006). Ideology and ideological state apparatuses (notes towards an investigation). *The Anthropology of the State: A Reader*, 9(1), 86–98.

Ariotti, L. (1999). Social construction of an Angu disability. *Australian Journal of Rural Health*, 7(4), 216–222.

Australian Human Rights Commission. (n.d.). An introduction to human rights. *Australian Human Rights Commission*. Retrieved January 28, 2025, from https://humanrights.gov.au/our-work/education/introduction-human-rights

Bagenstos, S. R. (2003). "Rational discrimination," accommodation, and the politics of (disability) civil rights. *Virginia Law Review*, 89(5), 825–923. https://doi.org/10.2307/3202421

Bagenstos, S. R. (2009). *Law and the contradictions of the disability rights movement*. Yale University Press.

Baharna, N. A. (2013). *A universal human rights model: A human rights handbook*. Outskirts Press.

Bayer, R. (1987). *Homosexuality and American psychiatry: The politics of diagnosis*. Princeton University Press.

Bickenbach, J. E., Chatterji, S., Badley, E. M., & Üstün, T. B. (1999). Models of disablement, universalism and the international classification of impairments, disabilities and handicaps. *Social Science & Medicine*, 48(9), 1173–1187.

Bolton, D., & Gillett, G. (2019). *The biopsychosocial model of health and disease: New philosophical and scientific developments* (p. 149). Springer Nature.

Brewster, B., & Althusser, L. (2001). *Lenin and philosophy and other essays*. New York University Press.

Cameron, C. (2014). Developing an affirmative model of disability and impairment. In J. Swain, S. French, C. Barnes, & C. Thomas (Eds.), *Disabling Barriers–enabling environments* (pp. 24–30). Sage Publications.

Chappell, A. L. (1998). Still out in the cold: People with learning difficulties and the social model of disability. In T. Shakespeare (Ed.), *The disability reader: Social science perspectives* (pp. 211–220). Cassell.

Disability Advocacy Resource Unit. (2019, January 31). Introducing the human rights model of disability. *Disability Advocacy Resource Unit*. https://daru.org.au/daru-publication/how-we-talk-about-disability-matters/introducing-the-human-rights-model-of-disability

Dolmage, J. T. (2017). *Academic ableism: Disability and higher education* (p. 244). University of Michigan Press.

Dorfman, D. (2021). Pandemic "disability cons". *Journal of Law, Medicine & Ethics*, 49(3), 401–409.

Drum, C., Meade, M., Serlin, D., Olkin, R., Scambler and Scambler, Scotch, R., Stiker, H.-J., & Hickel, K. W. (2010). Disability models. In *Disability in higher education* (pp. 54–56). Northern Arizona University. https://in.nau.edu/wp-content/uploads/sites/189/Disability-Models-Article.pdf

Engel, G. L. (1977). The need for a new medical model: A challenge for biomedicine. *Science*, 196(4286), 129–136. https://doi.org/10.1126/science.847460

Gatchel, R. J., Peng, Y. B., Peters, M. L., Fuchs, P. N., & Turk, D. C. (2007). The biopsychosocial approach to chronic pain: Scientific advances and future directions. *Psychological Bulletin*, 133(4), 581–624. https://doi.org/10.1037/0033-2909.133.4.581

Givens, L. D. (2019). [Review of the book Disability, health and human development, by S. Mitra]. *Critical Studies in Teaching and Learning*, 7(2), 134–137. https://doi.org/10.14426/cristal.v7i2.242
Goffman, E. (2009). *Stigma: Notes on the management of spoiled identity*. Simon and Schuster.
Goodley, D. (2014). *Dis/ability studies: Theorising disablism and ableism*. Routledge.
Gotto, G. S. (2009). Persons and nonpersons: Intellectual disability, personhood, and social capital among the Mixe of Southern Mexico. *Disabilities: Insights from Across Fields and Around the World*, 1, 193–209.
Guevara, A. (2021). The need to reimagine disability rights law because the medical model of disability fails us all. *Wisconsin Law Review*, 2021, 269–292.
Guevara, A. (2024). Not able enough, not disabled enough. *Texas Journal on Civil Liberties & Civil Rights*, 29(2), 147–195.
Hahn, H. (1988). The politics of physical differences: Disability and discrimination. *Journal of Social Issues*, 44(1), 39–47.
Hahn, H. (1996). Antidiscrimination laws and social research on disability: The minority group perspective. *Behavioral Sciences & the Law*, 14(1), 41–59.
Hevesi, D. (2008). Harriet Johnson, 50, activist for disabled, is dead. *New York Times*, A15.
Jenks, A. (2019). Crip theory and the disabled identity: Why disability politics needs impairment. *Disability & Society*, 34(3), 449–469.
Johnson, H. M. (2003). *Unspeakable conversations. The New York Times Magazine*, 50–55, 74–79. The New York Times Company.
Johnson, H. M. (2006). *Too late to die young: Nearly true tales from a life*. Macmillan.
Kanter, A. S. (2010). The law: What's disability studies got to do with it or an introduction to disability legal studies. *Columbia Human Rights Law Review*, 42, 403.
Linton, S. (1998). *Claiming disability: Knowledge and identity*. NYU Press.
Mace, L. R. (1998). Papers 1974–1998. *NC State University Libraries*. https://www.lib.ncsu.edu/findingaids/mc00260/
Mittenberg, W., Patton, C., Canyock, E. M., & Condit, D. C. (2002). Base rates of malingering and symptom exaggeration. *Journal of Clinical and Experimental Neuropsychology*, 24(8), 1094–1102. https://doi.org/10.1076/jcen.24.8.1094.8379
Nielsen, K. E. (2012). *A disability history of the United States*. Beacon Press.
Nussbaum, M. C. (2011). *Creating capabilities: The human development approach*. Harvard University Press.
Oliver, M. (1990). *The politics of disablement*. Palgrave Macmillan.
Piepzna-Samarasinha, L. L. (2018). Care work: Dreaming disability justice. https://openlibrary.org/books/OL26976977M/Care_work
Price, M. (2011). *Mad at school: Rhetorics of mental disability and academic life*. University of Michigan Press.
Price, M. (2015). The bodymind problem and the possibilities of pain. *Hypatia*, 30(1), 268–284.
Psych DB. (n.d.). Malingering. https://www.psychdb.com/teaching/malingering
Shakespeare, T. (1996). Disability, identity and difference. In C. Barnes & G. Mercer (Eds.), *Exploring the divide: Illness and disability* (pp. 94–113). The Disability Press.
Shakespeare, T. (2006). *Disability rights and wrongs*. Routledge.
Shakespeare, T. (2013). *Disability rights and wrongs revisited*. Routledge.
Shakespeare, T. (2016). The social model of disability. *The Disability Studies Reader*, 2(3), 197–204.
Sins Invalid. (2019). *Skin, tooth, and bone: The basis of movement is our people: A disability justice primer* (2nd ed.). Sins Invalid.
Stone, D. A. (1986). *The disabled state*. Temple University Press.

Swain, J., & French, S. (2000). Towards an affirmation model of disability. *Disability & Society*, 15(4), 569–582. https://doi.org/10.1080/09687590050058189
Tasca, C., Rapetti, M., Carta, M. G., & Fadda, B. (2012). Women and hysteria in the history of mental health. *Clinical Practice and Epidemiology in Mental Health: CP & EMH*, 8, 110.
Ursano, R. J. (2011). Disease and illness: Prevention, treatment, caring, and health. *Preventing Chronic Disease*, 8(6), Article A128. https://www.ncbi.nlm.nih.gov/pmc/articles/PMC3221570/.
United Nations. (2006). *Convention on the rights of persons with disabilities*. https://www.un.org/disabilities/documents/convention/convoptprot-e.pdf
Wendell, S. (2016). Unhealthy disabled: Treating chronic illnesses as disabilities. *The Disability Studies Reader*, 5, 160–172.
World Health Organization. (2001). International classification of functioning, disability, and health (ICF). *World Health Organization*. https://www.who.int/standards/classifications/international-classification-of-functioning-disability-and-health

Bibliography

Davis, L. J. (2016). *The disability studies reader*. Routledge.
Dorfman, D. (2019). Fear of the disability con: Perceptions of fraud and special rights discourse. *Law & Society Review*, 53(4), 1051–1091.

4

ABLEISM WITHIN ACADEMIA

Impact on the Lives of Disabled Persons

Rhoda Olkin

Introduction

Ableism is defined as: "A system that places value on people's bodies and minds based on societally constructed ideas of normalcy, intelligence, excellence, and productivity. This form of systemic oppression leads to people and society determining who is valuable and worthy based on a person's appearance and/or their ability to satisfactorily [re]produce, excel, and behave" (Lewis, 2020). Ableism results in discrimination and microaggressions, whether intentional or unconscious. In higher education, ableism can become a barrier to successful passage through the pipeline to graduation and careers.

Ableist assumptions in academia might include ideas such as that (a) there are no disabled students in a class, (b) everyone has the equal opportunity to do well, (c) some types of differing abilities are inferior, (d) accommodations give disabled students an unfair advantage, and (e) teachers should wait to be asked for accommodations before raising the issue of disability. Instead, it is recommended that the teacher take the lead in initiating this conversation.

There are several reasons to include a discussion of disability-prevalence in higher education in a book for therapists. First, the field needs to be accessible to trainees with disabilities. If 15% of students in kindergarten through college receive disability services (National Center for Education Statistics, 2023), we can expect some subset of these students to continue to graduate education. Reducing disability-related barriers to the profession is necessary to increase the representation of mental health counselors with disabilities. Second, many students at both undergraduate (25%) and graduate levels continue to live at home with their parent(s), meaning that therapy might include the family system. Third, disability is rarely included in the curriculum (e.g., Berrin, Olkin, & Taube, 2012; Bluestone,

DOI: 10.4324/9781003362586-7

Stokes, & Kuba, 1996; Deroche et al., 2020; Feather & Carlson, 2019; Heitzman, 2015; Olkin & Pledger, 2003), which further marginalizes disabled students. And fourth, improving therapy accessibility for disabled clients is incumbent on all mental health fields.

For ages 5–18, students with disabilities were covered by Education for All Handicapped Children Act (1975), later expanded to ages 3–21 and reauthorized as the Individuals with Disabilities Education Act (IDEA, 2004; 2011), and the Education for All Handicapped Children Act (1975). The IDEA is an entitlement law. Entitlement laws are about something to which one has the right. Students are entitled to a public education, and as such, there is more responsibility placed on the school to ensure successful completion of the grade or program. However, at the graduate level, the level at which we train therapists, students with disabilities are no longer covered by IDEA but by the Americans with Disabilities Act Amendments Act (ADAAA, 2008). The ADAAA is a civil rights law; such laws are about equity protected by the Federal Government. This law puts more responsibility on the student or trainee to identify as a disabled person and to request accommodations. Further, there is no "right" to a graduate education. Although students cannot be dismissed from a program solely for a disability, there are many ways that disability plays into the evaluations of students.

These laws are relevant in understanding the histories of disabled clients that come to us for therapy. Those who came of age before the IDEA (then called the Education of All Handicapped Children Act, PL94–142, 1975) had very different experiences in school and growing up compared to those who attended school with the IDEA in place. Without legal protections, one million disabled children were not in school at all. Disabled students were not provided any accommodations.

Once relevant education laws were passed, a generation of disabled young adults discovered their rights in college for the first time. However, only 13% of persons with disabilities over age 25 in the United States have a bachelor's degree, compared with 31% of the non-disabled (Dolmage, 2017).

Laws affecting education for disabled children were not a panacea. The federal government promised to reimburse states for 25% of costs but has never contributed more than about 5% of costs for accommodations. Therefore, the economics of the community often affect rates of identification of disabilities as well as number and types of accommodations. Unfortunately, racial bias seems to affect diagnosis, with Black male students being disproportionately placed into particular categories that are more stigmatized and have poorer outcomes (Shifrer , 2018). Further, in college, Black, indigenous, and people of color (BIPOC) students are less likely to self-identify and request accommodations.

In a study of 225 graduate students in professional programs, Olkin and Hanrahan (2023) found that more students (63%) were not registered with the office of disability services (ODS) than were registered. Responses to a survey showed many reasons for not registering with ODS, but the three main ones were (a) needing assistance with the process itself; (b) not being able to get or afford current documentation (especially international students), and (c) not having any idea what accommodations would be helpful. Another factor was intersectionality, with BIPOC students less willing to disclose a disability than White students. A key feature of disability-affirmative practices in higher education is assuming that at least one of every ten students has a disability.

The most frequent disability (65%) was psychological/emotional, such as depression, anxiety, post-traumatic stress disorder, and bipolar disorder (Olkin & Hanrahan, 2023). When students responded to an open-ended question about what they wish faculty knew about disability, responses included the desire to not be seen as less capable or professional due to the disability. This is especially important in mental health training, where trainees want to be acknowledged as professionals instead of clients. The most frequent category of what disabled graduate students in professional programs wanted faculty to know was about what a disability really entails. They wanted faculty to be aware of more than the obvious impairments and to understand the range and number of disability sequelae (Olkin & Hanrahan, 2023). For example: "ADHD is real and involves more than just being organized and not procrastinating." Another student wrote "Some days are better than others, while other days are a complete struggle."

It often is hard for those without disabilities to really grasp the considerable time and energy most disabilities demand. And many of those requirements are not covered by routine lists of reasonable accommodations. Some requirements are less tangible, such as management of mental fatigue, making time for multiple medical appointments, creating detailed calendars of all assignments and activities, and managing pain and exhaustion. Behaviors often are labeled as deficits rather than sequela of disabilities. For example, a student who requires additional days to turn in an assignment may be labeled as procrastinating, rather than struggling to juggle extra tasks due to disability. Additionally, there is often a "disability tax," i.e., the many meetings, committees, or discussions where disabled students have to represent disability issues because no one else will be aware or knowledgeable about them.

Statistics indicate that only 3.6% of tenure-track professors have disabilities (Dalmage, 2017). There could be many factors keeping this percentage low. First, disabled students have to navigate through k–12, then college, then graduate school, with each successive stage having an increased workload and higher standards. Second, disabled students are less likely to graduate from college (49.5%, compared with 68% for nondisabled students), take longer to finish, and emerge from college with higher debt load (National Center for Education Statistics; NCES, 2023). Third, there may not be disabled role models as instructors from kindergarten through graduate school. Accommodations are not the same as mentoring, and a lack of teachers and disabled professors can be a psychological barrier. Fourth, most curricula do not discuss disability even when focusing on diversity (Berrin et al., 2012; Olkin & Pledger, 2003), and when the topic of disability is included, it is viewed through a pathological lens of deficit and inability (Olkin, 2002).

Once a disabled person becomes a faculty member, there are more barriers. Generally, university budgets have line items for disabled student services, but not for faculty. Newer faculty are likely to start as adjuncts at two or more institutions. The average work week of a professor is 60 hours. Applications for retention, tenure, and promotion all require documentation and evidence of specific impairments, which many faculty may be unwilling to disclose. Those less likely to disclose are newer and BIPOC faculty and those needing to prove themselves for retention, tenure, and promotion.

Professors in graduate programs may see themselves as gatekeepers to the profession, and, as such, may confuse changes to processes as lowering of standards. For example, a blind student in an assessment course cannot independently administer test batteries. If we believe that all students must do the same activities, then no blind student could earn a degree that required assessment courses (e.g., clinical psychology). Suppose instead we ask what are the main functions of a psychologist? We know there are many psychologists who do not conduct testing. However, psychologists often read assessment reports written by others, and need to understand them. Then understanding test reports becomes the goal for the blind student, and the more involved the student is in the testing process, the better they are able to comprehend results. Having the student attend the testing sessions and following along with accessible materials (oral, Brailed, raised 3D pictures, descriptions of visual materials) will facilitate learning about testing procedures and the tests and make it more likely that they could even interpret the results, but at the least understand the resulting report. From this example, we see that equality—all students do the same things—does not work as well as equity—altering processes to achieve similar outcomes.

In mental health professions, the medical model of disability still prevails. This is a very pathologizing view of disability. In the medical model, the disability resides in the individual who needs special accommodations to gain access or to perform alongside non-disabled peers. Problems arise when disabled students are unable to utilize appropriate accommodations to mitigate their deficits. In contrast, the social model construes disability as a social construct, and problems arise due to a mismatch between the person and the environment. It is incumbent on those who control the environment to make it as universally accessible as possible. This does not obviate the need for some reasonable accommodations but does put more onus on those in positions of power.

A key ableist assumption is that there are no disabled students in the classroom unless they have a visible disability. Instead, we should assume that at least one of every ten students has a disability. If instructors make the assumption that disability is absent then they may not think about alternative ways of delivering materials and assessing learning. There is a corollary in therapy of failing to consider disability: (a) not inquiring if a new client needs any accommodations to come to therapy; (b) not having intake forms in any alternative formats; (c) failing to ensure your therapy website has disability accessibility features; (d) not providing any information on your website about accessibility of the office.

A second ableist assumption is that all disabilities are apparent and that those which are non-apparent are minor or even nonexistent. The first tenet of disability-affirmative therapy (Olkin, 2017) is that the person with the disability is the expert on the disability, and that we can only begin to understand by asking "What is your disability, and how does it affect you?" Interestingly, these are illegal questions in academia except when asked under limited circumstances by designated personnel. Thus, while therapists are free to ask all sorts of personal questions, in academia, the instructor is limited to the information provided in a list of reasonable accommodations. Although this restriction is designed to prevent intrusiveness, it prevents open exchange of ideas on best practices for accommodations between disabled students and faculty.

One aspect of disability-affirmative therapy is about models of disability (moral, medical, social, and biomedical and environmental). Olkin (2017) has argued that therapists should hold the social model but not insist that clients do so. Similarly, academia should create policies and procedures from a social model perspective. In the social model, the problem is a mismatch between the disabled person and the environment, and the failure to plan for disability in advance.

Universal Design for Learning

Universal design (UD) refers to making "products, environments, and communication to be usable by all people, to the greatest extent possible, without adaptation or specialized design" (Institute for Human Centered Design, 2017). Note how the definition of UD differs from reasonable accommodations, which are individualized. In contrast, UD endeavors to minimize the need for individualized accommodations, though it must be stressed that it does not erase the need for them. Common examples of UD are sensors on grocery store doors and close captioning options on televisions.

Universal design for learning (UDL) comes to higher education and especially graduate education circuitously. UDL began with grades K-12, simultaneously with the Education for All Handicapped Children Act (1975; reauthorized as the Individuals with Disabilities Education Act). A key aspect of UDL was putting the "disability" tag on the curriculum, not the learner. UDL began to enter post-secondary education in the 2000s but has not taken a firm hold. UDL helps all students, not just those with disabilities. However, there are numerous studies on faculty members' responses to UDL and "in multiple large studies since 1981, the emotional valence associated with accommodations is almost uniformly negative" (Tobin, 2019). Similarly, resistance to UDL mirrors that to accommodations. Push-back arguments against UDL include that it (a) takes too much time on the part of faculty; (b) requires specialized learning by faculty; (c) somehow advantages some students over others; (d) opens the gatekeeping door too widely; and (e) lowers standards. However, UDL and reasonable accommodations do not lower standards but do alter processes for demonstrating standards.

Not all of these objections are incorrect. Adopting principles of UDL does take time and learning on the part of faculty, beginning with the initial development of a course and the syllabus. However, not all steps have to be taken simultaneously. Small changes can make a big difference. Take one example: adopting use of untimed open-book tests taken at home, instead of in-class timed closed-book tests. This method obviates the need for finding separate rooms and proctors for students who need accommodations. It allows students to use their own accessibility features on their devices. It makes it difficult to cheat. It helps not only disabled students but those who are test anxious. And it serves as an excellent learning tool. Surprisingly, the ranking of students that was obtained from multiple homework assignments will remain roughly the same after this kind of testing; the better students will know where to look for answers and struggling students may not.

Example of Ableism in Academia

In the study by Olkin and Hanrahan (2023), students gave numerous examples of experiencing microaggressions and ableism, even outright discrimination. The most referenced experience was feeling invisible or disbelieved when the disability was not apparent to others. Refusal to provide accommodations ("I'm not doing this") was cited, even though this is illegal. Statements such as "people with ADHD shouldn't be in graduate school" or being asked personal questions were made. There were complaints about materials that were not in accessible formats (e.g., videos without captioning, PowerPoint slides that used 18-point font) or instructors interacting inappropriately with service animals. These events constitute discrimination and could be targeted for training on laws and risk management. There were more subtle occurrences of stereotyping, lack of representation of disability in curricula and faculty, being inflexible about how and when homework was completed, downgrading a dyslexic student's homework points for spelling errors, selecting textbooks unavailable in alternate formats, wanting American Sign Language interpreters to be in the back because they were "distracting," using only one type of assessment of learning, and equating disability with negative concepts such as deficit, deficiencies, pathology, and abnormality.

Levels of Advising

Disabled students in professional programs would benefit from three levels of advising. Unfortunately, colleges and universities generally only do level one. Full integration of students and graduates with disabilities requires an accomplishment of all three levels.

Level one: The student provides documentation of a diagnosis and impairments to an ODS. The ODS then determines what reasonable accommodations are appropriate and gives the student a completed form that can be shown to instructors. The reasonable accommodations generally come from an existing list of common accommodations, such as time and a half on tests, quiet rooms for testing, an extra 24–36 hours for homework, reading materials in advance, Braille copies of reading.

Level two: A faculty member who is very familiar with the program in which the disabled student is enrolled meets with the student individually. Together, they review the requirements of the program and anticipate any areas that may pose difficulties or barriers. For example, an incoming student with a learning disability related to reading might want a slower pace of the program, or to know which courses have high reading loads. A student with mobility limitations might want to know which practica sites are more accessible. A blind student would need all materials well in advance but need particular tailored accommodations in statistics courses. This kind of anticipation allows for removal of barriers to successful navigation through the pipeline. The best advisor is familiar with both the program and with various types of disabilities and their concomitant impairments.

Level three: Disabled students in graduate programs are budding professionals with disabilities. They need role models and mentors with disabilities who can help them navigate the program, interviews, placements, internships, licensing exams, etc., as professionals who both own and take charge of their own disabilities. They will undoubtedly have questions about whether to put information about the disability in an application to internships, how to talk about the disability in any interviews, ways to use the disability as a niche area of expertise that can become an advantage in a competitive market. Those with early onset disabilities may already be well versed in these areas, though many are not. Those with newer disabilities may not yet know well their own limitations, coping skills, work-arounds, or may not feel comfortable talking about the disability. And BIPOC and other minoritized disabled students may well need mentoring about all of their identities as an integrated whole.

Initial Steps to Take

Assessing the physical space should be undertaken to see both, what is readily accessible, but also for signs of attention to various disabilities. This is not about being "ADA compliant" but about truly integrating those with disabilities. Are there Braille signs on doors, automatic door openers to each area, smooth paths to places were students and/or faculty gather, wheelchair accessible water fountains, single use and gender-neutral bathrooms, sufficient handicapped parking spaces, lockers in which to stores backpacks, etc. These not only increase accessibility but are visible signs of attention to disability.

Another important initial step is to assess the current state of self-identification of disabilities and barriers that exist. A survey should go to all students, not just those registered with an office of disability services, as it may well be that there are more who were not registered than who were. Two questions that we found useful were to ask about reasons for not registering with ODS and an open-ended question about what information about disabilities they most wanted faculty to know. The answers can lead directly to the kinds of training that would be most helpful.

Many professional training programs include disability content as a part of pathology or deficit (e.g., so-called special needs children; autism spectrum disorder in the DSM-5). Consider places where disability information can be included in the curriculum, not as a deficit but as a difference that is inadequately accommodated. Disability should be part of every diversity course, preferably by addressing intersectionality (disability in the context of other demographic variables; for suggested activities to teach about disability from a social model perspective, see Olkin, 2021).

Another area to address is about the accessible delivery of teaching. Examples could include choosing only materials that are available in accessible formats, giving flexibility in assignments, using large fonts on Powerpoint slides, delivering information both orally and in writing, and allowing use of devices that contain students' accessibility features. Most instructors read portions of their syllabi to students on the first day of class. Faculty can use built-in accessibility checkers (e.g., *Office 365 accessibility checker*; *grackle* for google suite; *UDOIT*—universal design online content inspection tool; *file transformer* for Blackboard), *Bookshare* (for ebooks; *Webcaptioner*; *dictate.io*)

Issues that are harder to both assess and address are stereotypes, microaggressions, and biases. One place to start these conversations are to review basic models of disability and try to move faculty to the social model (Olkin, 2017) in which disability is centered in the mismatch between abilities and environment, with the emphasis on how the environment has to change. Discussing the language of disability can help faculty feel more comfortable talking about disability without being offensive, such as the use of person-first versus identity-first language—neither is incorrect; those with disabilities are likely to prefer one over the other, but it's the discussion about the language that is the important part. The word itself—disability—is not a dirty word; euphemisms are unnecessary, and offensive to many adults with disabilities. There also are antiquated terms that can be offensive (e.g., deaf and dumb; wheelchair bound; seeing eye dog).

Rooting out ableist assumptions and values is not easy, as most of us are unaware of these until we encounter a relevant situation. Growth can occur in forums that allow for mistakes, honest opinions and real feedback; multiple chances to explore disability; selected first person accounts of lived experience; readings that situate disability as part of diversity. If the 18% of individuals and 50% of families that include disabilities are to be fully included in all aspects of society, we need to do the work.

References

ADA Amendments Act of 2008, Public Law 110–325, 122 Stat. 3553 (2008).

Americans with Disabilities Act of 1990, 42 U.S.C. § 12101 (1990).

Berrin, S., Olkin, R., & Taube, D. (2012). What do graduate students think about their diversity courses? *The California Psychologist, 45*(2), 28.

Bluestone, H. H., Stokes, A., & Kuba, S. (1996). Toward an integrated program design: Evaluating the status of diversity training in a graduate school curriculum. *Professional Psychology: Research and Practice, 27*, 394–400.

DEA, 2004. Individuals with Disabilities Education Improvement Act of 2004, Pub. L. No. 108–446, 118 Stat. 2647.
Deroche, M. D., Herlihy, B., & Lyons, M. L. (2020). Counselor trainee self-perceived disability competence: Implications for training. *Counselor Education and Supervision, 59*(3), 187–199. https://doi.org/10.1002/ceas.12183
Dolmage, J. T. (2017). *Academic ableism: Disability and higher education.* Ann Arbor: University of Michigan Press.
Education for All Handicapped Children Act, Pub. L. No. 94–142, 89 Stat. 773 (1975). Individuals with Disabilities Education Improvement Act of 2004, Pub. L. No. 108–446, 118 Stat. 2647. Rehabilitation Act of 1973, Pub. L. No. 93–112, § 504, 87 Stat. 355.
Feather, K. A., & Carlson, R. G. (2019). An initial investigation of individual instructors' self-perceived competence and incorporation of disability content into CACREP-accredited programs: Rethinking training in counselor education. *Journal of Multicultural Counseling and Development, 47*(1), 19–36.
Heitzman, A. M. (2015). Disability awareness, knowledge, and skills: Developing foundational and functional competencies training for graduate psychology and counseling students. *Professional Psychology Dissertations, 2015–23.* Retrieved from https://ir.stthomas.edu/caps_gradpsycho_docdiss/23
Institute for Human Centered Design. (2017). *Universal design definition.* Institute for Human Centered Design. https://humancentereddesign.org/inclusive-design/principles
Lewis, T. A. (2020). *Ableism 2020: An updated definition.* Retrieved from https://www.talilalewis.com/blog/ableism-2020-an-updated-definition
National Center for Education Statistics (2023). Students with disabilities. *Condition of Education, U.S. Department of Education, Institute of Education Sciences.* Retrieved from https://nces.ed.gov/programs/coe/indicator/cgg
Olkin, R. (2002). Could you hold the door for me? Including disability in diversity. *Cultural Diversity and Ethnic Minority Psychology, 8*(2), 130–137.
Olkin, R. (2017). *Disability-affirmative therapy: A case formulation template for clients with disabilities.* New York: Oxford University Press.
Olkin, R. (2021). *Teaching disability: Activities for in class and homework.* New York: Oxford University Press.
Olkin, R., & Hanrahan, S. (2023). *Report on survey Part I and Part II* [Unpublished manuscript]. Available from the first author.
Olkin, R., & Pledger, C. (2003). Can disability studies and psychology join hands? *American Psychologist, 58*(4), 296–304.
Shifrer, D. (2018). Clarifying the social roots of the disproportionate classification of racial minorities and males with learning disabilities. *The Sociological Quarterly, 59*(3), 384–406. https://doi.org/10.1080/00380253.2018.1479198
Tobin, T. J. (2019). Reaching all learners through their phones and universal design for learning. *Journal of Adult Learning, Knowledge and Innovation, 4(*1), 9–19.
United States. (2011). Individuals with Disabilities Education Improvement Act, 20 U.S.C. § 1400, 2004.
U.S. Congress, Public Law 94–142, Education for All Handicapped Children Act (November 29, 1975). U.S. Congress, Senate, Education for All Handicapped Children Act S. 6, 94th Congress, 1st Session, June 2, 1975, Report No. 94–168.

Bibliography

National Center for Education Statistics (2022). Retrieved from https://nces.ed.gov/programs/coe/indicator/cgg
Olkin, R. (1999). *What psychotherapists should know about disability.* New York: Guilford Press.

Further Reading

Brown, N., Ed. (2021). *Lived experiences of ableism in academia: Strategies for inclusion in higher education*. Bristol: Policy Press.

Brown, N., & Leigh, J., Eds. (2020). *Ableism in academia: Theorising experiences of disabilities and chronic illnesses in higher education*. London: University College London.

Brown, R., Silny, M., & Brown, J. T. (2021). Ableism in the academy? A systematic review and meta-analysis of experiences of students with disabilities in US higher education. In W. Pearson Jr. & V. Reddy (Eds.), *Social justice and education in the 21st century: Research from South Africa and the United States* (pp. 293–307). Springer Nature Switzerland AG. https://doi.org/10.1007/978-3-030-65417-7_15

Lund, E. M., Wilbur, R. C., & Kuemmel, A. M. (2020). Beyond legal obligation: The role and necessity of the supervisor-advocate in creating a socially just, disability-affirmative training environment. *Training and Education in Professional Psychology*, *14*(2), 92.

Mireles, D. (2022). Theorizing racist ableism in higher education. *Teachers College Record*, *124*(7), 17–50.

Nieminen, J. H. (2023). Unveiling ableism and disablism in assessment: A critical analysis of disabled students' experiences of assessment and assessment accommodations. *Higher Education*, *85*(3), 613–636.

Olkin, R., & Taube, D. O. (2013). Disability in the ivory tower. In K. Johnson & K. Couture (Eds.), *Disability discrimination at work* (pp. 81–100). Williamstown, MA: Piraeus Books.

Singer, S., & Bacon, J. (2020). Ableism in the academy: A series about disability oppression and resistance in higher education. *Critical Education*, *11*(14), 1–13.

Wilbur, R. C., Kuemmel, A. M., & Lackner, R. J. (2019). Who's on first? Supervising psychology trainees with disabilities and establishing accommodations. *Training and Education in Psychology*, *13*(2), 111.

SECTION II

Contextualizing Disability through an Intersectional Lens

PART II

Held in Touch and Sound (Written in Braille)

Caitlin Hernandez

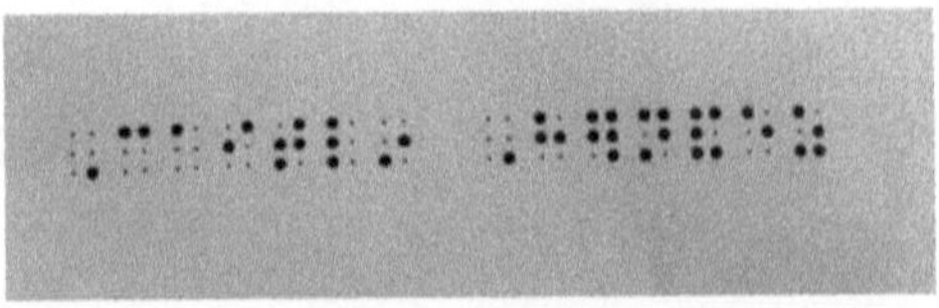

Throughout my life, people have asserted that my total blindness must make my remaining senses more acute than those of sighted people. My response is twofold. First, I admit that, without the distraction of sight, I may very well be able to give my other senses more attention. Next, however, I explain that having been born with only light perception, it's impossible to know where blindness and my personality intersect and diverge, and maybe it doesn't matter.

Touch, rather than hearing, as most people suspect, is my primary sense. It is my eye contact, my avenue for giving and receiving innumerable wordless exchanges. My fingers fly over Braille with ease. I feel most connected to my sighted students when they insist on sitting beside me, steer my fingers along their artwork, or endeavor to write and draw with me, hand over hand. I absorb facets of someone's essence in the way they touch, reach out to, and guide me.

My sensitivity to touch comes with drawbacks. As a female-identified, totally blind survivor of sexual assault who just barely scrapes five feet, nothing spikes my anxiety more than being grabbed without consent. I am pushed, pulled, and propelled multiple times daily. The paradox of fearing and craving touch is vulnerable and nearly impossible to explain.

As a child, I taught myself basic piano by ear, memorized and recreated complex harmonies, and identified touch tones by sound. Few things nourished my soul as much as being read to, playing, and replaying my beloved tape-recordings, and the singular sounds of my family's and friends' voices.

These days, however, my departure from singing has caused my once-perfect pitch to degrade. And though I love the sound of my partner, Martha, reading aloud

DOI: 10.4324/9781003362586-9

while our dog, Maíte, snores noisily at the foot of the bed, I value Martha's hand running through my hair, and the warm weight of Maíte sprawling across my legs, even more.

Despite the fact that its symptoms were present all my life, I was diagnosed with Avoidant/Restrictive Food Intake Disorder only recently. ARFID is common among neurodivergent people, who often prefer, or even require, the reliability of "safe," predictable foods.

Taste, smell, and mouth-feel combine with my inability to visually examine my food, making eating more of a chore than a pleasure. The upside is that, when I love a food, its familiarity brings me inexplicable comfort.

My greatest advantage is not heightened senses. Rather, it's my capacity for happiness, excitement, and joy, which enriches my days. Hugs, hand-holding, and the breeze on my skin as I skip; listening to close, resonant harmonies; the delightful amalgamation of darkly bitter ice cream and sugary-sweet Oreo cookies, these things, and so many others, can soothe the stings of ableism, condescension, and microaggressions.

I benefit from many privileges: my family's and friends' acceptance of my queerness; being a white-passing woman of color; my education; and my early exposure to blindness skills, to name a few. Yet, my ebullience remains my most steadfast gift, during even the most trying of times, and for that, I am, and will always be, tremendously grateful.

5

THE INTERSECTION OF OLDER ADULTHOOD, MENTAL HEALTH, AND DISABILITY

Pamela B. Teaster and Onyinye F. Mbanefo

Introduction

The United States, like most developed countries around the world, is an aging one. In fact, the U.S. population is older today than ever before in history. The number of individuals aged 65 and older is projected to increase from 58 million in 2022 to 82 million by 2050 (a 47% increase), and the share of the total population of the 65-and-older age group is projected to grow from 17% to 23% (Population Reference Bureau, 2024). Older Americans are far more likely than their younger counterparts to have some form of disability; nearly half (46%) of adults aged 75 and older and 24% of adults 65–74 report having at least one form of impairment. Common disabilities affecting older adults include foot problems, arthritis, cognitive impairment, heart problems, vision loss, and hearing impairment (U.S. Census Bureau, 2024). In addition, nearly 25% of adults 65 and older are living with a mental health condition such as anxiety or depression (National Council on Aging, 2024). Also, substance use among older people has been increasing for a number of years; unfortunately, fewer than half of older adults with mental health and/or substance use problems receive any treatment (Yarnell et al., 2020). The intersection of these egregious problems increases chronic and acute health problems overall and raises costs for care and treatment, significantly reducing the quality of life of older adults and their families. Given that a significant percentage of the disabled community consists of older adults, it would be negligent to overlook this crucial intersection in a handbook on disability-affirmative therapy.

The purpose of this chapter is to elucidate the intersection of old age, disability, and mental health problems from a strengths-based approach while emphasizing that individual aging is highly variable. Although we acknowledge that forms of loss can accompany aging, we stress that aging can also be accompanied by

DOI: 10.4324/9781003362586-10

resiliency, strength, and perspective. It is through this lens that we discuss issues that disabled older adults face and offer solutions for overcoming related challenges in order to enhance the quality of life for disabled clients and their families.

Terms and Concepts

In order to adequately address the intersection of older adulthood, disability, and mental health, we present terms and concepts to help frame possibilities for assistance that mental health providers, in particular, can provide. We underscore that we are in no way problematizing older adults, but rather, we offer ideas and strategies to help providers address the mental health and related challenges of disabled older adults.

Cumulative Advantage and Disadvantage

Problems associated with aging, disability, and mental health can arise suddenly and unexpectedly, or conversely, they may accumulate over time. One reason for the variance is cumulative advantage and cumulative disadvantage (Ferraro et al., 2016). The concept of cumulative advantage indicates that if a person is afforded advantages (e.g., money, location, education, good health), advantages will accumulate and increase over a lifetime. Conversely, cumulative disadvantage emphasizes that early life problems may become additive and explains how individuals become differentiated over a lifetime. Even early risk factors can shape a person's life trajectory, affecting both short-term and long-term outcomes (Ferraro & Kelly-Moore, 2003). Life course studies suggest that a wide range of biological and social forces can create differences in whole populations over time. Some people are able to surmount disadvantages, while others face an insurmountable mountain of additional and growing risks to health, income, and well-being.

Understanding the concepts of cumulative advantages and disadvantages is critical for mental healthcare providers. Because disabled older adults have had time in their lives to accrue many advantages or disadvantages, it is necessary for providers to peel back the layers and accumulations that affect them, in order to help assist and restore an individual being treated, especially when disability accompanies aging.

Ageism

When meeting a person for the first time, the first characteristic we often notice is their age, which is frequently used to categorize and define people. Defining a person by age can lead to harm, disadvantage, and injustice. This unique form of prejudice is ageism, which includes stereotypes (our thoughts), prejudice (our feelings), and discrimination (our actions) towards others or ourselves based on age (Ayalon & Tesch-Römer, 2018). Even into the past century and across most cultures, older adults were respected as wise and valuable contributors to their families and communities. Although many modern societies still hold positive views of older adults, ageism persists and festers, particularly in contemporary Western cultures, largely attributable to a society that places a high premium on productivity, acquisition, and individualism. Stereotypes about disability and aging present later life as a period marked by ill health, loneliness, dependency, and diminished physical and mental functioning, disregarding individual variability and possibility. Such stereotypes are deeply rooted culturally and historically and are negative and damaging. About half of the world's population holds ageist attitudes against older people, manifesting in prejudicial attitudes, discriminatory practices, and institutional biases (Gutterman, 2021). Efforts to address bias and discrimination often fall short, as ageism remains largely unnoticed and socially acceptable, impacting individuals of all ages and worsening over time. Discrimination against older adults is particularly evident in health care and the workplace, where older people may face patronizing communication, accusations of declining job performance, and limited access to services and opportunities.

The mental health workforce is poised to counter the narrative concerning ageism by recognizing its existence and promoting fairness and respect for people of all ages, particularly disabled older adults. Providers should work at individual and population levels to challenge deeply ingrained attitudes and advocate for comprehensive policies and practices that uphold the dignity and worth of every individual, regardless of age. One such tool for discerning inflection points is the Socio-Ecological Model explained below.

The Socio-Ecological Framework

The Socio-Ecological Model (Bronfenbrenner, 1986) provides a highly useful framework because of its explicability and applicability to complex problems such as the health of disabled older adults. Originally conceptualized for children, the model consists of micro through chrono system levels. The framework places the individual older adult at the center of nested rings, consistent with a "person-centered or person-directed" approach to understanding the phenomenon of disabled older adults' mental health.

The premise of the Socio-Ecological Framework is that older adults are embedded in a series of environmental systems that interact with one another and with the individual to influence all types of human development. Its focus is on the characteristics of the older adult and five influencing systems (see Figure 5.1): (a) the microsystem, which represents the individual within his or her environment; (b) the mesosystem, or the relationship between the older adult and those closest to them (e.g., relative; friend, caregiver); (c) the exosystem, which involves environments external to the older adult (e.g., community services) that may affect their well-being; (d) the macrosystem, or broad ideological values, norms, and cultural and institutional patterns; and the (e) chronosystem, which includes environmental changes that take place over an individual's life that influence their development and include major life transitions (e.g., adolescence, adulthood, retirement) and

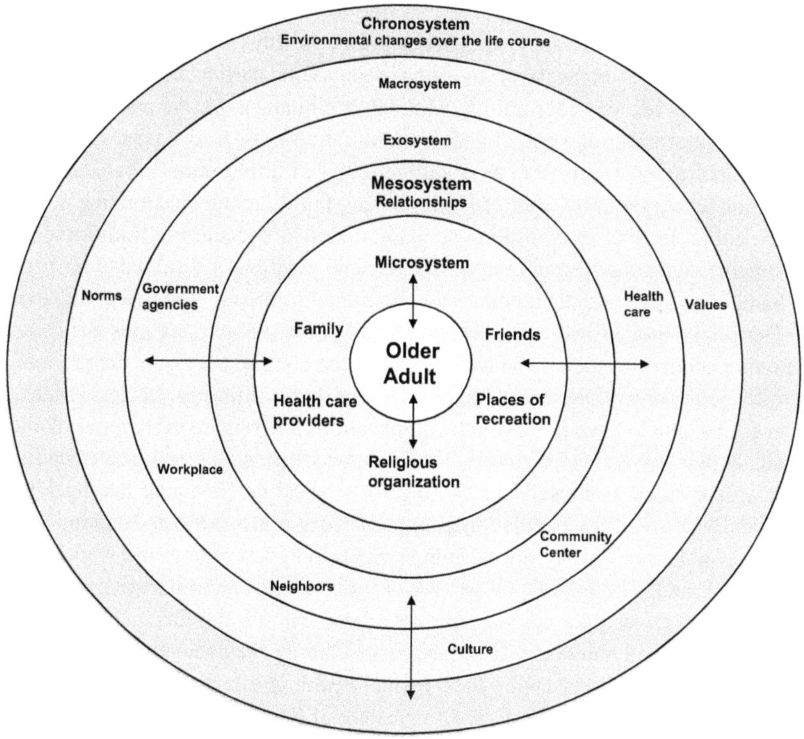

Figure 5.1 Socio-Ecological Framework for older adults.
Adapted from Bronfenbrenner (1986).

historical events (e.g., the Vietnam War and COVID-19). The framework helps amplify that disability and mental health in later life are multifaceted constructs requiring a nuanced understanding as well as coordinated responses involving multiple levels of interaction and intervention.

Systemic therapists, such as MFTs, often draw on the Socio-Ecological Framework when conceptualizing treatment, as it aligns with their focus on understanding complex, interrelated factors. This framework, widely used in research on older adults with disabilities and their mental health (Igarashi et al., 2022; Monetz et al., 2017), provides a comprehensive lens for examining the multiple variables influencing disability and mental health needs in this population.

Population Growth of Older Adults

As mentioned above, the proportion of individuals aged 65 and above will rise from 16% in 2019 to an anticipated 21.6% by 2040, with the population aged 85 and older expected to more than double during the same period (2020 Profile of

Older Americans, n.d.). This increase is due to factors such as decreased fertility, increased life expectancy, and better public health (Mondal & Shitan, n.d.). Notable challenges come with an aging population, particularly the well-being and quality of life of older adults (Mondal & Shitan, n.d.). As adults age, they may encounter mounting social and economic problems, health issues, and functional impairments (Samsudin & Abdullah, 2017). Furthermore, urbanization and migration have gradually removed many young family members from the midst of older people, leading to dwindling social networks and declining traditional family support that can adversely impact the societal position of disabled older people by hampering their social standing and communal influence (Fakoya et al., 2018).

The population growth of older adults has numerous implications for society, including economic, social, and healthcare-related consequences. As the proportion of older adults grows, there will be an increased demand for healthcare services, as older adults tend to have more health complications and require more medical attention than their younger counterparts. This increased demand for health care can strain healthcare systems and result in a shortage of medical professionals and healthcare facilities. Moreover, the population growth of older adults presents economic challenges, as older adults may not be able to work and contribute to the workforce as they once could. The population growth of older adults can impact the very social fabric of society, as older adults, especially those with disabilities, may experience social isolation and loneliness due to the loss of family members and friends, which can produce negative effects on their mental health and overall well-being (Committee on the Health and Medical Dimensions of Social Isolation and Loneliness in Older Adults et al., 2020; Hwang et al., 2020; Wu, 2020). The changing demographics of society will require a shift in societal norms and attitudes towards aging, including changes in policies and programs to better support older adults.

Disabled Older Adults

The intersection of aging and disability is dynamic and complex. According to the Centers for Disease Control and Prevention (2023), "one in four older individuals have some form of disability." Further, an estimated 40% of older adults aged 65 and over report at least one disability, with mobility limitations being the most common (Musich et al., 2018). In addition to mobility limitations, other types of disabilities prevalent among older adults include sensory impairments (e.g., vision and hearing impairments), which can significantly impact a person's ability to navigate the environment and communicate effectively. Cognitive disabilities, such as dementia, Alzheimer's disease, and other cognitive impairments, can affect memory, reasoning, and decision-making abilities, posing challenges for independence, particularly if they impede performing activities of daily living. This demographic shift, as highlighted by the CDC, underscores the need to understand and address issues germane to disabled older adults (Centers for Disease Control and Prevention, 2023).

Older Adults and Mental Health-Related Disabilities

Undoubtedly, mental health remains one of the most crucial aspects of individual well-being, regardless of age, gender, or origin/background. According to the World Health Organization (2022), optimal mental health is a state where a person can manage life's stressors, work and learn effectively, reach their potential, and give back to the community. Therefore, maintaining strong mental health is crucial as individuals progress through different life stages. This is especially true in the context of disabled, older adults, a demographic often vulnerable and struggling with mental health challenges that impact their overall health and well-being. Prioritizing the mental health and holistic well-being of disabled older adults is critical. According to the Committee on the Health and Medical Dimensions of Social Isolation and Loneliness in Older Adults et al. (2020), social isolation, anxiety, and depression are common among older adults due to the interconnection of their mental and physical health and the frequent impairments they experience.

Growing old brings with it a range of physiological, psychological, and social changes. In this context, a significant number of older adults experience mental health issues such as depression, anxiety, and cognitive disorders. Alternately, many older individuals with or without disabilities lead happy and rewarding lives. According to the Global Health Estimate (2019), depression and anxiety are the most common mental health challenges, affecting one in four older adults. A 2023 report by the World Health Organization indicates that older adults with mental health problems are projected to double by 2030 and triple by 2050.

In the United States, around 15 million older adults suffer from depression or anxiety (Reynolds et al., 2022). The economic burden of unaddressed mental health issues, including depression and anxiety among older adults, is substantial. According to the National Alliance on Mental Illness (NAMI, n.d.), the economic cost of untreated mental illness in the U.S. is over $100 billion annually, which includes costs related to health care, lost productivity, and disability support services. This cost emphasizes the persistent need for effective mental health interventions and support systems for older adults, particularly those with disabilities, in order to alleviate their suffering and reduce the economic burden on individuals and society.

Despite the increasing prevalence of mental health challenges among some older adults, mental health services are undervalued in the healthcare system. This under-prioritization of older adults' mental health has led to the poor management of the aging population, exacerbating ageism, which significantly affects the health and overall quality of life for disabled older adults.

Older Adults with Dementia

While the incidence of dementia is declining in the United States, the number of individuals and families affected by dementia is rising. This increase is primarily due to the aging population, as simply living to an older age is a significant risk factor for dementia (Aufill et al., 2021). If racial and ethnic patterns related to Alzheimer's Disease and Related Dementias (ADRD) are predictive, then their occurrence is more likely predicated on health disparities than on biological predisposition. Thus, in many cases, the problem is a remediable one. Also, although there are commonalities related to the progression of some dementias, disabled older adults and, concomitantly, their families, experience dementia in diverse ways (Aufill et al., 2021). To address the problem of physical and mental health, therapists and other healthcare professionals must understand that the incidence, risk factors, impact on dementia care, and economic costs associated with ADRD can provide clues to target risk and protective factors for all older people as well as addressing health disparities. Personal and economic costs for persons living with dementia and their care-providing families are high and affect future generations (Aufill et al., 2021). Providing affordable and appropriate mental health care remains an important solution for the often debilitating problem of dementia.

Intersectional Factors

Intersectionality concerns how societal categories such as disability, race, class, and gender, as applied to individuals or groups, create overlapping and interdependent systems of discrimination or disadvantage (Carbado et al., 2013). Although intersectionality affects all age groups, it is particularly problematic in the disabled older adult population because of the years the discrimination may have accumulated, which reflects the concept of cumulative disadvantage mentioned earlier. In addition, due to accrued health problems and other injustices, older adults may be least able to surmount them. Consequently, and particularly pertinent to this chapter, the accumulation of a lifetime of mental and physical health problems can quickly escalate into an acute situation extremely difficult for providers to disentangle, one with lethal consequences if the situation continues unabated.

While some situations can become dire, it is also inappropriate, inaccurate, and ageist to conclude that problems of older adults with disabilities are unresolvable and that such efforts are unreasonable or simply too late to administer. Instead, older adults stand to benefit the most from counseling and other interventions even compared to any other age group (Kampfe, 2015). They have longevity and resilience on their side; simple interventions may easily net significant gains.

Older Adult Caregivers and Caregiver Burnout

The increase in the older adult population also has implications for caregivers who provide assistance, healthcare management, and emotional support to disabled older adults. The number of caregivers for older adults has been increasing in many countries due to the aging population and changes in family structures. In the United States alone, there were approximately 53 million caregivers providing care to adults and older adults in 2020 (Schulz et al., 2020), a number expected to continue rising along with the aging population. This statistic is salient to consider for systemic therapists, as more families turn to therapists for support with optimal navigation of caregiving experiences.

Caregivers perform various tasks to support disabled older adults, including assistance with activities of daily living such as bathing, dressing, feeding, toileting, and mobility. They may also help with instrumental activities of daily living such as meal preparation, medication management, transportation, shopping, and household chores. Additionally, caregivers manage healthcare needs, including coordinating medical appointments, managing medications, monitoring health conditions, and providing emotional support. Companionship and emotional support are also vital aspects of caregiving, especially for disabled older adults who may be socially isolated. Costs associated with caregiving can be substantial, both in terms of financial expenses and the physical and emotional toll on caregivers themselves. These costs include direct financial expenses such as medical care, medications, home modifications, and assistive devices. Indirect costs may involve lost wages or reduced work hours for caregivers who must balance caregiving responsibilities with their own employment. There are also intangible costs of caregiving related to the stress, burden, and health consequences experienced by caregivers, including an increased risk of depression, anxiety, and other health issues. According to a report by the Reinhard et al. (2023), the estimated economic value of unpaid caregiving provided by family and friends of older adults in the United States was approximately $470 billion in 2017. This underscores the significant contribution of caregivers to the healthcare system and the economy.

Sometimes caregiving is too long and too intense and leads to caregiver burnout (Gérain & Zech, 2019), which can result from caregiving without adequate support or respite. Factors contributing to caregiver burnout include the intensity of care required, lack of social support, financial strain, and personal health issues (Schulz et al., 2020). It is challenging to estimate the number of caregivers experiencing burnout at any given time due to factors such as individual coping mechanisms, the fluctuating nature of caregiving responsibilities, and differences in access to support services. However, research indicates that caregiver burnout is a widespread issue with significant implications for both caregivers and care recipients. Studies suggest that a substantial proportion experience symptoms of burnout at some point during their caregiving journey, with approximately 40% of caregivers reporting high levels of emotional stress (AARP, 2023). A survey conducted by the Alzheimer's Association (2021) found that more than one-third of dementia caregivers experience symptoms of depression. The prevalence of burnout underscores the need for effective support mechanisms and resources to help caregivers manage their responsibilities and maintain their well-being (Aufill et al., n.d.). Access to respite care, counseling services, support groups, and educational programs can play an important role in mitigating burnout and supporting caregivers' overall health and resilience, assistance for which mental health providers should be especially mindful.

Dispersion of Mental Health Providers Who Work with Disabled Older Adults

A review of mental health providers on the website of *Psychology Today* reveals a list of qualified therapists in every state in the country. Many professionals advertise that they serve individuals with mental health concerns across the lifespan, with some noting that they specialize in serving older adults. Still, a shortage of qualified providers exists overall, especially in rural areas (Health Resources & Services Administration, 2023), and especially in relation to disability expertise. This shortage is analogous to the lack of health providers in rural areas overall and, more specifically, a lack of physicians and nurses who specialize in caring for disabled, older persons (Weinhold & Gurtner, 2014). An overall lack of mental health providers qualified to work with older adults is exacerbated by disparities in mental healthcare for disabled older adults. Chief among these issues are ageism and its effects on extending care to older adults, as well as societal and individual attitudes toward older adults experiencing mental health issues. Additional attention is needed to address these disparities and ensure equitable access to mental health services for disabled older adults.

Guidance for Mental Health Practitioners Working with Disabled Older Adults

Mental health practitioners working with disabled, older adults should be aware of the multiple comorbidities that many clients may have accumulated and should be taken into account when developing treatment plans. Because the genesis of the problems vary, practitioners should adopt a person-directed, holistic approach (reference the Bronfenbrenner Framework discussed earlier) in addressing the mental health concerns of disabled older people. Reasons for mental health struggles may have a biological etiology and could be attributed to poor diet, lack of transportation, inadequate finances, loneliness, social isolation, unmet support for disabling conditions, and medication interactions. Excellent mental healthcare practitioners should investigate how these problems co-exist and take steps to remedy them. In addition, in every encounter, mental healthcare practitioners should consider whether disabled, older people feel safe in their homes and whether they have the assistance that they need to have the highest quality of life possible.

A number of older adults struggle with mental health concerns, but they also struggle with a general distrust of mental healthcare providers, many of whom are decades younger than their clients. Mental healthcare providers must attempt to dispel these concerns – one important way to do so is to become ingratiated into the fabric of the community in which disabled older adults and their families dwell.

Therapists must be aware that some disabled older adults struggle with becoming a burden on family members should they require extra assistance in their daily lives. Mental healthcare providers need to approach the older person's apprehension through validation, active listening, and creative and helpful problem-solving performed if possible, in collaboration with the older adult client.

Conclusion and Looking to the Future

With a rising population of disabled older people in the United States, now is an important and necessary time to place the mental health concerns of older adults on equal footing with their physical health concerns. In doing so, mental health providers must include not only the disabled older adults themselves but also family members who are helping them. Training that includes learning about how disabled, older people function in the world is essential to providing quality mental health care, improving older adults' quality of life, and promoting their dignity. One policy action that prioritizes the mental health of older adults is implementing changes in reimbursement patterns (Schmidt et al., 2024). These changes can significantly improve access to affordable, high-quality mental health care for this group, leading to positive outcomes not only for families but, most importantly, for disabled older adults themselves.

References

AARP. (2023). AARP research insights on caregiving. https://www.aarp.org/pri/topics/ltss/family-caregiving/aarp-research-insights-caregiving.html#:~:text=Roughly%20one%2Dfifth%20of%20U.S.,quarter%20between%2018%20and%2034.

Administration for Community Living. (2021). *2020 profile of older Americans*. U.S. Department of Health and Human Services. https://acl.gov/sites/default/files/aging%20and%20Disability%20in%20America/2020ProfileOlderAmericans.Final_.pdf

Aufill, J., Aranda, M. P., Kremer, I. N., Hinton, L., Zissimopoulos, J., Whitmer, R. A., Hummel, C. H., Trejo, L., & Fabius, C. (2021). Impact of dementia: Health disparities, population trends, care interventions, and economic costs. *Journal of the American Geriatrics Society*, *69*(7), 1774–1783. https://doi.org/10.1111/jgs.17345

Aufill, J., Burgdorf, J., & Wolff, J. (n.d.). *In Support of Family Caregivers: A Snapshot of Five States* [Technical report]. Milbank Memorial Fund; The John A. Hartford Foundation. https://www.milbank.org/wp-content/uploads/2019/06/MMF_Caregiver_Report_6.19.pdf

Ayalon, L., & Tesch-Römer, C. (Eds.). (2018). *Contemporary Perspectives on Ageism* (Vol. 19). Springer International Publishing. https://doi.org/10.1007/978-3-319-73820-8

Bronfenbrenner, U. (1986). Recent advances in research on the ecology of human development. In R. K. Silbereisen, K. Eyferth, & G. Rudinger (Eds.), *Development as Action in Context: Problem Behavior and Normal Youth Development* (pp. 287–309). Springer-Verlag Berlin Heidelberg. https://doi.org/10.1007/978-3-662-02475-1_1

Carbado, D. W., Crenshaw, K. W., Mays, V. M., & Tomlinson, B. (2013). Intersectionality: Mapping the movements of a theory. *Du Bois Review: Social Science Research on Race*, *10*(2), 303–312.

Centers for Disease Control and Prevention. Disability and Health Data System (DHDS) [Internet]. [updated 2023 May; cited 2023 May 15]. Available from: https://dhds.cdc.gov

Committee on the Health and Medical Dimensions of Social Isolation and Loneliness in Older Adults, Board on Health Sciences Policy, Board on Behavioral, Cognitive, and Sensory Sciences, Health and Medicine Division, Division of Behavioral and Social Sciences and Education, & National Academies of Sciences, Engineering, and Medicine.

(2020). *Social Isolation and Loneliness in Older Adults: Opportunities for the Health Care System* (p. 25663). National Academies Press. https://doi.org/10.17226/25663

Fakoya, O. O., Abioye-Kuteyi, E. A., Bello, I. S., Oyegbade, O. O., Olowookere, S. A., & Ezeoma, I. T. (2018). Determinants of quality of life of elderly patients attending a general practice clinic in Southwest Nigeria. *International Quarterly of Community Health Education, 39*(1), 3–7. https://doi.org/10.1177/0272684X18781781

Ferraro, K. F., Schafer, M. H., & Wilkinson, L. R. (2016). Childhood disadvantage and health problems in middle and later life: Early imprints on physical health? *American Sociological Review, 81*(1), 107–132. https://doi.org/10.1177/0003122415619617

Ferraro, K. F., & Kelley-Moore, J. (2003). Cumulative disadvantage and health: Long-term consequences of obesity? *American Sociological Review, 68*(5), 707–729. https://doi.org/10.2307/1519759

Gérain, P. & Zech, E. (2019). Informal caregiver burnout? Development of a theoretical framework to understand the impact of caregiving. *Frontiers in Psychology, 10*, Article 1748. https://doi.org/10.3389/fpsyg.2019.01748

Gutterman, A. (2021). Ageism: Where it comes from and what it does. *SSRN Electronic Journal*. https://doi.org/10.2139/ssrn.3849022

Health Resources & Services Administration. (2023). *Behavioral health workforce shortage designations summary 2023* [Data dashboard]. U.S. Department of Health and Human Services. https://data.hrsa.gov/topics/health-workforce/health-workforce-shortage-areas

Hwang, T.-J., Rabheru, K., Peisah, C., Reichman, W., & Ikeda, M. (2020). Loneliness and social isolation during the COVID-19 pandemic. *International Psychogeriatrics, 32*(10), 1217–1220. https://doi.org/10.1017/S1041610220000988

Igarashi, H., Kurth, M. L., Lee, H. S., Choun, S., Lee, D., & Aldwin, C. M. (2021). Resilience in older adults during the COVID-19 pandemic: A socioecological approach. *The Journals of Gerontology, Series B: Psychological Sciences and Social Sciences, 76*(6), e59–e64. https://doi.org/10.1093/geronb/gbab058

Kampfe, C. M. (2015). *Counseling older people: Opportunities and challenges.* Alexandria, VA: American Counseling Association.

Mondal, N. I., & Shitan, M. (n.d.). Impact of socio-health factors on life expectancy in the low and lower middle income countries. *42*(12), 1354–1362. https://www.ncbi.nlm.nih.gov/pmc/articles/PMC4441932/.

Montez, J. K., Hayward, M. D., & Wolf, D. A. (2017). Do U.S. states' socioeconomic and policy contexts shape adult disability? *Social Science & Medicine, 178*, 115–126. https://doi.org/10.1016/j.socscimed.2017.02.012

Musich, S., Wang, S. S., Ruiz, J., Hawkins, K., & Wicker, E. (2018). The impact of mobility limitations on health outcomes among older adults. *Geriatric Nursing, 39*(2), 162–169. https://doi.org/10.1016/j.gerinurse.2017.08.002

National Alliance on Mental Illness. (n.d.). *Mental health by the numbers.* https://www.nami.org/about-mental-illness/mental-health-by-the-numbers

National Council on Aging (2024). Mental health stigma: Changing the conversation. https://www.ncoa.org/article/mental-health-stigma-changing-the-conversation

Population Reference Bureau. (2024). *Fact sheet: Aging in the United States*. https://www.prb.org/resources/fact-sheet-aging-in-the-united-states/

Reinhard, S. C., Feinberg, L. F., Houser, A., Schulz, R., & Choula, R. (2023). *Valuing the invaluable 2023 update: Strengthening supports for family caregivers* [Report]. AARP Public Policy Institute. Retrieved from https://archrespite.org/wp-content/uploads/2023/03/valuing-the-invaluable-2023-update.doi_.10.26419-2Fppi.00082.006.pdf

Reynolds, C. F., Jeste, D. V., Sachdev, P. S., & Blazer, D. G. (2022). Mental health care for older adults: Recent advances and new directions in clinical practice and research. *World Psychiatry, 21*(3), 336–363. https://doi.org/10.1002/wps.20996

Samsudin, S., & Abdullah, N. (2017). Healthcare utilization by older age groups in Northern States of Peninsular Malaysia: The role of predisposing, enabling and need factors. *Journal of Cross-Cultural Gerontology*, *32*(2), 223–237. https://doi.org/10.1007/s10823-017-9318-4

Schmidt, N. E., Carpenter, B., & Steffen, A. M. (2024). Brief aging education affects continuing education preferences and behaviors of mental health providers. *The Gerontologist, 64*(9), Article gnae085. https://doi.org/10.1093/geront/gnae085

Schulz, R., Beach, S. R., Czaja, S. J., Martire, L. M., & Monin, J. K. (2020). Family caregiving for older adults. *Annual Review of Psychology*, *71*(1), 635–659. https://doi.org/10.1146/annurev-psych-010419-050754

U.S. Census Bureau. (2024). *Disability status by age group: 2022 one-year estimates.* Retrieved from https://www.census.gov/library/visualizations/2024/comm/disability-status-age-group.html

Yarnell, S., Li, L., MacGrory, B., Trevisan, L., & Kirwin, P. (2020). Substance use disorders in later life: A review and synthesis of the literature of an emerging public health concern. *The American Journal of Geriatric Psychiatry*, *28*(2), 226–236.

Weinhold, I., & Gurtner, S. (2014). Understanding shortages of sufficient health care in rural areas. *Health Policy, 118*(2), 201–214. https://doi.org/10.1016/j.healthpol.2014.07.018

World Health Organization. (2021, June 17). *Mental health of older adults* [Fact sheet]. WHO. https://www.who.int/news-room/fact-sheets/detail/mental-health-of-older-adults

World Health Organization. (2022, June 17). Mental health: *Strengthening our response* [Fact sheet]. https://www.who.int/news-room/fact-sheets/detail/mental-health-strengthening-our-response

Wu, B. (2020). Social isolation and loneliness among older adults in the context of COVID-19: A global challenge. *Global Health Research and Policy*, *5*(1), 27. https://doi.org/10.1186/s41256-020-00154-3

Bibliography

Bainbridge, H. T. J., Cregan, C., & Kulik, C. T. (2006). The effect of multiple on caregiver stress outcomes. *Journal of Applied Psychology*, *91*(2), 490–497. https://doi.org/10.1037/0021-9010.91.2.490

6

THE INTERSECTION OF RACE AND DISABILITY

Redefining Inclusive Therapeutic Practice

Angélica Guevara

Introduction

To effectively meet the mental health needs of clients, particularly those with marginalized identities, providers must adopt a holistic approach that acknowledges the social contexts and critical intersections within which they exist. Failure to do so undermines the potential for comprehensive healing and perpetuates existing disparities in care. In the United States, those providing care to racial minorities cannot ignore the complex struggles that clients must endure on multiple systemic levels. It is essential to recognize that identities are socially constructed and shaped by their specific historical and sociopolitical contexts-particularly within the United States, where the legacy of eugenics and racial discrimination continues to influence how identities are perceived and treated. Failing to address these marginalized identities and their intersections would significantly reduce the effectiveness of care. This 'partial' care diminishes the importance of healing the entire self. Not addressing this intersection would only treat parts of the self rather than the whole self, leading to poor therapeutic alliances and unhelpful outcomes in therapy.

For instance, if a therapist was providing services to a client who has an apparent disability and identifies as Black, the clinician should have a working knowledge and understanding of the racist and ableist history in America that inevitably impacts the daily lived experiences of this client. If this engagement is not actively practiced by the clinician, the lack of cultural competence and critical reflection will further marginalize the client's existence and compound their struggles. This chapter addresses this critical intersectionality of race and disability, specifically in the provision of therapeutic care.

DOI: 10.4324/9781003362586-11

Prevalence

According to the 2019 American Community Survey, approximately 12.6% of the U.S. population has a disability, and this rate is disproportionately higher among BIPOC communities. Ongoing research continues to explore these disparities in greater detail (Goodman et al., 2017). African Americans have the highest disability prevalence rate (14%), compared to White (11%), Latino (8%), and Asian (5%) populations in the United States. The likelihood of having a disability increases with age (Goodman et al., 2017). Disabled individuals generally have lower educational levels, affecting job prospects and income. Only 13% of disabled adults have a college degree (Goodman et al., 2017). The poverty rate for disabled people is significantly higher (27%) than for those without (12%). African Americans with disabilities face the highest poverty rate at 37% (Goodman et al., 2017). Only one-third of working-age disabled adults are employed. In fact, African Americans with disabilities have the lowest employment rate at 25% (Goodman et al., 2017). In addition, a third of disabled adults struggle to pay medical bills. This challenge is more pronounced for African Americans at 33% (Goodman et al., 2017). Sadly, disabled individuals are also more likely to forgo medical care due to cost, with 16% unable to afford necessary care, when faced with illness. Race and disability intersect in important ways, leading to compounded disadvantages reinforced through structural racism and ableism.

Healthcare Access and Care Inequality

Similar to the structural inequalities people of color have encountered in education (Talbert-Johnson, 2004; Darling-Hammond, 2001), housing (Vargas et al., 2023; Bailey et al., 2017), and employment, so too have they experienced disparities in healthcare access and quality of care (Lopez et al., 1998). An important part of the cultural competency of a therapist lies in recognizing that structural racism contributes to health inequalities (Bailey et al., 2017). Structural racism persists, resulting in racial inequalities in wealth, employment, income, and health care between African Americans and White Caucasians (Yearby, 2018). The structural racism that causes these social determinants of health largely contributes to the disparities in access to health care and overall health status (Williams et al., 2019; Yearby, 2018). This became particularly clear during the COVID-19 pandemic, prompting a call to action as it highlighted that structural racism may be the primary cause of health disparities (Churchwell et al., 2020). Regardless of an individual's disability, a provider becomes most equipped and effective in assisting a disabled person of color if they recognize the ways in which structural racism impacts access and quality of care.

In the United States, at times (though not always accurately so), race and ethnicity, although different, are used interchangeably. Both are historically othered identities. Othered identities are those identities that have been historically marginalized, placing the individual who belongs to these marginalized groups as an outsider because of the stigma associated with these them (Goffman, 2009). The U.S. Census contributes to the conflating dynamic between race and ethnicity by placing them in the same grouping. Traditionally, race has been understood as a biological category, while ethnicity is more cultural. Today, the definition of race has changed, given that some individuals identify with more than one race or ethnicity. The U.S. Census encapsulates the social definition of race rather than "attempting to define race biologically, anthropologically, or genetically" (U.S. Census, 2024). Theoretical frameworks are offered here to assist in understanding these types of complexities that continue to plaque large groups of minoritized individuals in the United States.

Historical Context of Racism and Ableism

It is vital that clinicians understand the historical context of the eugenics movement (Jackson et al., 2005; Allen, 1997) that devalued people of color and disabled people. Eugenics largely contributed to racialized identities (Winfield, 2007) and the exclusion of disabled individuals (Pfeiffer, 2006). All of these processes were compounded by the many years of segregation people of color experienced during Jim Crow, the system of laws that enforced racial segregation and reinforced racial hierarchy (Packard, 2003). Therefore, it becomes even more challenging to exist in America as a person of color while also being disabled (Jiang et al., 2021).

The school-to-prison pipeline effect due to racial disparities within school discipline practices has been well-established in the literature (Raufu, 2017; Losen, 2011; Kim et al., 2010; Alexander, 2010; Lewis & Solorzano, 2006; Noguera, 2003). Socioeconomic factors and racial disparities, along with criminalizing behavior and discipline policies, contribute to the school-to-prison pipeline. Thus, a competent provider should be aware that this social travesty exists, rather than dismissing this phenomenon and inadvertently criminalizing behavior. The provider should understand that general education and inclusion are challenging for students of color living in poor neighborhoods, but all the more so for disabled students of color (Cooc, 2022).

Just as systems like public education are shaped by structural 'isms,' the medical field is similarly impacted by the oppressive forces of racism and ableism, which distort epistemic frameworks and influence how knowledge is formed and valued (Reynolds & Peña-Guzmán, 2019). This is especially an inescapable reality when working with issues of mental health (Legha & Miranda, 2020). Unfortunately, epistemic errors rooted in identity-based biases, especially those of disability, are undertheorized in the literature on medical errors (Reynolds & Peña-Guzmán, 2019). Multiple cultural barriers would prevent an individual from obtaining access to mental health services, from ideological to financial (Leong & Kalibatseva, 2011). Developing cultural competence to better understand the struggles of these communities is a good place to start (Hernandez et al., 2009). Accounting for the medical racism and ableism, researchers can dig deeper to understand why, in a 2018 study, among non-Hispanic, Black, and Hispanic adults, nearly 30% of disabled people forewent services due to cost, compared to persons without disabilities (Dorsey Holliman et al., 2023). Since further research is still needed, it is critical for therapists to adopt frameworks that avoid perpetuating oppression and marginalization of disabled, people of color to ensure effective treatment. To begin, here are two major frameworks that can help contextualize this crucial intersection of our clients' identities.

Framing Perspectives on Race and Disability

The prevalence of implicit bias and its impacts has been well-established (Morehouse & Banaji, 2024; Banaji et al., 2015). Even well-informed clinicians are seldom immune to implicit biases; even in the case of implicit intergroup bias (Lai & Banaji, 2020). However, individuals can reshape their beliefs and attitudes towards each other by remaining mindful of this implicit bias and reframing their perspective when needed (Lai & Banaji, 2020). Thus, it is important to re-frame perspectives on race and disability to eliminate damaging and limiting beliefs about disabled, BIPOC people. The following sections will explore two theoretical frameworks, DisCrit and Sins Invalid, to provide a perspective on race and disability that fosters a more empowering and supportive view of disabled, people of color. Clinical examples will be provided at the end of the section to illustrate these frameworks.

The theoretical framework of DisCrit, also known as Disability Studies and Critical Race Theory, is particularly appropriate as it integrates key elements of both perspectives. The first ideology helps to frame the intersection of disability and race, while the second helps frame the importance of acknowledging all body types and embracing all disabilities, apparent and non-apparent. By incorporating the two, the provider eradicates racist and ableist language and subconscious attitudes. It has the potential to prevent inadvertent medical racism for those interested in ensuring such a negative dynamic is not present in their therapeutic sessions (Hoberman, 2012). Furthermore, since this is an educational handbook to assist providers in providing affirmative therapy, the theoretical framework found in DisCrit may be the most beneficial. This is especially true since it is used to deconstruct oppressive systems and better understand people's unique social locations, a priority for many systemic therapists.

DisCrit

DisCrit, a groundbreaking theoretical framework that merges Disability Studies and Critical Race Theory, offers critical insights for practitioners by illuminating how the intertwined forces of racism and ableism shape the lived experiences of marginalized individuals. It also helps inform more inclusive and effective therapeutic practices. This framework has helped to dismantle problematic systems by adopting seven central tenets. The seven tents are first named and then applied in the context of providing therapeutic care. The seven tents of the DisCrit framework are as follows:

1 Focuses on ways that the forces of racism and ableism circulate interdependently, often in neutralized and invisible ways, to uphold notions of normalcy.
2 It values multidimensional identities and troubles singular notions of identity such as race or dis/ability, class, gender or sexuality, and so on.
3 Emphasizes the social construction of race and ability while recognizing the material and psychological impacts of being labeled as raced or dis/abled, which sets one outside of the Western cultural norms.
4 Privileges the voices of marginalized populations, traditionally not acknowledged within research.
5 Considers legal and historical aspects of dis/ability and race and how both have been used separately and together to deny the rights of some citizens.
6 Recognizes Whiteness and ability as a form of "property" owned by some.
7 Requires activism and supports all forms of resistance (Annamma, 2016, p. 19).

There are a few important ways in which these tenants can be translated into clinical care with disabled clients. Primarily, by addressing how racism and ableism circulate in invisible ways to uphold notions of normalcy, a therapist can begin to help a client normalize their existence in a society that has made them feel "abnormal". It also signals to the client that the therapist is socially aware of additional factors that impact their life experiences and potentially, their presenting issues. Next, the therapist can effectively serve and care for clients by acknowledging their multidimensional identities. Addressing how race and ability were socially constructed, acknowledges the psychological impacts of such identities in daily interactions.

Sins Invalid

While DisCrit helps therapists recognize marginalized identities within broader social systems, the Sins Invalid framework deepens this understanding by highlighting how these identities can be further erased or overlooked without deliberate care and intentionality in clinical practice. Disabled people have had to learn how to achieve their liberation amidst oppressive environments. Therefore, disabled clients can benefit significantly from reassurance that they are not the 'wrong' way of being, despite society's attempt to make them feel less than the abled-bodied norm. Healing begins when therapists recognize the whole person-not fragmented parts. By fully acknowledging all aspects of a client's identity, clinicians create the conditions for transformative healing rooted in being truly seen.

Sins Invalid is a disability justice primer for all. It defines disability justice as an evolving definition that changes and grows with the movement (Invalid, 2016, p 10). Although the disability rights movement helped establish civil rights for disabled people, it fell significantly short of achieving equity and justice. It prioritized disability rights as "a single-issue identity, focusing exclusively on disability at the expense of other intersections of race, gender, sexuality, age, immigration status, religion, etc." (Invalid, 2016, p. 13). The leadership of the movement primarily "centered White experiences and does not address the ways in which White disabled people can still wield privilege" (Invalid, 2016, p. 13). The movement also centered on "people with mobility impairments, marginalizing other types of disability and/or impairment" (Invalid, 2016, p. 13). As a result, a person of color with a non-apparent disability often faces dismissive attitudes from those who fail to grasp the compounded oppression arising from the intersection of these marginalized identities. Sins Invalid attempts to address these issues in the larger society and within the disability community. Therapists can best assist clients by acknowledging that they "are powerful not despite the complexities of [their] identities, but because of them" (Invalid, 2016, p. 14). Past "rights-based strategies often addressed the symptoms of inequality but not the root" (Invalid, 2016, p. 15). Therapists are uniquely positioned to address both the symptoms and the root causes of inequality through the ways they engage with disabled clients holding intersecting identities – beginning with how they are perceived in the therapy room.

Intersectionality

The concept of Intersectionality has become an invaluable topic of discussion in the field of couple and family therapy. Intersectionality is an invaluable framework that underscores the criticality of recognizing and addressing individuals' multiple, overlapping identities, enabling therapists to deliver more nuanced and effective care through a recognition of the complex ways these identities interact. Kimberlé Crenshaw first coined the term "Intersectionality" in the legal field (Crenshaw, 1991), later adopted by other disciplines because of its functionality. The provision of care for clients with mental health challenges can vary significantly based on an individual's race and/or ethnic background. Depending on the unique intersection, a client may experience different spaces where one marginalized identity is more central than another.

Consider the example of a disabled, Black woman who is navigating the healthcare system. When this woman visits a physician for a physical health issue related to her disability, her experience may be predominantly shaped by her physical disability. In this context, the provider might focus primarily on her disability, potentially overlooking the unique challenges she faces as a Black woman. For instance, the provider may assume her assertiveness in advocating for her care is due to her disability, rather than recognizing that systemic biases based on race may also influence how her concerns are perceived and addressed. Different aspects of her identity can become more pronounced, highlighting the importance of recognizing and addressing the interplay between these marginalized identities.

Asian American and Pacific Islanders (AAPIs) have suffered from the oversight of being understood from an Intersectionality lens, also known as disregarding the "Asian other" (Hasnain et al., 2020; Cooc & Yang, 2017). As a result, the literature on Asian Americans and Pacific Islanders with disabilities is scarce (Mereish, 2012). However, a study did find that AAPIs with a learning, emotional, or physical disability reported more experiences of everyday discrimination, greater psychological and physical distress, and poorer physical and mental health ratings than AAPIs without a reported disability (Mereish, 2012).

Thus, therapists should regularly engage in self-reflection regarding their biases and assumptions. Therapists must resist racializing trauma in ways that frame people of color and disabled individuals through a deficit lens (Alvarez, 2023). Ongoing professional development regarding systemic racism and ableism is vital for maintaining awareness of how these issues persist in the healthcare landscape.

Clinical Examples

To effectively support clients with marginalized identities, therapists must actively engage in continuous, reflective practices that minimize racist and ableist language and scenarios, fostering a therapeutic environment that validates and respects the complexities of each client's lived experience. In addition to consistent self-reflection and professional development, the following are examples of ways a therapist can avoid racist and ableist language and practices. Here are a few recommendations for clinically competent care with disabled, clients of color.

1. Avoid dismissive language when caring for a person of color with a mental health condition. Avoid making insinuations generalizing their marginalized identity group, such as, "I thought people in your community were strong." Doing so, implies there is a deficiency in the client's behavior, and perpetuates racism by suggesting that they must conform to a specific cultural standard. The following statement also captures another example of this, "you seem to be letting your disability define you," suggesting that embracing an aspect of one's identity is a weakness or a flaw.
2. Avoid being dismissive of Intersectionality, such as "if you just focus on getting better, your racial identity might not have as much of a role in all of this". This ignores the complex interplay of race and disability in a client's life experiences and the challenges they face as a result. It also places the onus on the client, rather than on the systems that disable them.
3. Avoid stereotyping by making assumptions about resilience. For example, avoid statements such as "I have seen from my experience that people from

your culture tend to be less emotionally fragile". This statement invalidates a client's experiences while also implying that expressing emotional vulnerability is unhealthy. Also, avoid assuming that "members of this community should be 'strong enough' to overcome these issues" since this perpetuates the stereotype of racial groups as overly resilient while dismissing the mental health needs of the individual.

4 Avoid implicitly attributing behavior to disability – for example, saying, 'your anger may just be the disability itself'. Such statements dismiss legitimate emotions as mere symptoms, undermining the client's cultural context and lived experience.
5 Avoid over-pathologizing; this is often seen when a doctor overdiagnoses a client from a racially marginalized group based on behaviors, saying, "your assertiveness is due to your anxiety." There are two layers to this scenario; it is an ableist attitude towards an emotional expression and racial bias towards behavior norms.
6 Avoid invalidating cultural expressions that may be perceived as being culturally insensitive. For example, saying, "past traumas faced by your community should not affect your outlook". This minimizes the impact of historical and systemic racism on mental health while also implying that a client's response to trauma is a sign of weakness. Alternatively, refrain from statements such as "your mental illness should not affect you as much, given the history of your community". This trivializes the client's struggles and suggests that their feelings are less valid due to their racial or cultural background. This demonstrates cultural ignorance and insensitivity, damaging the client's trust toward the care provider.

Ideally, a therapist should consistently monitor their implicit biases and prejudices, even outside of sessions. For example, when encountering a person of color with a physical disability, especially wheelchair users, a therapist may benefit from asking themselves, what do I think about the individual? Am I stereotyping? A therapist can identify if they are stereotyping by asking themselves, "Would my perspective change if the individual were White?" Often, the reaction toward a White disabled wheelchair user is one of pity, while the reaction toward a person of color may be one of disgust, shame, or sometimes even fear. This disgust or feelings of disappointment arise from the stereotypical belief that the reason why the BIPOC wheelchair user is in the wheelchair must have been a result of their own actions, either because of their negligence or because they were involved in nefarious activity. Recognizing and resisting initial stereotypical thoughts is a critical first step for therapists. The next step involves examining how they interact with the person of color who uses a wheelchair, ensuring they are treated with the same respect and engagement as non-disabled clients. This progression requires intentional introspection, but it holds the potential for profoundly transformative outcomes in therapy.

Conclusion

Addressing the intersection of race and disability is not merely a theoretical exercise; it is an essential practice for therapists who aim to deliver holistic and effective care. As highlighted throughout this chapter, the identities of individuals are complex and multifaceted, composed of various social, cultural, and historical influences that cannot be disentangled. The incorporation of frameworks such as DisCrit and Sins Invalid empowers providers to recognize the unique challenges faced by clients who navigate both racial and disability-related identities, ensuring that their healing journeys are validated and supported. Therapists play a crucial role in dismantling harmful stereotypes and biases. By consciously acknowledging the whole person, therapists can foster a deeper understanding of their clients' lived experiences and the systemic barriers that they frequently encounter. This understanding is vital for creating safe, affirming spaces that honor and respect a person's entire identity.

Additionally, recognizing and challenging personal biases enhances the therapist's clinical effectiveness, cultivating trust and building a stronger rapport with clients. Therapy must transcend the treatment of symptoms to encompass the broader implications of racism and ableism in a client's life. Through this comprehensive approach, providers can facilitate genuine healing, allowing individuals to reclaim their narratives and navigate complexities without experiencing shame or stigma within the therapy room.

Ultimately, the journey toward equity and justice in mental health care demands collective accountability and a commitment to continuous learning. As we strive to dismantle the barriers created by intersecting systems of oppression, we move closer to realizing the promise of holistic care-one that embraces all aspects of client identity, acknowledges the weight of societal constructs, and honors the resilience of those who courageously confront these challenges. Only then can we hope to co-construct meaningful change in the lives of those we serve. This comprehensive approach benefits individual clients and contributes to broader systemic change within healthcare systems, while meaningfully strengthening the field of psychotherapy.

References

Alexander, M. (2010). *The new Jim Crow: mass incarceration in the age of colorblindness*. The New Press.

Allen, G. E. (1997). The social and economic origins of genetic determinism: a case history of the American Eugenics Movement, 1900–1940 and its lessons for today. *Genetica*, *99*, 77–88.

Alvarez, A. J. (2023). Disrupting three prominent racialized trauma tropes. *Educational Researcher*, *52*(4), 238–243.

Annamma, S. A. (2016). *DisCrit: disability studies and critical race theory in education*. Teachers College Press.

Bailey, Z. D., Krieger, N., Agénor, M., Graves, J., Linos, N., & Bassett, M. T. (2017). Structural racism and health inequities in the USA: evidence and interventions. *The Lancet*, *389*(10077), 1453–1463.

Banaji, M. R., Bhaskar, R., & Brownstein, M. (2015). When bias is implicit, how might we think about repairing harm?. *Current Opinion in Psychology*, *6*, 183–188.
Churchwell, K., Elkind, M. S., Benjamin, R. M., Carson, A. P., Chang, E. K., Lawrence, W., … & American Heart Association. (2020). Call to action: structural racism as a fundamental driver of health disparities: a presidential advisory from the American Heart Association. *Circulation*, *142*(24), e454–e468.
Cooc, N. (2022). Disparities in general education inclusion for students of color with disabilities: understanding when and why. *Journal of School Psychology*, *90*, 43–59.
Cooc, N., & Yang, M. (2017). Underrepresented and overlooked: a review of Asian American children with disabilities. *Multiple Voices for Ethnically Diverse Exceptional Learners*, *17*(1), 3–19.
Crenshaw, K. 1991. Mapping the margins: Intersectionality, identity politics and violence against women. *Stanford Law Review*, *43*, 1241.
Darling-Hammond, L. 2001. Inequality in teaching and schooling: how opportunity is rationed to students of color in America. In B. D. Smedley, A. Y. Stith, L. Colburn, & C. H. Evans (Eds.), *The right thing to do, the smart thing to do: enhancing diversity in the health professions – Summary of the Symposium in Honor of Herbert W. Nickens, M.D.* (pp. 208–233). National Academies Press. https://doi.org/10.17226/10186
Dorsey Holliman, B., Stransky, M., Dieujuste, N., & Morris, M. 2023. Disability doesn't discriminate: health inequities at the intersection of race and disability. *Frontiers in Rehabilitation Sciences*, *4*, 1075775.
Goffman, E. 2009. *Stigma: notes on the management of spoiled identity*. Simon and Schuster.
Goodman, N., Morris, M., Boston, K., & Walton, D. 2017. *Financial inequality: disability, race, and poverty in America*. National Disability Institute.
Hasnain, R., Fujiura, G. T., Capua, J. E., Bui, T. T. T., & Khan, S. 2020. Disaggregating the Asian "other": heterogeneity and methodological issues in research on Asian Americans with disabilities. *Societies*, *10*(3), 58.
Hernandez, M., Nesman, T., Mowery, D., Acevedo-Polakovich, I. D., & Callejas, L. M. 2009. Cultural competence: a literature review and conceptual model for mental health services. *Psychiatric Services*, *60*(8), 1046–1050.
Hoberman, J. 2012. *Black and blue: the origins and consequences of medical racism*. University of California Press.
Jackson, J. P., Weidman, N. M., & Rubin, G. (2005). The origins of scientific racism. *The Journal of Blacks in Higher Education*, *50*(50), 66–79.
Jiang, C., Vitiello, C., Axt, J. R., Campbell, J. T., & Ratliff, K. A. (2021). An examination of ingroup preferences among people with multiple socially stigmatized identities. *Self and Identity*, *20*(4), 569–586.
Kim, C. Y., Losen, D. J., & Hewitt, D. T. (2010). *The school-to-prison pipeline: structuring legal reform*. NYU Press.
Lai, C. K., & Banaji, M. R. (2020). The psychology of implicit intergroup bias and the prospect of change. In G. Hull (Ed.), *Difference without domination: pursuing justice in diverse democracies* (pp. 151–173). University of Chicago Press.
Legha, R. K., & Miranda, J. (2020). An anti-racist approach to achieving mental health equity in clinical care. *Psychiatric Clinics*, *43*(3), 451–469.
Leong, F. T., & Kalibatseva, Z. (2011, March). Cross-cultural barriers to mental health services in the United States. In *Cerebrum: the Dana forum on brain science* (Vol. 2011). Dana Foundation.
Lewis, T., & Solorzano, E. V. (2006). Unraveling the heart of the school-to-prison pipeline. In C. A. Rossatto, R. L. Allen, & M. Pruyn (Eds.), *Reinventing critical pedagogy: Widening the circle of anti-oppression education* (pp. 63–76). Routledge.
Lopez, G. E., Gurin, P., & Nagda, B. A. (1998). Education and understanding structural causes for group inequalities. *Political Psychology*, *19*(2), 305–329.

Losen, D. (2011). *Discipline policies, successful schools, and racial justice*. National Education Policy Center. https://nepc.colorado.edu/publication/discipline-policies

Mereish, E. H. (2012). The intersectional invisibility of race and disability status: an exploratory study of health and discrimination facing Asian Americans with disabilities. *Ethnicity and Inequalities in Health and Social Care*, *5*(2), 52–60.

Morehouse, K. N., & Banaji, M. R. (2024). The science of implicit race bias: evidence from the Implicit Association Test. *Dædalus*, *153*(1), 21–50.

Noguera, P. A. (2003). Schools, prisons, and social implications of punishment: rethinking disciplinary practices. *Theory into Practice*, *42*(4), 341–350.

Packard, J. M. (2003). *American nightmare: the history of Jim Crow*. Macmillan.

Pfeiffer, D. (2006). Eugenics and disability discrimination. In *Overcoming disabling barriers* (pp. 80–100). Routledge.

Raufu, A. (2017). School-to-prison pipeline: impact of school discipline on African American students. *Journal of Education and Social Science*, *7*(1), 47–53.

Reynolds, J. M., & Peña-Guzmán, D. (2019). The harm of ableism: medical error and epistemic injustice 1. In F. Allhoff & S. Borden (Eds.), *Ethics and error in medicine* (pp. 167–199). Routledge.

Sins Invalid. 2016. Skin, tooth, and bone. The basis of movement is our people: a disability justice primer (2nd ed., pp. 1–34). *Sins Invalid*. Retrieved from https://static1.squarespace.com/static/58d3f955d2b857698e8dfff2/t/5c9930b508522954e2d3059a/1553543364713/Disability+Justice+Primer.pdf

Talbert-Johnson, C. (2004). Structural inequities and the achievement gap in urban schools. *Education and Urban Society*, *37*(1), 22–36.

U.S. Census Bureau. (2024, December 20). *About the Topic of Race* [Webpage]. U.S. Department of Commerce. https://www.census.gov/topics/population/race/about.html

Vargas, E. A., Scherer, L. A., Fiske, S. T., Barabino, G. A., & National Academies of Sciences, Engineering, and Medicine. (2023). The historical and contemporary context for structural, systemic, and institutional racism in the United States. In *Advancing antiracism, diversity, equity, and inclusion in STEMM organizations: beyond broadening participation*. National Academies Press (US).

Williams, D. R., Lawrence, J. A., & Davis, B. A. (2019). Racism and health: evidence and needed research. *Annual Review of Public Health*, *40*(1), 105–125.

Winfield, A. G. (2007). *Eugenics and education in America: institutionalized racism and the implications of history, ideology, and memory* (Vol. 18). Peter Lang.

Yearby, R. (2018). Racial disparities in health status and access to healthcare: the continuation of inequality in the United States due to structural racism. *American Journal of Economics and Sociology*, *77*(3–4), 1113–1152.

Bibliography

Rahman, Labib. *Disability language guide*. Stanford University. https://disability.stanford.edu/sites/g/files/sbiybj26391/files/media/file/disability-language-guide-stanford_1.pdf

7

INTERSECTING IDENTITIES

Supporting 2SLGBTQ+ Disabled People

Alan Santinele Martino, Melissa Miller, Jordan Parks, and Eleni Moumos

Introduction

This chapter serves as a primer and an essential conversation starter for clinicians seeking to navigate the complexities of being a disabled, gender and/or sexual minority, with sensitivity and competence. It provides a comprehensive exploration of the unique experiences and challenges faced by individuals at this critical intersection. We examine specific barriers to mental health and overall well-being, such as societal stigma, discrimination, and systemic inequities, while also celebrating the resilience and strengths that are often overlooked. We aim to highlight the criticality of leveraging these strengths in therapeutic settings by focusing on these positive aspects. For many, this intersection is not merely a theoretical construct, but a lived reality, making the need for informed, sensitive, and effective clinical approaches more pressing than ever.

Intersectional Realities: A "Double Minority" Experience

Kimberlé Crenshaw's (1989) introduction of the term "Intersectionality," highlighted a pivotal insight: social categorizations such as race, gender, and disability do not exist in isolation but interact in complex, multifaceted ways that shape individual and collective experiences. This intersectional perspective is crucial for understanding the lives of 2SLGBTQ+ (Two-Spirit, Lesbian, Gay, Bisexual, Transgender, Queer or Questioning and additional sexual orientations and gender identities) disabled people, whose experiences of discrimination, stigma, and systemic inequality are not merely additive but exponential. "Two-Spirit" is a term used by some Indigenous people to describe a person who embodies both masculine and feminine spirits, encompassing a wide range of gender identities, sexual orientations, and roles

 DOI: 10.4324/9781003362586-12

within their communities (López, 2023). These unique challenges cannot be fully appreciated through single-axis frameworks, which often overlook the compounded nature of intersecting identities (Nakkeeran & Nakkeeran, 2018; Santinele Martino, 2017). At times, the label of disability can dominate, overshadowing other intersecting identities (Santinele Martino & Schormans, 2018). This overshadowing often leads to the erasure of intersectional experiences, compelling disabled individuals to navigate issues of gender and sexuality, independently. Their experiences may go unrecognized by families, caregivers, and service providers, adding further challenges to their identity exploration and expression (Santinele Martino, 2017; Santinele Martino & Moumos, 2023).

The concept of "double minority" underscores the particular experiences and challenges faced by 2SLGBTQ+ disabled people (Howarth & Abbott, 2005). As identified by Howarth and Abbott (2005), and further explored by Santinele Martino (2017), individuals at this intersection occupy a uniquely marginalized position-they are not only discriminated against based on their sexual orientation or gender identity but also based on their disability. This dual layer of minority status often intensifies feelings of isolation, as these individuals might struggle to find complete acceptance or belonging within either the 2SLGBTQ+ or disability communities, which are themselves shaped by distinct norms and expectations (Santinele Martino & Moumos, 2023; Wilson et al., 2018).

A common societal perception, as noted by Stoffelen et al. (2013), labels 2SLGBTQ+ disabled people as "going too far" (p. 265). This reflects a broader societal discomfort with deviation from the norm, where either being disabled or queer may already situate an individual outside mainstream societal acceptance; the combination of these identities tends to amplify marginalization. Such perceptions can limit individuals from fully expressing their identities and experiences, as they might restrain themselves to mitigate further marginalization (Dinwoodie et al., 2020; Howarth & Abbott, 2005; Kafer, 2003; Santinele Martino & Moumos, 2023).

Additionally, many disabled individuals may not have the language necessary to articulate their experiences, identities, or needs. This is often exacerbated by inadequate sex education that fails to encompass the diversity of human sexuality and the specific needs of disabled individuals, thus leaving out crucial perspectives of 2SLGBTQ+ people (Charley et al., 2023; Hobaica & Kwon, 2017; Hughes & Santinele Martino, 2023). The scarcity of representation in media, literature, and public discourse further deprives 2SLGBTQ+ disabled people of the language and images that might help them articulate and affirm their identities, presenting additional barriers to self-expression and visibility.

Challenges in Gender and Sexual Exploration for Disabled Individuals

Power dynamics play a crucial role in relationships involving disabled people, their families, caregivers, and service providers, shaping opportunities for gender and sexual exploration. Some disabled people may depend on others for daily support, resulting in power imbalances. This need for support can lead caregivers or therapists to impose their own beliefs and values, heavily influencing or even restricting aspects of gender expression and sexual exploration (Frawley & Wilson, 2016; Gill 2015). Often, therapists may skirt discussions about sexuality and sexual identity, viewing these topics as uncomfortable or outside their professional responsibilities, thus denying access to crucial information or discussions (Santinele Martino & Perreault-Laird, 2019; Sommarö et al., 2020). Additionally, there is resistance from some caregivers and healhcare providers towards non-heterosexual identities, leading to the denial or invalidation of 2SLGBTQ+ identities (Abbott & Burns, 2007; Santinele Martino, 2022a, 2022b; Sommarö et al., 2020).

For 2SLGBTQ+ disabled people, these dynamics introduce specific challenges that hinder their opportunity to freely explore and express their gender and sexual identities. They may face strict rules about relationships, limited access to inclusive sexual and gender education, and censorship of materials that could aid in their exploration of identity (Davies et al., 2023; Mitchell, 2023; O'Shea et al., 2020; Santinele Martino, 2022a, 2022b). These restrictions not only limit personal freedom but also perpetuate harmful myths that certain aspects of identity are inappropriate or taboo for disabled people (Azzopardi-Lane, 2022; Björnsdóttir & Stefánsdóttir, 2020; Ferrante & Oak, 2020). While intended to protect, these boundaries often undermine the autonomy and rights of disabled individuals to explore their identities and make informed choices (Benoit et al., 2023; Björnsdóttir & Stefánsdóttir, 2020; Horner-Johnson et al., 2022).

Contrary to the assumption that disabled people are not having sex, let alone having queer forms of sex, there is ample research that shows otherwise (Okotie & Jolly, 2024; Santinele Martino & Moumos, 2023). These individuals often assert that they seek, enjoy, or are interested in sex, demonstrating that they are active agents in their own sexual experiences. Overlooking this sexual agency not only denies them the rights associated with sexual citizenship (Bahner, 2020) but also fails to recognize their capability to engage in and enjoy sexual activities (Gill, 2015).

Furthermore, disabled people frequently encounter a "limited menu of options" when it comes to gender and sexual identity exploration (Azzopardi-Lane & Santinele Martino, 2024; Santinele Martino, 2022a, 2022b). This metaphorical menu often mirrors and reinforces the societal norms of compulsory heterosexuality (McRuer, 2011), presenting it as the default and expected orientation with little room for deviation. As a result, disabled people may feel pressured to conform to these restrictive norms, suppressing or denying parts of their identity that do not align with societal expectations.

Addressing these challenges requires a paradigm shift towards more inclusive, empathetic, and empowering practices that respect the individuality and rights of disabled people, affirming their capacity to make decisions about their own lives, including their sexual and gender identities.

Redefining Vulnerability

Research consistently demonstrates that disabled people are at least twice as likely to experience sexual abuse and harassment compared to their non-disabled peers (Klebanov et al., 2024; Sullivan & Knutson, 2000; Withers & Morris, 2012). This risk remains elevated into adulthood, unlike for non-disabled individuals, where it typically decreases (Amborski et al., 2022). Contributing significantly to this increased vulnerability is the lack of inclusive and accessible sex education tailored to the needs of disabled individuals. This educational gap leaves them inadequately prepared to navigate their sexual health and interpersonal relationships (Campbell et al., 2020; Hollomotz, 2011). The consequences of this gap are severe, including increased risks of sexually transmitted infections, unintended pregnancies, and vulnerability to sexual exploitation (Bernert, 2011; Sandberg et al., 2021).

Furthermore, the concept of vulnerability is often misapplied as a rationale to restrict sexual expression and withhold critical information from disabled people (Azzopardi-Lane & Santinele Martino, 2024; Fish, 2016). Hollomotz (2011) importantly argues that vulnerability should not be seen merely as a result of individual limitations but should be understood as arising from structural inequities that systematically disadvantage disabled individuals. A key structural barrier is the limited opportunities for these individuals to engage in decision-making across various life domains. This restriction severely impacts their capacity to navigate their sexual lives autonomously. When disabled people are excluded from making independent choices in education, employment, and community engagement, they are also deprived of essential experiences that are crucial for developing the skills necessary for managing their sexual and intimate lives.

While ensuring the safety of disabled individuals is paramount, an excessively protective approach can undermine their autonomy and obstruct their ability to engage in intimate relationships, make personal choices, and learn from these experiences, just as their non-disabled counterparts do (Santinele Martino, 2022a, 2022b). It is critical to find a balance that provides necessary support while also promoting an environment that empowers disabled individuals to explore and express their sexuality freely. They deserve equitable opportunities to form intimate connections, take personal risks, and benefit from their interactions, contributing to their overall growth and self-determination. However, prevailing societal norms and misconceptions frequently curtail their sexual agency, restricting their full participation in this vital aspect of human life.

Bridging Educational Support for 2SLGBTQ+ Disabled People

The intersectional experiences of 2SLGBTQ+ disabled people are frequently marked by a lack of adequate support and information, particularly in terms of access to sex education (Charley et al., 2023; Hobaica & Kwon, 2017). Traditional sex education curricula often adhere to heteronormative frameworks, overlooking the diverse experiences and needs of 2SLGBTQ+ individuals (Hobaica & Kwon, 2017). This neglect leaves many, especially those with disabilities, devoid of crucial information about their bodies, relationships, and sexual health (de Heer et al., 2021). The absence of inclusive sex education not only perpetuates stigma and misinformation but also hampers the ability of disabled 2SLGBTQ+ individuals to confidently manage their sexual health, understand consent, and foster relationships (Hole et al., 2022). A paradigm shift towards inclusive, comprehensive sex education is crucial to address these shortcomings (Campbell et al., 2020). Such curricula should cover the broad spectrum of human sexuality and gender identities, with explicit attention to accessibility for disabled people. Beyond basic sexual health and preventative measures, there is a vital need for sex-positive education that celebrates the enjoyable aspects of sexuality, such as love, romance, and pleasure, empowering disabled 2SLGBTQ+ individuals to make informed choices and develop healthy relationships (Azzopardi-Lane & Santinele Martino, 2024; Frawley & O'Shea, 2019).

Similarly, service providers within the disability sector face significant challenges in adequately supporting 2SLGBTQ+ disabled people (Santinele Martino, 2017). Many lack the necessary training and resources to provide inclusive, comprehensive support services that cater to the nuanced needs at the intersection of disability and 2SLGBTQ+ identities (Hogan, 2023; O'Shea et al., 2020). This shortfall often results in suboptimal care, further marginalizing this population within healthcare and social service settings. To overcome these challenges, service providers in the disability sector must receive specialized training and access resources that are specifically tailored to the needs of 2SLGBTQ+ disabled people. This might include developing inclusive resources, establishing partnerships with 2SLGBTQ+ health organizations, and implementing training programs that enhance cultural competence and sensitivity. By equipping service providers with the necessary knowledge and tools, they can deliver more effective and affirming support services (Santinele Martino, 2017).

Moreover, the valuable insights from disabled 2SLGBTQ+ individuals' lived experiences should be integral to the development of educational and support structures. Frawley and O'Shea (2019) recognize the profound potential of disabled people to contribute to creating sex education materials that reflect their desires and experiences. This involvement not only facilitates learning and connection but also strengthens their identity as 2SLGBTQ+ disabled people. It is essential for curricula and supports to acknowledge and champion the sexual agency and capacity of disabled people. This approach not only empowers, but also affirms the identity of the individual as a knowledgeable sexual being. Moving away from the traditional protectionist approach in sexuality education for disabled people, there is an opportunity to "crip" sex education, making it more inclusive and reflective of diverse experiences (Campbell et al., 2020; Frawley & O'Shea, 2019).

By addressing the educational and support gaps within both sex education and disability services, and advocating for inclusive approaches, we can create environments that truly affirm the diverse identities and needs of this population.

Intersectional Exclusion: Seeking Inclusion in 2SLGBTQ+ and Disabled Communities

Individuals who identify as both 2SLGBTQ+ and disabled frequently navigate environments that inadequately address their distinct needs and experiences (Santinele Martino et al., 2023; Vassallo & Azzopardi-Lane, 2022). Research shows that these individuals face significant barriers to full participation in traditional 2SLGBTQ+ environments, including social venues, support groups, and service providers (Santinele Martino et al., 2023; Vassallo & Azzopardi-Lane, 2022). Despite a professed commitment to inclusivity, such spaces frequently cater predominantly to the needs of white, male, gay, middle-class, and non-disabled individuals, neglecting a broader spectrum of the community (Santinele Martino et al., 2023; Vo, 2021). A common issue is the focus on nightlife and alcohol-centric activities, which can alienate those who are uncomfortable or unable to engage in such environments due to sensory, physical, or other disabilities. The predominance of loud music and flashing lights creates environments that are inaccessible and exclusionary for many, exacerbating feelings of isolation and detachment from their community (Noonan & Taylor Gomez, 2011; Santinele Martino, 2017; Santinele Martino et al., 2023).

Conversely, within disabled communities, there is often an oversight regarding the experiences of 2SLGBTQ+ individuals within these spaces (Kempapidis et al., 2024; Santinele Martino, 2017). This neglect results in diminished visibility and support for 2SLGBTQ+ individuals, perpetuating their feelings of erasure and making it challenging for them to find acceptance and understanding within these circles (Vassallo & Azzopardi-Lane, 2022). By focusing predominantly on disability, without integrating an understanding of gender and sexual diversity, these communities inadvertently uphold exclusionary practices.

To dismantle these systemic barriers, both 2SLGBTQ+ spaces and disabled communities must embrace truly inclusive practices. Queer spaces can improve accessibility by providing clear information, offering necessary accommodations, and choosing venues equipped with accessibility features (Santinele Martino et al., 2023; Simić Stanojević et al., 2023). Disabled communities should strive to incorporate 2SLGBTQ+ perspectives in their activities and advocacy efforts, ensuring that all identities are acknowledged and valued (Egner, 2019; Toft, 2020). Additionally, both queer and disabled spaces could benefit from implementing mentorship or partnered experience programs. Recruiting and training peer mentors who understand these intersecting identities can foster a sense of belonging, enhance comfort, and encourage interactions within these communities (Simić Stanojević et al., 2023). Fostering inclusivity within both 2SLGBTQ+

and disabled communities requires a comprehensive approach that includes clear communication, proactive efforts to create better access, careful venue selection, intentional integration of diverse perspectives, and ongoing education. By actively embracing and celebrating the intersections of identities, these communities can create supportive environments where every individual feels empowered, valued, and fully included.

Reimagining Sexuality through a "Crip" Lens

The concept of "cripping" emerged from disability activism and scholarship, symbolizing a transformative process of reframing conventional views through a disability lens (Sandahl, 2003). In the context of sexuality, cripping entails a critical re-evaluation and reshaping of traditional understandings of sexual practices, relationships, and identities to include the diverse experiences of disabled individuals (McRuer & Cassabaum, 2021). Similar to the term "queer," "crip" has been reclaimed by some in the disability community as an empowering act of self-identification. Originally a derogatory term used to demean disabled people, crip has been transformed within disability activism to confront ableism and promote disability pride.

The act of cripping sexuality involves recognizing that disabled individuals possess sexual rights comparable to anyone else. It emphasizes that these disabled people's desires can be expressed in varied forms that may not align with mainstream societal norms (McRuer, 2011). Cripping sex highlights the creativity, adaptability, and resilience that disabled individuals bring to their sexual lives. It calls for a broader, more inclusive understanding of sexuality that validates all experiences, including those traditionally marginalized (Egner, 2017).

According to McRuer and Mollow (2012), disability can "transform sex, creating confusion about what and who is sexy and what counts as sex" (p. 32). This reimagining of disabled sexuality actively questions the normative definitions of sex. For instance, it challenges why sexual exploration should be limited to reproductive organs when numerous other erogenous zones offer pleasure (Siebers, 2010). It critiques the traditional sexual script which suggests that sex must follow a specific pattern or exclude the involvement of support partners (Azzorpadi-Lane & Santinele Martino, 2024; Simon & Gagnon, 1984). Research by Santinele Martino and Moumos (2023) further challenges ableist assumptions by demonstrating that disability does not reduce intimacy or pleasure. Instead, it introduces a unique, transformative dimension to intimate relationships, enhancing them through required openness in communication and a diversity of expressions of sexuality and desire. Normative sexual scripts often exclude disabled individuals by promoting a narrow, typically non-disabled, heteronormative view reliant on certain physical abilities and performances. By cripping these scripts, advocates assert that sexuality encompasses a spectrum of experiences and expressions beyond traditional binaries and standards (Löfgren-Mårtenson, 2013).

This approach not only encourages a reassessment of what constitutes sexual intimacy, pleasure, and connection but also advocates for the inclusion of multiple forms of embodiment, desire, and pleasure (Cohen, 2015; Santinele Martino & Schormans, 2018). It promotes a more holistic understanding of human sexuality, utilizing crip theory to deconstruct binary categorizations of normal/abnormal and able/disabled. In doing so, it amplifies a less dominant discourse centred on pleasure, enjoyment, and intimacy from a disabled perspective, pushing for a broader, inclusive narrative that celebrates the full spectrum of human sexual expression (Cohen, 2015; Löfgren-Mårtenson, 2013).

As clinicians working with disabled individuals, it is crucial to recognize the limitations and biases inherent in societal norms about sexuality. The traditional approach often focuses on normalization and conformity, pushing individuals towards a narrow understanding of sexual expression that aligns with mainstream societal expectations. This approach not only limits the sexual autonomy of disabled individuals but also perpetuates a restrictive narrative of what is considered "normal" or "acceptable." Instead of enforcing these conventional standards, there should be space for disabled individuals to challenge and redefine normative expressions of sexuality. This involves acknowledging and facilitating a diverse range of sexual experiences and identities that reflect the unique perspectives and needs of disabled individuals. By doing so, clinicians can help dismantle the barriers that prevent disabled people from fully expressing their sexual identities.

Cripping sexuality, in this context, serves a dual purpose. Firstly, it empowers disabled individuals by validating their sexual experiences as legitimate and valuable. This validation is essential for fostering self-esteem and a positive sexual identity. Secondly, cripping sexuality challenges and expands the existing frameworks of sexual expression for society as a whole. By questioning the rigidity of traditional sexual norms, everyone can benefit from a richer array of possibilities when it comes to sexual expression. This broader perspective not only benefits disabled individuals by creating a more inclusive and accepting environment but also enriches the general population's understanding of sexuality. It promotes a culture where diverse sexual expressions are recognized and celebrated, leading to greater acceptance and empathy across all societal sectors. Ultimately, reimagining sexuality through a crip lens can catalyse a cultural shift towards a more expansive and inclusive view of human sexuality.

Intersectional Activism: QueerCrip Mobilizing

QueerCrip mobilizing represents a dynamic collective effort by individuals and groups at the intersection of queer and disabled identities to challenge societal norms, advocate for rights, and foster more inclusive environments. The term, blending queer and crip, highlights the rich array of sexual and gender identities among disabled people. This mobilization serves as a formidable catalyst for social transformation, promoting solidarity, intersectional advocacy, and the dismantling of oppressive systems that disproportionately affect marginalized communities. QueerCrip activists emphasize the interconnectedness of struggles against ableism, queerphobia, racism, sexism, and other forms of discrimination, advocating that liberation for one group is intertwined with freedom for all oppressed groups.

One area where QueerCrip activists are particularly influential is in the arts and media, where they leverage their creativity to subvert mainstream perceptions of disability, gender identity, and sexual orientation. Through tools like filmmaking, writing, performance art, and other creative mediums, they explore themes of identity, body politics, and inclusivity, thus increasing the visibility of their experiences (Santinele Martino, 2020). Their artistic endeavours not only facilitate self-expression but also serve as vital instruments for societal change, engaging wider audiences and deepening public understanding of the complexities at the nexus of queerness and disability (Santinele Martino, 2020).

QueerCrip activists also extend their influence through educational endeavours, leading workshops, delivering talks, and developing content that raises awareness. They provide training sessions for clinicians on 2SLGBTQ+ cultural competency and disability-informed care, offering strategies to create welcoming environments for 2SLGBTQ+ disabled individuals and addressing biases and discrimination in practice. Such efforts are crucial in breaking down stereotypes and cultivating a comprehensive understanding of diverse identities.

On social media, QueerCrip influencers like Annie Segarra and Andrew Gurza have spearheaded movements using hashtags such as #HotPersonInAWheelchair and #DisabledPeopleAreHot, sparking widespread engagement, and reframing perceptions of sexuality through a crip lens (Santinele Martino, 2020). Digital platforms such as YouTube feature influencers like Annie Elainey and Jessica Kellgren-Fozard, who provide advice and perspectives on navigating life as disabled members of the 2SLGBTQ+ community. Influential crip bloggers like Bethany Stevens and Eva Sweeney explore topics related to crip and queer sexuality, offering realistic and candid discussions on disabled 2SLGBTQ+ sex and desire, thereby enriching the discourse on sexuality and identity. By harnessing the power of digital platforms, QueerCrip activists create virtual communities that foster belonging and solidarity, especially for those feeling isolated by their intersecting identities. These online spaces are pivotal in amplifying marginalized input and advocating for systemic change. Through creative expression, educational advocacy, and digital community building, QueerCrip activists are not just participating in social change; they are at the forefront of driving a more equitable and inclusive society for all.

Fostering Intentional Support Systems for 2SLGBTQ+ Disabled People

Creating intentional support systems for 2SLGBTQ+ disabled people demands a comprehensive approach that prioritizes empowerment, inclusivity, and collaboration. Central to this empowerment is language: equipping 2SLGBTQ+ disabled people with the vocabulary to articulate their identities, experiences, and needs is fundamental. More than merely offering terminology, it involves validating their unique perspectives and facilitating self-advocacy. Collaborative development of accessible workshops, educational programs, and resources is essential to disseminate this vocabulary effectively. Creating materials that explain terms related to gender, sexuality, and disability in plain language empowers individuals to better understand and express their identities.

Bridging gaps between service providers, queer spaces, and disabled communities is crucial for building a cohesive support network that comprehensively addresses their intersecting needs. Networking and partnerships between queer and disabled service providers are vital for facilitating resource sharing and joint initiatives. Implementing cross-training sessions can significantly enhance competency in understanding intersectionality and providing inclusive services. Developing comprehensive, accessible directories of queer-friendly and disability-knowledgeable resources can streamline access to needed support. Additionally, community forums and panels that bring together diverse stakeholders can foster dialogue, share experiences, and explore opportunities for deeper collaboration.

Peer support networks and community spaces where 2SLGBTQ+ disabled people can connect with others who share similar experiences, challenges, and identities are invaluable. These spaces offer validation, solidarity, and a sense of belonging, creating environments where individuals can thrive. For instance, in Canada, SprOUT Toronto serves as an exemplary model by providing a gathering space for lesbian, gay, bisexual, trans, and questioning adults living with intellectual disabilities.

Walmsley and Johnson (2003) and other scholars like Frawley and O'Shea (2019) argue that disabled people are unequivocal experts in their own experiences, including their sexual identities. They advocate for their peers and for their right to be sexual and have membership within sexual fields. The principle of "nothing about us without us" is widely acclaimed within disability services, yet there remains a significant gap in recognizing and utilizing the capacity of disabled people to contribute to the creation of sex education materials that acknowledge and represent their desires and experiences (Gill, 2015; Frawley & O'Shea, 2019).

Presuming competence and challenging prevailing narratives about vulnerability are imperative steps towards true empowerment. Rejecting over-protectionist paradigms is crucial; often, withholding language and information, rather than providing it, renders individuals more vulnerable. By reframing certain language as empowering rather than taboo, we can shift the narrative towards empowerment. This shift fosters environments that are conducive to forming healthy relationships and enhancing empowerment for disabled 2SLGBTQ+ individuals. Collaboration between service providers and communities is essential to dismantle outdated notions and create a more inclusive, supportive framework for all.

Conclusion

Recent policy changes in Alberta, along with similar developments in other provinces across Canada, have raised significant concerns among members and allies of the 2SLGBTQ+ community. Specifically, in Alberta, new regulations require parental consent for students under 15 years old who wish to modify their names or pronouns, and necessitate notification for parents of 15–17-year-old students regarding pronoun changes. Furthermore, the implementation of an opt-in system for sex education could disproportionately affect disabled and/or 2SLGBTQ+ individuals, who already encounter substantial barriers to accessing relevant sex education. This policy approach suggests a troubling misconception: that withholding information can change beliefs or feelings, or reduce vulnerability. Instead, such measures only serve to heighten the vulnerability of marginalized groups, especially disabled 2SLGBTQ+ individuals, reinforcing the institutional and structural barriers that increase their exposure to harm.

In response to these challenges, clinicians must develop more effective support systems for disabled individuals grappling with questions about gender and sexuality. Recognizing, understanding, and competently addressing these intersecting identities is crucial for providing effective, compassionate care that supports diverse needs and affirms all identities. Continuous education is essential to ensure healthcare professionals are well-informed about the latest research, theories, and best practices relevant to serving 2SLGBTQ+ disabled people.

Therapists may play a pivotal role, particularly in times when other systems fail to provide safe spaces to disabled, 2SLGBTQ+ people. Healthcare providers need to create welcoming environments where individuals feel empowered to disclose their identities and experiences without fear of judgment. Therapists must avoid presumptions about the sexual or gender identities of disabled individuals and be mindful of the implications of intersecting minority statuses. Implementing inclusive practices, such as using gender-affirming language and respecting chosen names and pronouns, is crucial in establishing clinical settings as safe havens of acceptance and understanding.

Ultimately, acknowledging and valuing the dual identities of being a disabled member of the 2SLGBTQ+ community is essential for fostering a culture that supports and affirms disabled individuals' rights to a sexual life. This approach contributes to a broader, more inclusive definition of sexuality that validates all experiences, promoting a society that appreciates diversity in all its forms.

References

Abbott, D., & Burns, J. (2007). What's love got to do with it?: Experiences of lesbian, gay, and bisexual people with intellectual disabilities in the United Kingdom and views of the staff who support them. *Sexuality Research & Social Policy, 4*(1), 27–39. https://doi.org/10.1525/srsp.2007.4.1.27

Amborski, A. M., Bussières, E.-L., Vaillancourt-Morel, M.-P., & Joyal, C. C. (2022). Sexual violence against persons with disabilities: A meta-analysis. *Trauma, Violence, & Abuse, 23*(4), 1330–1343. https://doi.org/10.1177/1524838021995975

Azzopardi-Lane, C. (2022). "It's not easy to change the mentality": Challenges to sex education delivery for persons with intellectual disability. *Journal of Applied Research in Intellectual Disabilities, 35*(4), 1001–1008. https://doi.org/10.1111/jar.12947

Azzopardi-Lane, C., & Santinele Martino, A. (2024). We are sexual too: Sexuality in the lives of disabled adolescents. In B. E. Angharad & A.-M. Callus (Eds.), *The lives of children and adolescents with disabilities* (pp. 207–225). Routledge. https://doi.org/10.4324/9781003102915-15

Bahner, J. (2020). *Sexual citizenship and disability: Understanding sexual support in policy, practice and theory*. Routledge. https://doi.org/10.4324/9780429488993

Benoit, C., Mellor, A., & Premji, Z. (2023). Access to sexual rights for people living with disabilities: Assumptions, evidence, and policy outcomes. *Archives of Sexual Behavior, 52*(8), 3201–3255. https://doi.org/10.1007/s10508-022-02372-x

Bernert, D. J. (2011). Sexuality and disability in the lives of women with intellectual disabilities. *Sexuality and Disability*, *29*(2), 129–141. https://doi.org/10.1007/s11195-010-9190-4

Björnsdóttir, K., & Stefánsdóttir, G. V. (2020). Double sexual standards: Sexuality and people with intellectual disabilities who require intensive support. *Sexuality and Disability*, *38*(3), 421–438. https://doi.org/10.1007/s11195-020-09643-2

Campbell, M., Löfgren-Mårtenson, C., & Santinele Martino, A. (2020). Cripping sex education. *Sex Education*, *20*(4), 361–365. https://doi.org/10.1080/14681811.2020.1749470

Charley, C., Tureson, A., Wildenauer, L., & Mark, K. (2023). Sex education for LGBTQ+ adolescents. *Current Sexual Health Reports, 15*(3), 180–186. https://doi.org/10.1007/s11930-023-00361-2

Cohen, J. J. (2015). Queer crip sex and critical mattering. *A Journal of Lesbian and Gay Studies, 21*(1), 153–162. https://doi.org/10.1215/10642684-2818552

Crenshaw, K. W. (1989). Demarginalizing the intersection of race and sex: A Black feminist critique of antidiscrimination doctrine, feminist theory and antiracist politics. *University of Chicago Legal Forum, 1,* Article 8. Retrieved April 23, 2024, from https://chicagounbound.uchicago.edu/uclf/vol1989/iss1/8

Davies, A. W. J., Bryan, M. K., Martin, T., Shay, B., Akers, T., Soud, R., Balter, A.-S., O'Leary, S., & Neustifter, R. (2023). Dismantling barriers to access: The necessity of cripping sexuality education in Canadian schools. *The Canadian Journal of Human Sexuality*, *32*(1), 1–19. https://doi.org/10.3138/cjhs.2022-0031

de Heer, B., Brown, M., & Cheney, J. (2021). Sexual consent and communication among the sexual minoritized: The role of heteronormative sex education, trauma, and dual identities. *Feminist Criminology, 16*(5), 701–721. https://doi.org/10.1177/15570851211034560

Dinwoodie, R., Greenhill, B., & Cookson, A. (2020). 'Them two things are what collide together': Understanding the sexual identity experiences of lesbian, gay, bisexual and trans people labelled with intellectual disability. *Journal of Applied Research in Intellectual Disabilities, 33*(1), 3–16. https://doi.org/10.1111/jar.12252

Egner, J. (2017). A messy trajectory: From medical sociology to crip theory. In S. E. Green & S. N. Barnartt (Eds.), *Sociology looking at disability: What did we know and when did we know it* (pp. 159–192). Emerald Group Publishing Limited. https://doi.org/10.1108/S1479-354720160000009009

Egner, J. E. (2019). "The disability rights community was never mine": Neuroqueer disidentification. *Gender & Society, 33*(1), 123–147. https://doi.org/10.1177/0891243218803284

Ferrante, C. A., & Oak, E. (2020). "No sex please!" We have been labelled intellectually disabled. *Sex Education, 20*(4), 383–397. https://doi.org/10.1080/14681811.2020.1719479

Fish, R. (2016). "They've said I'm vulnerable with men": Doing sexuality on locked wards. *Sexualities*, 19(5–6), 641–658. https://psycnet.apa.org/doi/10.1177/1363460715620574

Frawley, P., & O'Shea, A. (2019). "Nothing about us without us": Sex education by and for people with intellectual disability in Australia. *Sex Education, 20*(4), 413–424. https://doi.org/10.1080/14681811.2019.1668759

Frawley, P., & Wilson, N. J. (2016). Young people with intellectual disability talking about sexuality education and information. *Sexuality and Disability, 34*(4), 469–484. https://doi.org/10.1007/s11195-016-9460-x

Gill, M. C. (2015). *Already doing it: Intellectual disability and sexual agency*. University of Minnesota Press.

Hobaica, S., & Kwon, P. (2017). "This is how you hetero:" Sexual minorities in heteronormative sex education. *American Journal of Sexuality Education, 12*(4), 423–450. https://doi.org/10.1080/15546128.2017.1399491

Hogan, J. A. (2023). Having a disability and identifying as LGBTQ+: Are educational professionals prepared for this intersectional experience? *Journal of LGBT Youth, 21*(4), 1–22. https://doi.org/10.1080/19361653.2023.2231921

Hole, R., Schnellert, L., & Cantle, G. (2022). Sex: What is the big deal? Exploring individuals' with intellectual disabilities experiences with sex education. *Qualitative Health Research, 32*(3), 453–464. https://doi.org/10.1177/10497323211057090

Hollomotz, A. (2011). *Learning difficulties and sexual vulnerability: A social approach*. Jessica Kingsley Publishers.

Horner-Johnson, W., Klein, K. A., Campbell, J., & Guise, J.-M. (2022). "It would have been nice to have a choice": Barriers to contraceptive decision-making among women with disabilities. *Women's Health Issues, 32*(3), 261–267. https://doi.org/10.1016/j.whi.2022.01.001

Howarth, J., & Abbott, D. (2005). Breaking the silence: Service providers could do far more to help people with learning disabilities who are lesbian, gay and bisexual to engage in the relationships of their choice, say Joyce Howarth and David Abbott. *Learning Disability Practice, 8*(5), 10–11. https://doi.org/10.7748/ldp2005.06.8.5.10.c1625

Kafer, A. (2003). Compulsory bodies: Reflections on heterosexuality and able-bodiedness. *Journal of Women's History, 15*(3), 77–89. https://doi.org/10.1353/jowh.2003.0071

Kempapidis, T., Heinze, N., Green, A. K., & Gomes, R. S. M. (2024). Queer and disabled: Exploring the experiences of people who identify as LGBT and live with disabilities. *Disabilities, 4*(1), 41–63. https://doi.org/10.3390/disabilities4010004

Klebanov, B., Friedman-Hauser, G., Lusky-Weisrose, E., & Katz, C. (2024). Sexual abuse of children with disabilities: Key lessons and future directions based on a scoping review. *Trauma, Violence, & Abuse, 25*(2), 1296–1314. https://doi.org/10.1177/15248380231179122

Löfgren-Mårtenson, L. (2013). "Hip to be crip?" About crip theory, sexuality and people with intellectual disabilities. *Sexuality and Disability, 31*(4), 413–424. https://doi.org/10.1007/s11195-013-9287-7

López, Quispe. (2023, November 21). What does it mean to be Two-Spirit? *Them*. https://www.them.us/story/what-does-two-spirit-mean-according-to-indigiqueer-people

McRuer, R. (2011). Disabling sex: Notes for a crip theory of sexuality. *A Journal of Lesbian and Gay Studies, 17*(1), 107–117. https://doi.org/10.1215/10642684-2010-021

McRuer, R., & Cassabaum, E. (2021). Crip theory. Oxford Bibliographies: Literary and Critical Theory. https://doi.org/10.1093/obo/9780190221911-0109

McRuer, R., & Mollow, R. (2012). *Sex and disability*. Duke University Press.

Mitchell, C. (2023). Censorship, cultural expectations and transformations: The role of genitalia in disabled lives. *Northern Lights, 21*(1), 25–36. https://doi.org/10.1386/nl_00036_1

Nakkeeran, N., & Nakkeeran, B. (2018). Disability, mental health, sexual orientation and gender identity: Understanding health inequity through experience and difference. *Health Research Policy and Systems, 16,* Article 97. https://doi.org/10.1186/s12961-018-0366-1

Noonan, A., & Taylor Gomez, M. (2011). Who's missing? Awareness of lesbian, gay, bisexual and transgender people with intellectual disability. *Sexuality and Disability, 29*(2), 175–180. https://doi.org/10.1007/s11195-010-9175-3

O'Shea, A., Latham, J. R., McNair, R., Despott, N., Rose, M., Mountford, R., & Frawley, P. (2020). Experiences of LGBTIQA+ people with disability in healthcare and community services: Towards embracing multiple identities. *International Journal of Environmental Research and Public Health, 17*(21), 8080. https://doi.org/10.3390/ijerph17218080

Okotie, E. S., & Jolly, S. (2024). Feeling 'happy, loved, cherished, desired' and 'hopeful for the future': Disabled women in Nigeria talk about sex and pleasure. *Sexuality and Disability, 42*(1), 85–99. https://doi.org/10.1007/s11195-023-09830-x

Sandahl, C. (2003). Queering the crip or cripping the queer?: Intersections of queer and crip identities in solo autobiographical performance. *A Journal of Lesbian and Gay Studies, 9*(1–2), 25–56. https://doi.org/10.1215/10642684-9-1-2-25

Sandberg, L. J., Rosqvist, H. B., & Grigorovich, A. (2021). Regulating, fostering and preserving: The production of sexual normates through cognitive ableism and cognitive othering. *Culture, Health & Sexuality, 23*(10), 1421–1434. https://doi.org/10.1080/13691058.2020.1787519

Santinele Martino, A. (2017). Cripping sexualities: An analytic review of theoretical and empirical writing on the intersection of disabilities and sexualities. *Sociology Compass, 11*(5), e12471. https://doi.org/10.1111/soc4.12471

Santinele Martino, A. (2020). Also here, also queer: The work of LGBT+ disabled activists/scholars in 'cripping' sexualities. In A. Toft & A. Franklin (Eds.), *Young, disabled and LGBT* (pp. 13–28). Routledge. https://doi.org/10.4324/9780429198458-3

Santinele Martino, A. (2022a). "I don't want to get in trouble": A study of how adults with intellectual disabilities convert and navigate intellectual disability sexual fields. *Culture, Health & Sexuality, 24*(9), 1230–1242. https://doi.org/10.1080/13691058.2021.1942552

Santinele Martino, A. (2022b). The intersection of sexuality and intellectual disability: Shattering the taboo. In N. Fischer & L. Westbrook (Eds.), *Introducing the new sexuality studies* (4th ed., pp. 460–469). Taylor & Francis Group. https://doi.org/10.4324/9781003163329-57

Santinele Martino, A., & Fudge Schormans, A. (2018). When good intentions backfire: University research ethics review and the intimate lives of people labelled with intellectual disabilities. *Forum: Qualitative Social Research, 19*(3), 1–18. https://doi.org/10.17169/fqs-19.3.3090

Santinele Martino, A., & Moumos, E. (2023). "Cripping" intimate relationships: The experiences of 2SLGBTQ+ adults with developmental and/or intellectual disability. *Sexuality & Culture, 28*, 1446–1466. https://doi.org/10.1007/s12119-023-10185-w

Santinele Martino, A., & Perreault-Laird, J. (2019). "I don't know if I can talk about that": An exploratory study on the experiences of care workers regarding the sexuality of people with intellectual disabilities. *Disability Studies Quarterly, 39*(3), Article ID: 6383. https://doi.org/10.18061/dsq.v39i3.6383

Siebers, Tobin. (2010). *Disability aesthetics.* University of Michigan Press. https://doi.org/10.3998/mpub.1134097

Simić Stanojević, I., Baugh, M., Greer, K. M., Piatt, J., & Yarber, W. (2023). Increasing opportunities for healthy sexual socialization in LGBTQ+ people with IDD: The role of LGBTQ+ organizations and community. *Sexuality and Disability, 41*, 531–541. https://doi.org/10.1007/s11195-023-09789-9

Simon, W., & Gagnon, J. H. (1984). Sexual scripts. *Society, 22*(1), 53–60. https://doi.org/10.1007/BF02701260

Sommarö, S., Andersson, A., & Skagerström, J. (2020). A deviation too many? Healthcare professionals' knowledge and attitudes concerning patients with intellectual disability disrupting norms regarding sexual orientation and/or gender identity. *Journal of Applied Research in Intellectual Disabilities, 33*(6), 1199–1209. https://doi.org/10.1111/jar.12739

Stoffelen, J., Kok, G., Hospers, H., & Curfs, L. M. G. (2013). Homosexuality among people with a mild intellectual disability: An explorative study on the lived experiences of homosexual people in the Netherlands with a mild intellectual disability. *Journal of Intellectual Disability Research, 57*(3), 257–267. https://doi.org/10.1111/j.1365-2788.2011.01532.x

Sullivan, P. M., & Knutson, J. F. (2000). Maltreatment and disabilities: A population-based epidemiological study. *Child Abuse & Neglect, 24*(10), 1257–1273. https://doi.org/10.1016/S0145-2134(00)00190-3.

Toft, A. (2020). Identity management and community belonging: The coming out careers of young disabled lgbt+persons. *Sexuality & Culture, 24*(6), 1893–1912. https://doi.org/10.1007/s12119-020-09726-4

Vassallo, M., & Azzopardi-Lane, C. (2022). *Intersectionality and people with disability*. Commission for the rights of persons with disability. Retrieved March 16, 2024, from https://www.crpd.org.mt/wp-content/uploads/2022/09/Intersectionality-and-Disability-Report-Final-Version-May-2022.docx.pdf

Vo, T. D. (2021). The whiteness of 'safe' spaces: Developing a conceptual framework to critically examine the well-being of racialized 2SLGBTQ+ people within 2SLGBTQ+ leisure spaces. *The Canadian Journal of Human Sexuality, 30*(2), 219–231. https://doi.org/10.3138/CJHS.2021-0016

Walmsley, Jan, & Johnson, K. (2003). *Inclusive research with people with learning disabilities past, present, and futures*. Jessica Kingsley Publishers.

Wilson, N. J., Macdonald, J., Hayman, B., Bright, A. M., Frawley, P., & Gallego, G. (2018). A narrative review of the literature about people with intellectual disability who identify as lesbian, gay, bisexual, transgender, intersex or questioning. *Journal of Intellectual Disabilities, 22*(2), 171–196. https://doi.org/10.1177/1744629516682681

Withers, P., & Morris, J. (2012). Sexual exploitation of people with intellectual disabilities. In E. Emerson, C. Hatton, K. Dickson, R. Gone, A. Caine, & J. Bromley (Eds.), *Clinical psychology and people with intellectual disabilities* (2nd ed., pp. 273–292). Wiley. https://doi.org/10.1002/9781118404898.ch13

Bibliography

Arora, S., Gonzalez, K. A., Abreu, R. L., & Gloster, C. (2022). "Therapy can be restorative, but can also be really harmful": Therapy experiences of QTBIPOC clients. *Psychotherapy (Chicago, Ill.), 59*(4), 498–510. https://doi.org/10.1037/pst0000443

Freeman-Coppadge, D. J., & Langroudi, K. F. (2021). Beyond LGBTQ-affirmative therapy: Fostering growth and healing through intersectionality. In K. L. Nadal & M. R. Scharrón-del Río (Eds.), *Queer psychology* (pp. 159–179). Springer. https://doi.org/10.1007/978-3-030-74146-4_9

Grzanka, P. R. (2020). From buzzword to critical psychology: An invitation to take intersectionality seriously. *Women & Therapy, 43(3–4)*, 244–261. https://doi.org/10.1080/02703149.2020.1729473

Santinele Martino, A., Moumos, E., Ulicki, N., & Robbins, M. (2023). The experiences of 2SLGBTQ+ adults labeled with intellectual and/or developmental disabilities when navigating mainstream queer social spaces. *Journal of Homosexuality, 71*(13), 1–20. https://doi.org/10.1080/00918369.2023.2276320

Toft, A., Franklin, A., & Langley, E. (2020). 'You're not sure that you are gay yet': The perpetuation of the 'phase' in the lives of young disabled LGBT+people. *Sexualities, 23*(4), 516–529. https://doi.org/10.1177/1363460719842135

SECTION III

Foundations of Disability-Affirmative Therapy

PART III

Becoming Dyslexic

Catherine Kapphahn

Alarm bells ring inside my body. Breathless, reeling, heart racing, nauseous, and shaky, I'm hit with overwhelming panic. I'm a graduate student of creative writing, lying on my back on campus grass, trying to breathe. My first brief stint in therapy has unleashed a tsunami of anxiety. After a long line of schools, I am getting close to the finish line and the learning identity I have worked so hard to create—is about to collapse.

After this experience, non-stop anxiety and out-of-body sensations send me into therapy again, which becomes another classroom where I mistrust myself. I'm familiar with going unnoticed, holding my breath, bracing myself, failing, and then feeling furious with myself. In J's office, as we sit across from each other, I have the impulse to plan, troubleshoot and predict what's needed, but unexpectedly I slide into silence again and again. It's maddening! In fact, the harder I try to be a good student in this room that magnifies every emotion, the quieter things get. In therapy, I navigate a minefield of chronic self-doubt, self-hatred and self-blame, which is how I survived school. In therapy, I watch myself withhold when I know—if I could only let go—she could help me. Time rushes at me; the session is over before I've even begun. I walk out feeling like a failure, again and again.

In therapy and in life, I move in and out of disappearing spells. Over time, I'm able to describe to my therapist the unnerving sensation of floating outside my body, feeling unmoored and living in suspension. I truly believe nothing huge or terrible has ever happened to me, other than losing my mom to cancer when I was 22. I am a mystery, and I push J to tell me what is wrong. "Let's not pathologize," she says like she's closing a drawer. And I sense what she thinks is bad might not be bad for me. "Let's not put a label on things," she says cryptically. But I long for a name for what's happening to me.

DOI: 10.4324/9781003362586-14

By chance, as I finish my thesis, I find someone to do an educational evaluation on me, and the diagnosis is: dyslexia. The first time I say, "I am dyslexic," I choke up. I look back at my life and my entire history shifts. I've been keeping a secret I didn't know I was keeping. Finally, I have a name for how I learn. Still, it will be years before I recognize my disappearing, my anxiety and tough mindset is directly linked to my learning traumas. I will have to untangle myself from a learning identity I created in order to fit an educational system that didn't value my intelligence.

Now it's clear how important it was for me to make the invisible, visible, to solidify the suffering and name my dyslexia. The process of making something real is complicated, and even when you have a name, it doesn't happen right away. I'd spent so long trying to fix, wrestle, prevent, and destroy the way I learned, so it would take years to embrace becoming dyslexic. I had to face the magnitude of my learning shame in order to expand the meaning of intelligence to include dyslexic thinking, seeing and being. I may have failed 3rd grade, gotten Fs on high school essays, and been placed in college remedial English and math, but that same person wrote this essay. I hold up the infinite magic of the dyslexic brain and begin to see the intelligence of interconnections. I wonder if even now, as I write this, I am trying to prove my worth. Or maybe, I'm opening the door to dyslexia for you. When I was lying on the grass in grad school, reeling from my first panic attack, I'd pushed so hard for so long—my body collapsed. Now through the process of embracing the way my brain works; the reclamation of my dyslexic self is possible. I sit beside that woman lying on the grass, holding her ribs, trying to breathe, and I tell her, "You are a storyteller; you have always been a storyteller."

8

THINKING PSYCHOANALYTICALLY ABOUT THERAPY WITH DISABLED PEOPLE

The Need to Begin with Ourselves

Brian Watermeyer

Introduction

In this chapter, I explore a range of key ideas and principles, which I have accumulated over more than two decades as a psychoanalytic psychotherapist working with disabled people. Across society, disability aversion and prejudice are ubiquitous, and it therefore stands to reason that we need to begin by uncovering and processing how these dynamics appear in the therapy room. A glance at the history of psychoanalytic psychotherapy reveals a distinct avoidance of engagement with disability, which betrays the presence of emotional unease and aversion which we all feel. To approach disability as a psychotherapist, it is essential to first examine your own complex counter-transference responses with humility. This is because the reactions that disability evokes in others (including ourselves), often have greater impact than the disability itself. But first, we need to draw members of the disability community into psychotherapeutic inquiry – as we shall see, a range of factors have contributed to an understandable ambivalence in this regard. There is much that needs to change in both training and practice if psychotherapy is to justify being described as 'disability-affirmative'. Disabled people continue to be subjected to stigma, control, marginalisation and, above all, silencing. Creating an environment within psychotherapy where this silence can be broken is no easy matter and demands an exceptional level of human engagement from the practitioner. This involves challenging deeply ingrained social conditioning in a world that often devalues life with disability, which can significantly shape how one understands both themselves and others. At the heart of the endeavour is, as

DOI: 10.4324/9781003362586-15

always, simple listening. But this requires that we, as practitioners, first overcome our own disability-related silences.

Anxious to avoid the risk of new ways for disabled people to be pathologised, 'mainstream' disability studies, driven by the social model approach (Oliver, 1996), was historically avoidant of any form of psychological analysis of disability. This was understandable, since 'traditional' psychological and psychoanalytic work on disability has typically viewed marginality as the consequence of individual, impairment-based factors, leading to a depoliticising, and hence victim-blaming account (Asch & Rousso, 1985; Harris & Wideman, 1988; Watermeyer, 2012a). Yet, a psychological conceptualisation of disablism, and the effects it may have on individuals, is essential if we are to develop ways to disrupt its often intricate, ideologically obscured mechanisms. As a psychotherapist, one has the opportunity to unpack disability as an experience of lifelong socialisation within discourses, which dehumanise, demean, conceal, discipline, and marginalise people with impairments, uncovering how ideology has taken up residence in the intrapsychic realm. There is much to undo, and layers of oppression are often cemented with trauma.

The area of disability and psychotherapy remains, in my view, relatively under-theorised. While some important contributions have emerged (Olkin, 1999; 2014), as a reader, one has at times had to find useful principles buried within discourses which are by now anachronistic, even harmful (e.g. De Groef & Heinemann, 1999; Blotzer & Ruth, 1995). Here, I contribute to the discussion by describing key learnings that have emanated from my own work, as therapist, clinical supervisor, and researcher in disability and mental health. The approach is informal, discursive, and applied, seeking to promote a sense of what I term a 'generosity of engagement' (Watermeyer, 2013) between practitioners and others working in the disability arena who may well have differing skills and political leanings. At the heart of my analysis is the idea that, because of its profound symbolic power and emotional evocativeness (Watermeyer, 2006), disability is, for most of us, hard to think about. And the work of 'thinking about' is, as we shall see, the essence of containment (Rustin, 1991) – the basis of depth-oriented psychotherapy. Because of deeply held, universal anxieties, learning to think about disability is a challenge for most of us. I hope that what is to follow provides some useful signposting on this journey.

Psychotherapy and the Disability Community

It will be familiar to readers of this book that a reluctance, even suspicion, regarding entering psychotherapy has historically been commonplace in the disability community (Reeve, 2004; Goodley & Lawthom, 2006). During my career, I have had countless conversations with disabled people who have felt unheard, pathologised, infantilised, blamed or otherwise misunderstood by psychotherapists. Clinical psychology and psychoanalysis have a history of attributing distress to individual factors, while paying little attention to contexts of material and cultural oppression (Asch & Rousso, 1985; Watermeyer, 2012a). This is dangerous in any context, but especially so in the disability arena, where it enacts relationships supporting self-blame which are pervasive in the lives of disabled people.

Developments in disability studies research and clinical training have, over recent times, begun to address this problem, but there remains a long road ahead. A key concern is the stubborn under-representation of disabled people in the professional therapeutic community, which obviously misses the opportunity to infuse discussions among both trainees and practitioners with first-hand knowledge of the psychosocial positioning of disabled people (Watermeyer, 2012a).

My own teaching of both trainees and professionals has made it clear to me that promoting receptivity and insight surrounding work with disabled clients requires not only social justice-oriented knowledge but, more significantly, an emotional shift in one's personal relationship with the notion of disability (Broderick & Lalvani, 2017; Watermeyer, McKenzie & Kelly, 2024). This is because oppressive social responses to disabled people at all levels of society – from disability-related laws and policies, and the nature of the material environment, to cultural representations and interpersonal relationships – are all, to some extent, shaped by unconsciously held anxieties which are evoked by exposure to disability (Marks, 1999; Watermeyer, 2006; 2013). Disability has come to represent universal existential anxieties we all struggle with, including insecurity about our intellect and ability, fears about our attractiveness and acceptability, and our struggles with the reality of dependency, the impermanence and frailty of the body, and the fact of mortality (Watermeyer, 2013). The need to defend against these evocations supports projections to do with damage, vulnerability, dependency, and shame, which are familiar stereotypes directed at the disability community (Hughes, 2019). Until we have recognised and processed our anxiety-ridden fantasies about disability, we will remain unable to hear the unique experience of disabled clients (Watermeyer, 2012b). We need to clear away our own emotional noise to create the stance of 'not knowing' (Casement, 2014), which is essential to the psychotherapeutic method.

Responding to Disability in the Therapy Room

Clinicians who I have trained and supervised tend, in response to disability, to either dismiss or overestimate its importance in the aetiology of distress. To some, disabled people are 'just like anyone else', and the disability can be all but ignored. Of course, in essence, there is truth to this – disabled people are human in just the same way as anyone else. Yet, what is occurring here is often a denial in the clinician of the fact that the life-worlds of disabled people may be starkly different, incorporating the reality of multiple, layered barriers to participation, as well as stigma, discrimination, and functional limitation due to impairment. As we shall see later, developing insight into the mechanisms of exclusion – both the tangible and cultural/relational barriers to participation – experienced by persons with a range of impairments, is essential for therapists working with disabled clients. Without this, a disabled client is likely to feel that the layer of their experience which connects closely to disability remains unheard (Wendell, 1996; Watermeyer, 2014).

The alternative, more common response involves therapists who are so mesmerised by corporeal difference, that the disability becomes the dominant, if not sole, factor to which mental states are attributed (Lussier, 1980). For practitioners who have not done the work of processing their own unconscious evocations, and hence projections, surrounding disability, the impairment can act as a lightning rod, monopolising attention in a way which, again, overpowers the client's voice. The result is a pathologising view of the client, whose struggles become constructed as the inevitable consequences of impairment, ignoring or minimising the often-defining influence of contextual and relational factors (Watermeyer, 2013). As noted, this can add the therapist's voice to that of an external social world which, overtly and symbolically, signals to disabled persons that 'the problem' is with their own 'flaws', rather than with an unjust, exclusionary environment. In the face of ongoing life struggles engendered by occupying environments designed exclusively for nondisabled people, self-blaming attributions are a very common part of the inner lives of disabled people (Watermeyer & Swartz, 2008). For example, a university campus and its media of education may create immense, stress inducing problems of access to a disabled student, yet ideas such as 'if I just tried harder … was better prepared, better organised … if I communicated better, made better choices' are never far away, provoking guilt rather than self-advocacy.

Being Subversive

In my view, all meaningful psychotherapeutic inquiry is subversive (Frosh, 2006) in the best possible sense; in fact, from a psychoanalytic viewpoint, Samuels (1993, p. 52) describes psychotherapy as 'a bridge between depth psychology and politics'. It is the work of uncovering and debunking hidden assumptions about the self - about worth, potential, entitlement, and the capacity for love and hope. In any life, the combination of problems in formative relationships and the early environment, along with experiences of physical and emotional trauma, can bury or pervert healthy expression of these parts of self, rendering defences which may be more or less adaptive. Invisible, hegemonic myths about one's value and place in the world cemented by love as well as trauma, must be dislodged through a painful revisiting of the experiences at their source (McWilliams, 1994). In the lives of disabled people, this is, if anything, even more true. This is because disability, in how it is culturally represented and popularly understood, has the power to elicit a host of emotionally charged ideas (i.e. projections), regarding what disabled people need, what their potentials are, where they belong, whether they are able to engage in fulfilling relationships, and much else. This means that the developmental milieu of disabled people (at least those living with impairment since birth or early childhood) is likely to have been shaped by feelings evoked in others by disability, and the defences which these provoke (Watermeyer, 2002).

Parenting a disabled child is often challenging, and in many contexts, families do not receive the support they need. For this reason, we need to hold compassion for such parents, in the present as well as in the formative years of our adult disabled clients (Ferguson, 2001). The birth of a baby who, unexpectedly, has some form of impairment may be traumatic for parents, bringing a host of anxieties about caring for their child, possible health complications, issues surrounding education, and hopes for a fulfilling future (Parens, 2006). As products of disablist segregation, such parents have probably had little experience of adults with the same impairment as their child, who may be living successful and fulfilled lives in the community. This position of not knowing what to expect, or how best to care for their child, can understandably create a climate of anxiety around the child, as adults struggle to manage painful fantasies about what the future may hold (Watermeyer & McKenzie, 2014). In these circumstances, it may be less likely that a child has opportunities to internalise from others an authentic, felt sense of faith in their ability to grow-develop, achieve, and belong. This support of healthy narcissism is crucial in the formation of a self, which is at once hopeful and secure about its potential, while not needing to resort to excessive, maladaptive narcissism to maintain its stability (Kohut, 1972). In sum, if psychotherapy is to achieve its goal of subverting taken-for-granted, oppressive assumptions, it must expose social contradictions implicit in disability inequality, thereby harnessing anger and healthy entitlement to inclusion, and leading to the 'giving back' of unconsciously held imputations of damage, inability, and shame (Samuels, 1993; Marks, 2002).

Looking Back on Early Life

In response to the emotionally loaded confusion of becoming the parent of a disabled child, parents may respond in different ways. Again, it is essential that we consider their experience in a compassionate way, while also recognising how feelings about disability may affect the developmental milieu. Some parents' natural emphasis on empathy may lead to a permissiveness with boundaries, as they are able to see little but vulnerability in their child, therefore possibly underestimating potential for resilience, growth and development. As noted, this may inadvertently communicate to the child a lack of faith in their potential, leaving her with a precarious sense of her ability to cope in the world. Alternatively, parents may, again quite understandably, hold a prominent concern about how unwelcoming they believe the world will be to their child, therefore creating for her an environment which emphasises discipline, spartanism and the need to continually strive to become stronger. This, in turn, may communicate to the growing child that her future belonging in the world is uncertain and contingent, while also placing responsibility upon her to 'make up' for the ways in which her body and its functioning diverge from an imagined norm.

In this vein, disability studies literature and my own clinical experience are replete with accounts from adult disabled persons of how, through childhood, long-term rehabilitation regimes contributed to an imperative to constantly try harder to become 'more normal'. Time and energy which might otherwise have been spent on play is instead sacrificed to what is felt to be a duty to 'overcome' impairment, as the child grows into an experience of self as a broken thing needing repair, or a problem to be solved (Swain & French, 2001; Goodley & Runswick-Cole, 2010). In the life of a child with cerebral palsy, for example, parents and practitioners may, with the best intentions, set rehabilitation goals and incentives which communicate that the child's natural state is not acceptable, even shameful, possibly manifesting in an imperative to learn to walk unaided, rather than with the use of an assistive device. These deeply held feelings may persist throughout adulthood, to be repeatedly confirmed by a social world which demonstrates time and again that there is no place for disability here. Micro-aggressions, bullying at school, and possible social isolation are among common life experiences which may embed such negative messaging, making it harder to grow a secure sense of self. Under the influence of medical professionals who are driven to cure, parents, and society as a whole, may put a large amount of personal and material resources into correction, while neglecting to address the challenge of creating a social world more welcoming of disability-difference (Davis, 1997).

'Disability Issues?'

A commonly held assumption among psychotherapists is that, in order to 'deal with' disabled clients, one needs to understand 'disability issues' – in other words, a reductive, decontextualised sense of 'what it feels like' to live with impairment. On examination, the implication here is that disabled people are somehow intrinsically different to 'us'; so different, that we need tuition in a new, unknown subjective world. This is a dangerous misapprehension, often borne of a defensive need to distance ourselves from what we imagine life with disability to be. Rather than creating 'disability issues', what disability does is take universal human issues and place them front and centre in the life experiences of persons living with impairment (Watermeyer & Swartz, 2016). For example, it is incontrovertible that dependency is a human universal, yet in our modern, narcissistic world, we have the luxury of pretending that it is not (Kittay, 2011). Indeed, showing evidence of our need for care or assistance is regarded as shameful, and to be avoided, contributing to its associated feelings and memories being internally split off and denied by most of us (Lourens, Watermeyer & Swartz, 2018).

For someone who, say, lives with a severe physical disability, the luxury of such deception is not available, meaning that, unlike their nondisabled counterparts, they must face and process those parts of themselves that struggle with showing need and accepting physical assistance, and emotionally grow beyond them. Other examples of universal human struggles which disabled people are forced to face include feelings about the frailty or 'imperfection' of the body, the challenge of surrendering control, managing the necessary transgression of physical boundaries, the foregoing of privacy, and much else. All of this is hard emotional work with which disabled people are confronted, requiring the development of stable inner foundations independent of the trappings of narcissism on which most of us rely. Having to confront the reality of vulnerability and non-control means shedding commonly held narcissistic illusions, thereby moving towards a point where the fact of our shared human vulnerability becomes not just an idea but also a reality (Watermeyer, 2013).

Reaching this point means being freed from the shame of difference produced by the 'modern man's' fantasy of his own perfection, as it places all of us in the same frail, flawed and quintessentially human position. But the journey towards such a point is very hard indeed and is often a significant aspect of the therapeutic task. As a clinician, this means working very closely with the phenomenology of self – with how one feels about oneself, one's entitlements, one's lovableness, and so forth – and relating this to experiences of mirroring and socialisation in the formative years and beyond. In the life of a child with a visible disability, continual othering in the family, school and community, combined with the 'evidence' of difference implicit in ongoing needs for assistance, can make it impossible to avoid internalising the myth that one is intrinsically different, damaged, an outlier (Harris & Wideman, 1988). Part of that othering will involve projections of vulnerability and dependency, which explicitly locate the disabled child or adult as the sole custodian of these characteristics, as they are denied by the observer. Overcoming this split means 'giving back' these imputations and moving towards a deep recognition of the need and vulnerability in others, which also overcomes the myth of intrinsic difference. For clinicians, moving past this same fantasy allows for the development of accurate empathy for a disabled client. This involves (carefully) identifying with the person 'inside' a world of impairment and disablist treatment, recognising them as a human who responds emotionally in ways not fundamentally different from oneself. I add the qualifier of 'carefully' for two reasons. First, one never *completely* gets over the urge to project vulnerability into disabled people, and so thinking continually about the basis of one's empathic reflections is essential. Second, it is important to remember that disabled people adjust to functional limitations (such as the inability to walk, see, communicate) over time, and therefore their experience of impairment, as well as of a discriminatory world, is almost always not what we imagine. As always, listening is key.

Disability and Social Justice

As I noted previously, while training in disability as a social justice issue is not in itself sufficient to promote empowering psychotherapy, it is nevertheless essential. Alongside exploration of one's own emotional relationship with disability, psychotherapists require a degree of knowledge about the social machinery which maintains the over-representation of disabled people among the poor, unemployed and marginal. Systemic exclusion means that disabled people are often under-educated, have poorer health care, lack essential services such as transportation and communications, and have reduced opportunities for participation in cultural, recreational and social activities (Shakespeare, 2014). Around the world, the medical pathologisation, and hence othering, of disabled people is evidenced by a sustained drive to segregate, institutionalise, conceal, correct, or otherwise 'deal with' impairment; or rather, with the 'tissue of myths, fears and misunderstandings' (Murphy, 1987, p. 113) which attach to it. At the level of relationships, disabled people are likely to experience stigmatisation, and be harmed by the assumption that they are not interested in or capable of sexual intimacy (Rohleder et al., 2019). Moving around in the material world, life with a physical, sensory, communication, or neurodevelopmental disability means continually bumping up against hidden barriers to participation, in the nature of the built environment, the technologies we use, our bureaucratic procedures, our ways of communicating, and much more.

At its root, a human rights view of disability inequality recognises that the social destiny of disabled people is far more the consequence of how societies are organised, than of the nature of individual impairments, and this principle is the key to an inquiry into the multimodal ways in which a disabled individual may, on a daily basis, be pushed to the margins. Developing insight into these mechanisms of exclusion is important, opening a space within the therapist's mind for experiences of exclusion which are invisible to most. What the human rights view tells us is that the systemic disadvantage experienced by disabled people amounts to social injustice, and a contravention of citizenship rights. In other words, public transport that is inaccessible to people with physical impairments, libraries without materials accessible to visually impaired persons, university lectures without sign language interpreters, and a host of other such examples represent ways in which institutions, and society as a whole, have failed to provide equitably for people with a range of impairments, amounting to illegal and indefensible discrimination. Recognition of this is essential for therapists working with disabled clients, yet it is also knowledge which needs to be used carefully (Watermeyer, 2012b).

In psychotherapy with disabled persons, one will often be confronted with individuals who, by virtue of being socialised in a disablist world, are unaware that their rights are being contravened. If one grows up in a family or school which continually signalled that disability was something shameful, that the problem was 'with you', and that disabled people need to do everything they can to make up for the ways in which their bodies and minds do not fit the shape and nature of the social environment, then one's excluded, marginal position may appear inevitable, even just. For example, a disabled sibling may feel pain at the fact that her brother and sister attend school, while she does not, but that is very different to feeling, in an authentic way, that she is also entitled to an education. For disabled as well as non-disabled people, the ubiquity of exclusion means that we are all constitutionally 'impaired' in our ability to imagine an inclusive society which welcomes and provides for the needs of all. When faced with such unawareness of rights in a disabled client, it may be tempting, especially for the therapist to whom disability oppression is a new discovery, to point out all of the ways in which citizenship rights have been contravened. In fact, scholars promoting the 'social model of disability' mistakenly believed that simply knowing one's rights was sufficient for liberation (Thomas, 1999). In truth, such a politically oriented approach in the therapy room can often backfire. The reason is this: simply identifying how rights have been contravened does not in any way contribute to processing the feelings associated with lifelong experiences of exclusion, and, in fact, may hamstring such work (Watermeyer, 2012b). Moving towards a secure inner foundation from which to exercise self-advocacy requires the deep unpacking and processing of hidden, emotionally laden forms of discrimination. It is through such work that healthy entitlement can be not only enacted, but also felt.

The journey to this point will involve grief, which is the basis for self-compassion (Cheng, 2000; Watermeyer, 2009; 2017). This is grief for a child who felt not good enough, for an adolescent who was told that they could no longer attend the same school as their friends, for a young person who faced discrimination in higher education, for the painful recognition that one over years internalised denigrating ideas about one's value, for experiences of bullying and stigma, for loneliness engendered by a prejudiced social world, and much more. All of these experiences can be traced to injustice – to institutional discrimination, an inaccessible environment and prejudice in relationships – and this understanding is important. But without the work of grief, a therapist overly, and perhaps defensively, preoccupied with political contradictions may inadvertently move further and further away from the lifeworld of the client. Unlike these political ideals, the client's life remains dominated by palpable exclusion which, historically as well as currently, does not simply dissolve away because of its wrongness. As is the case in many circumstances involving a fight against oppression, political principles can act as a defence for both client and practitioner, drawing the therapist into the comfortable, yet unhelpful, role of champion of the 'downtrodden'. Based on the foregoing, having the opportunity and support to process grief is an essential foundation for appropriate feelings of anger and healthy entitlement, which can drive social change. Perhaps because of this, oppressive ideologies place restrictions on expressions of grief among marginal groups, serving to silence the emotional consequences of mistreatment, while compounding domination. This phenomenon has been termed *melancholic suspension* (Cheng, 2000), which I explore elsewhere in relation to disability (Watermeyer, 2017; Watermeyer & McKinney, 2022).

Trauma

Both acute and ongoing trauma are almost always uncovered in psychotherapy with disabled people. Some individuals will have acquired disability through accident, violent crime or illness, bringing an abrupt and profound change to their world. As already explained, the impressions created by health professionals at such times are often powerful, filling spaces of confusion and uncertainty about identity and social belonging (Botha & Watermeyer, 2024). It is in the nature of trauma that it perforates one's view of the world and the self, while also cementing new, potentially harmful understandings and defences; in the case of disability, these may be oppressive beliefs about potential, entitlement, and belonging. But trauma is also to be found in the ongoing barrage of micro-aggressions, demeaning treatment, unnecessary material hardship and symbolic denigration experienced daily in the lives of disabled people. These are experiences which may be so commonplace to a disabled client as to generally go unproblematised, or simply not be noticed at all, instead settling unseen into a sense of self as defective. The work of meticulously tracking the emotional experience of these events, where emotion will often be at least partially hidden, is very important indeed.

Understanding ongoing, socially engendered emotional trauma requires thinking about the psychological substrate into which it settles (Watermeyer, 2013). Reflecting on the reality of how human development is hard for everyone reminds us that fears and feelings of being unacceptable, unlovable, unattractive, burdensome or otherwise damaged dwell in all of us. For most, allowing the mind to rest relies on populating our worlds with fantasies, experiences and objects which contradict this reality. For example, the experiences of control and mastery offered by a combination of middle-class privilege and non-disabled status (such as freedom of movement, access to technology, the enjoyment of amenities, and so forth) can serve to keep the 'fearsome reality' that we have no control over our physical and existential destiny well at bay (Watermeyer & Swartz, 2008). At the same time, our defences against deeply personal memories and feelings about the opposite of such control - of vulnerability, pain and fear, as well as the malignant views of self which these may have engendered - are repeatedly reinforced. By this, I refer to the truism that, to some extent, trauma will always resolve psychically into some version of self-blame; ultimately, the problem, the shortcoming, is within you. While non-disabled people may remain reassured by a world which continually reiterates its attunement to their needs, disabled people face very different messaging. The social positioning of disabled people, which reiterates a message of not belonging, not 'fitting', can selectively enliven and confirm one's most malignant aspects of self. Here, a world which rejects both material and relational ways can re-aggravate constitutional wounds we all have, siding with self-blaming and damaged internal objects.

Containment and Silence

Moving through a world which repeatedly ignores one's needs may be akin to the experience of a misattuned parental object, demonstrating again and again that it was unable or unwilling to think about one's subjective reality. Building on

Bion's (1962) concept of maternal reverie, Rustin (1991) describes containment as the experience of being thought about – that is, being shown that someone else is willing and able to 'take in' and accept the difficult parts of my inner world, including both needs and thorny emotions. It is through this experience of having one's feelings accepted and held by another, that one grows the capacity for self-compassion, which is an essential foundation for a secure sense of self. The combination of an inaccessible material world and the prohibition of expressing negative emotion to which disabled people are subject can recapitulate to the disability community that there is no compassionate place in human exchange for their experiences of embodiment and disablism. In the lives of disabled people, a web of relational forces and cultural messaging signals that feelings and experiences to do with impairment and social oppression are not permissible and should be kept to oneself (Watermeyer & Swartz, 2008; Watermeyer, 2009; Olkin, 1999; Ahmed, 2010). This means that disabled people are likely to have less access to that most precious commodity – experiences of feeling truly seen, understood and accepted by another. These moments are essential for the integration of one's own experiences, especially those involving trauma, and part of this process is the processing of grief. Until this work is made possible by care, understanding and acceptance – what we hope to provide in the therapeutic frame – the 'problems of living' associated with disability are likely to remain tinged with self-blame. After all, this is the essence of the medical model – that the 'problem', and cause for your marginality, is 'inside you'.

Auto-ethnographic accounts from disabled scholars reflect an awareness, sometimes from early childhood, of a social imperative to protect others from the lived realities of one's impairment (French, 1993; Watermeyer, 2018; Murphy, 1987; Wendell, 1996; Linton, 1998). Attempts to share one's experience may result in responses of helplessness, guilt, anxiety, anger or awkwardness, threatening the security of relationships. For many disabled people, secure belonging is felt to be contingent on bracketing off the messy reality of life with impairment in a disablist world. But this means living with minimal experiences of being truly seen, with the intimacy and trust which this can engender (Watermeyer, 2013). In her 1993 classic essay, Sally French notes how, from her earliest childhood, she was aware that talking about her visual impairment would simply 'spoil other people's fun', and so she managed her vision-related difficulties alone. Such silencing can relegate that layer of experience which pertains to both functional limitation and aversive social responses to a shadowy inner realm, limiting the likelihood of its associated feelings being explored and understood, and its potentially self-harming assumptions debunked. If we, as psychotherapists, are to create an environment which allows for the exploration of such hidden material, it is essential that our conscious and unconscious associations with disability – both cognitive and emotional – have been humbly and courageously explored. If we have not done this work, our ambivalences will certainly be sensed, constraining development of trusting, authentic relating.

Concluding Reflections

In the ongoing socialisation of disabled people, a continual message from both the human and material environment is that it is simply 'not OK' to be disabled (Watermeyer & Swartz, 2008). The all-pervading assumption that the able body is, in some way, the only legitimate body, is something that exists in ongoing conflict with the development of a secure and integrated sense of self among persons who live with impairment. There is, therefore, a trope at the very heart of modernist, neoliberal ideology which must be dislodged, opening the way for an authentic embracing of the universality of human vulnerability, and with it, the foundations of self-love. This is a hard path, but one with potentially rich rewards. As I noted earlier, what the onset of disability tends to do is confront an individual with existential dilemmas from which most people are, at least for part of their lives, shielded. For anyone seeking wholeness and self-compassion in psychotherapy, the same ideals of self-acceptance pertain, achieved through the processing of trauma and the integrating of malignant or self-harming objects. Disability can be a motivator which pushes one firmly down this road, acting as a tough teacher, but also beckoning towards a place of human commonality and care which is there for all to share, whether disabled or not. As clinicians, we, too, stand to learn a great deal from this work.

References

Ahmed, S. (2010). *The promise of happiness.* Duke University Press. https://doi.org/10.1515/9780822392781

Asch, A. & Rousso, H. (1985). Therapists with disabilities: Theoretical and clinical issues. *Psychiatry*, *48*, 1–12. https://doi.org/10.1080/00332747.1985.11024263

Bion, W. (1962). *Learning from experience*. Maresfield.

Blotzer, M. & Ruth, R. (1995). *Sometimes you just want to feel like a human being.* Paul H Brookes Publishing Co.

Botha, M. & Watermeyer, B. (2024). Metanarratives of visual impairment rehabilitation: The discursive positioning of disabled service users in South Africa. *Disability & Society*, *39*(2), 381–399. https://doi.org/10.1080/09687599.2022.2071232

Broderick, A., & Lalvani, P. (2017). Dysconscious ableism: Toward a liberatory praxis in teacher education. *International Journal of Inclusive Education, 21*(9), 894–905. https://doi.org/10.1080/13603116.2017.1296034

Casement, P. (2014). *On learning from the patient.* Routledge.

Cheng, A. A. (2000). *The melancholy of race: Psychoanalysis, assimilation, and hidden grief.* Oxford University Press.

Davis, L. J. (1997). Introduction: The need for disability studies. In L. Davis (Ed.), *The disability studies reader* (pp. 1–6). Routledge.

De Groef, J. & Heinemann, E. (Eds.). (1999). *Psychoanalysis and mental handicap.* Free Association Books.

Ferguson, P. M. (2001). Mapping the family: Disability studies and the exploration of parental response to disability. In G. Albrecht, K. Seelman, & M. Bury (Eds.), *Handbook of disability studies* (pp. 373–395). Thousand Oaks: Sage Publications.

French, S. (1993). "Can you see the rainbow?" The roots of denial. In J. Swain, V. Finkelstein, S. French, & M. Oliver (Eds.), *Disabling barriers – enabling environments* (pp. 69–77). Sage Publications.

Frosh, S. (2006). *For and against psychoanalysis* (2nd ed.). Routledge.
Goodley, D. & Lawthom, R. (Eds.). (2006). *Disability and psychology: Critical introductions and reflections*. Palgrave Macmillan.
Goodley, D. & Runswick-Cole, K. (2010). Emancipating play: Dis/abled children, development and deconstruction. *Disability & Society*, *25*(4), 499–512. https://doi.org/10.1080/09687591003755914
Harris, A. & Wideman, D. (1988). The construction of gender and disability in early attachment. In M. Fine & A. Asch (Eds.), *Women with disabilities: Essays in psychology, culture and politics* (pp. 115–138). Temple University Press.
Hughes, B. (2019). *A historical sociology of disability: Human validity and invalidity from antiquity to early modernity*. Routledge.
Kittay, E. F. (2011). The ethics of care, dependence, and disability. *Ratio Juris*, *24*(1), 49–58. https://doi.org/10.1111/j.1467-9337.2010.00473.x
Kohut, H. (1972). Thoughts on narcissism and narcissistic rage. *The Psychoanalytic Study of the Child*, *27*(1), 360–400. https://doi.org/10.1080/00797308.1972.11822721
Linton, S. (1998). *Claiming disability: Knowledge and identity.* NY University Press.
Lourens, H., Watermeyer, B., & Swartz, L. (2018). Ties that bind, and double bind: Visual impairment, help, and the shaping of relationship. *Disability & Rehabilitation*, *41*(16), 1890–1897. https://doi.org/10.1080/09638288.2018.1450454.
Lussier, A. (1980). The physical handicap and the body ego. *International Journal of Psycho-Analysis*, *61*, 179–185.
Marks, D. (1999). *Disability: Controversial debates and psychosocial perspectives.* Routledge.
Marks, D. (2002). Introduction: Counselling, therapy and emancipatory praxis. *Disability Studies Quarterly*, *22*(3), 1–5.
McWilliams, N. (1994). *Psychoanalytic diagnosis.* The Guilford Press.
Murphy, R. F. (1987). *The body silent: The different world of the disabled.* Henry Holt & Company.
Oliver, M. (1996). The social model in context. In *Understanding disability: From theory to practice* (pp. 30–42). Palgrave Macmillan. https://doi.org/10.1007/978-1-349-24269-6_4
Olkin, R. (1999). *What psychotherapists should know about disability.* The Guilford Press.
Olkin, R. (2014). *Disability-affirmative therapy: A case formulation approach.* Oxford University Press.
Parens, E. (Ed.) (2006). *Surgically shaping children: Technology, ethics, and the pursuit of normality*. Johns Hopkins University Press.
Reeve, D. (2004). Counselling and disabled people: Help or hindrance? In J. Swain, V. Finkelstein, S. French & M. Oliver (Eds.), *Disabling barriers - enabling environments* (2nd ed., pp. 233–238). Sage Publications.
Rohleder, P., Watermeyer, B., Hunt, X., Braathen, S., & Swartz, L. (2019). Impairment, socialization and embodiment: The sexual oppression of people with disabilities. *Psychoanalysis, Culture & Society*, *24*(3), 260–281. https://doi.org/10.1057/s41282-019-00128-6
Rustin, M. (1991). *The good society and the inner world: Psychoanalysis, politics and culture*. Verso.
Samuels, A. (1993). *The political psyche.* Routledge.
Shakespeare, T. (2014). *Disability rights and wrongs revisited.* Routledge.
Swain, J., & French, S. (2001). The relationship between disabled people and health and welfare professionals. In G. L. Albrecht, K. D. Seelman, & M. Bury (Eds.), *Handbook of disability studies* (pp. 734–746). Thousand Oaks, CA: Sage Publications.
Thomas, C. (1999). *Female forms: Experiencing and understanding disability.* University Press.
Watermeyer, B. (2002). Blindness, attachment and self: Psychoanalysis and ideology. *Free Associations*, *49*, 335–352.

Watermeyer, B. (2006). Disability and psychoanalysis. In B. Watermeyer, L. Swartz, M. Schneider, T. Lorenzo, & M. Priestley (Eds.), *Disability and social change: A South African agenda* (pp. 31–43). HSRC Press.

Watermeyer, B. (2009). Claiming loss in disability. *Disability & Society*, *24*(1), 91–102. https://doi.org/10.1080/09687590802535717

Watermeyer, B. (2012a). Is it possible to create a politically engaged, contextual psychology of disability? *Disability & Society*, *27*(2), 161–174. https://doi.org/10.1080/09687599.2011.644928

Watermeyer, B. (2012b). Disability and countertransference in group psychotherapy: Connecting social oppression with the clinical frame. *International Journal of Group Psychotherapy*, *62*(3), 393–417. https://doi.org/10.1521/ijgp.2012.62.3.392

Watermeyer, B. (2013). *Towards a contextual psychology of disablism.* Routledge.

Watermeyer, B. (2014). Disability and loss: The psychological commodification of identity. *Psychology Journal*, *11*(2), 99–107.

Watermeyer, B. (2017). 'I don't have time for an emotional life': Marginalization, dependency and melancholic suspension in disability. *Culture, Medicine, and Psychiatry*, *41*(1), 142–160. https://doi.org/10.1007/s11013-016-9503-x

Watermeyer, B. (2018). Growing up disabled: Impairment, familial relationships and identity. In K. Runswick-Cole, T. Curran, & K. Liddiard (Eds.), *The Palgrave handbook of disabled children's childhood studies* (pp. 443–460). Palgrave.

Watermeyer, B. & McKenzie, J. (2014). Mothers of disabled children: In mourning or on the march? *Journal of Social Work Practice*, *28*(4), 405–416. https://doi.org/10.1080/02650533.2014.889103

Watermeyer, B., McKenzie, J., & Kelly, J. (2024). Dealing with disability as 'matter out of place': Emotional issues in the education of learners with visual impairment. *International Journal of Inclusive Education*, *1*(1), 1–16. https://doi.org/10.1080/13603116.2022.2092780

Watermeyer, B. & McKinney, V. (2022). Disability, relationship, and the negotiation of loss. *BMJ Medical Humanities*, *48*(1), 2–8. https://doi.org/10.1136/medhum-2020-011860

Watermeyer, B. & Swartz, L. (2008). Conceptualising the psycho-emotional aspects of disability and impairment: The distortion of personal and psychic boundaries. *Disability & Society*, *23*(6), 599–610. https://doi.org/10.1080/09687590802328477

Watermeyer, B. & Swartz, L. (2016). Disablism, identity and self: Discrimination as a traumatic assault on subjectivity. *Journal of Community & Applied Social Psychology*, *26*(3), 268–276. https://doi.org/10.1002/casp.2266

Wendell, S. (1996). *The rejected body: Feminist philosophical reflections on disability.* Routledge.

Bibliography

Gibson, B. E. (2016). *Rehabilitation: A post-critical approach.* CRC Press.

9

THE COUNTERACTIVE VALUE OF DISABILITY-AFFIRMATIVE THERAPY

How Well-Meaning Assumptions ("I don't see disability") Impact Disabled Clients

Katy Evans and Mel Halacre

Introduction

We chose a title that includes the statement "I don't see disability" because at first glance, this phrase seems positive and empowering, but when we dig a bit deeper, we immediately realise it is not. It is a common statement made, or thought about, by therapists in relation to their disabled clients. Providing access and support to disabled people is so often seen as a positive practice, couched in kindness, so it can be difficult to access the hidden assumptions and uncomfortable feelings that lie underneath these words. We hope to uncover some of these hidden processes in this chapter and explore how we can provide more positive, empowering disability affirming therapy, or DAT as we will call it hereafter.

Note on Language

Throughout this chapter, we will use the term 'disabled' instead of 'impairment'. Both terms are often used interchangeably. In the absence of more suitable alternatives, we will use 'disabled' to reflect the idea that "the disadvantage or restriction caused by a contemporary social organisation which takes no or little account of people who have impairments, excludes them from the mainstream of social activities" (Barnes, 2012). This belief system is in line with the social model of disability described in several other parts of this handbook.

Both authors recognise that impairments vary widely, and our aim is to provide some sort of overview of disability-affirmative therapy (DAT), whilst acknowledging that it may not reflect everybody's experience, and therefore this chapter

DOI: 10.4324/9781003362586-16

is not a complete guide. We also recognise that many disabled people classified as disabled by the Equality Act of 2010 do not consider themselves thus or prefer the people-first term 'person with a disability'. We also recognise that impairments can be apparent, non-apparent, congenital, acquired, or a combination of these.

The Need for Specialist Services

Specialist disability-affirmative services are needed because many disabled people struggle to find accessible services, and experience iatrogenic harm in the process of doing so. Individuals that do manage to find an accessible service, often have negative experiences of the process. Of course, in an ideal world, specialist services would not be needed; a disabled client could pick a therapist from a directory, be certain they were accessible, and experience a non-prejudiced understanding of client experiences.

However, like all humans, many therapists are unaware of their own hidden attitudes and beliefs towards disability. Without this awareness, therapists reproduce societal oppression in the therapy room (Reeve, 2002; Hunt, 2023). Common responses that we may experience as therapists surround feelings of shame or guilt for our reactions, which lead to us then trying to 'fix' the client. We may, in therapy, mistakenly assign someone's issues to an impairment. On the other hand, we may instead deny the existence of an impairment. It is also common to feel overwhelmed by the complexity of people's situations (Wright, 1960, p. 113; Marini and Stebnicki, 2012). In this chapter, we explore why therapy with disabled people needs to be different, the need for affirmative therapy, and how affirmative practices can have an impact on both the therapist and the client experience. We will conclude this chapter with some strategies that therapists can learn to work more affirmatively in their practice.

Disabled Clients' Experiences of Therapy

Not much is changing within the therapy field because there are few disabled therapists, supervisors, and trainers (Parritt, 2012; Hunt, 2023). Many disabled people state that emotional stress stems from their relationship with others, not the impairment itself (Oliver, 1995; Thomas, 2012; Reeve, 2014b; Liddiard, 2018). Yet, the focus within training programs remains on the individual impairment rather than the impact of society's treatment of disabled people, causing further psychological harm to clients (Hunt, 2023). Therapy models were developed during an era of segregation (Barnes, 1991) and this history, combined with the universal fear of difference, further perpetuates exclusion. In fact, there are indications that a preference for 'able bodied' over 'disabled' may already exist by the time children begin primary school (Weinberg, 1978). The authors believe that this has created a stronger power imbalance than what already exists in the therapy room by way of the provider-client dynamic (McLeod, 1998; Watermeyer, 2012).

Therapists are subject to the prevalent negative connotations, images and symbols around disability and impairment as others in society (Olkin, 1999). There is some evidence that therapist's attitude towards disability affects the services rendered (Reeve, 2014a; Watermeyer, 2013; Fish 1986). Of particular interest is the study by Smart and Smart (2006) which demonstrated that few therapists considered impairment and disability as a strength or a resource for fulfilling one's potential. If we as therapists do not see disability as a resource and have little hope for our clients' lives, how can a positive outcome for therapy be reached?

There are many authors highlighting examples of this oppression in the therapy room. Some of these forms of oppression include understanding anger as a denial of impairment rather than a valid reaction to society's response to disability, expressing disbelief at the refusal to undergo medical treatment, thereby making assumptions about someone's needs or preferences. Other examples include assuming a disabled client cannot have children, the client educating the therapist about what it means to be disabled, or endorsing the 'supercrip' stereotype of 'overcoming in spite of impairment'. (Olkin, 1999; Reeve, 2002, 2014; Withers, 1996; Hunt, 2023). Some clients express that their therapist simply did not understand the complexity of the lived experience of disability (Reeve, 2014), which has certainly been this author's personal experiences as well. In 2019, Ashley Cox, a disabled person with a visual impairment, described in a newspaper article, the experience of being turned down from therapy eight times, with many therapists directly citing his visual impairment as the reason ('Dilemma: Disabled access', 2019). Ashley is still searching in 2023 and has contacted over 100 therapists to date, as per a personal conversation between this author and Ashley.

If a therapist does not understand the disempowering impacts of the systematic exclusion of disabled people, it is nearly impossible to provide effective therapy. One needs knowledge of internalised oppression; when repeated negative messages, and microaggressions, are internalised and believed by the recipient:

> We harbour inside ourselves the pain and the memories, the fears and the confusions, the negative self-images and the low expectations, turning them into weapons with which to re-injure ourselves, every day of our lives.
>
> (Mason, 1992)

If one does not understand how cumulative ongoing traumatic experiences contribute to low self-esteem, learned helplessness, and hopelessness, disabled clients may seem "too challenging" to work with. Trying to hold on to power, choice and control, a person may appear difficult, controlling, and angry (Olkin, 2017). Yet, through a disability affirmative approach, we see that these reactions are understandable in the context and complexities of disabled people's lives.

The Impact of Ableism/Disablism

Although ableism and disablism are often used interchangeably, they have slightly different meanings. Within this chapter, the authors take the viewpoint that ableism refers to the multifaceted privileging of non-disabled people and disablism relates to the resultant oppression and exclusion of disabled people. Liddiard (2018) notes that both oppression and exclusion frequently work in conjunction, driving each other. In recent times, this was seen painfully clearly in global reactions to the COVID-19 pandemic and the scant prioritisation of disabled people, sometimes going as far as questioning their right to life-saving treatment (Evans, Whitney-Mitchell, and Liddiard, 2022).

Disablism sits within other social oppressions such as sexism, racism, and homophobia. However, it is interesting to note that whilst these inequalities are being increasingly addressed in therapy training, disability as a result of oppression continues to be overlooked (Reeve, 2014; British Psychological Society, 2017; Murphy, 2017). Linking back to the phrase used in this chapter title 'I don't see disability', this takes quite a literal meaning, yet it does not hold the beneficial impact that the speaker thinks it does. Whilst other minorities continue to experience oppression in therapy despite advancements in training, a therapist openly saying they ignore someone's minority status is unlikely to be declared in such an overt way of assumed beneficence.

People's opportunities can be limited by disablism which can in turn affect their mental health and their sense of self. The often imposed 'sick role' of the medical model (Devore and Schlesinger, 1999) has prevented many disabled adults from taking the same risks and learning from mistakes as other adults (Mackelprang and Salsgiver, 2016). In addition, reduced opportunities are frequently imposed on disabled people. The UK's period of austerity has particularly affected disabled people through reduced welfare support and budget cuts (Ryan, 2019; Clifford, 2020). How can disabled people have the same opportunities as everyone else if they do not have the required support to dress and eat, let alone leave their homes? Understandably, the impact this has on their mental wellbeing is significant and circles back to Hunt's (2023) call that therapy with disabled people must recognise the socio-political factors which complicate their lives beyond individual impairment.

The impact of this disablism can be the client experiencing internalised oppression whereby a disabled person feels worthless, unattractive, and disgusting as a result of external attitudes (Thomas, 2004). The combination of this external and internal oppression leads to psycho-social disablism which can have significant impacts on disabled people's mental wellbeing. It can also lead to them exerting labour to counteract this by attempting to enable their social inclusion (Reeve, 2014). Reeve (2004) notes that disablism is often perpetuated by those closest to the person whom they trust the most, causing a greater degree of hurt. She goes on to highlight that therapists who adhere to individual models of disability can fall into the trap of pathologising disabled people's understandable reactions. For example, if a wheelchair user expresses frustration about not being able to access public spaces, they are unlikely to find meaningful support from a therapist who views this to be denial of their impairment as opposed to a reaction to discrimination. This is why DAT is needed so that therapists avoid perpetuating the harmful messages often encountered in society.

Although acknowledgement of external factors in disabled people's lives is vital, there is also space and a need in DAT to acknowledge embodied experiences of disability. Whilst the social model focuses on the external factors of disability, many disabled scholars have critiqued the social model for overlooking the need to also make space to discuss impairment effects (Crow, 1996; Lonsdale, 1990; Thomas, 1999; Wendell, 1996; Liddiard, 2018). The consequence of this is that embodied effects of impairment are silenced despite often continuing beyond the removal of external barriers. Therapists practising DAT need to navigate the delicate balance of holding both, whilst not colluding with the individualisation of the medical model. The degree of navigation provided on the part of the therapist will depend on where the client is in their disability journey, and this is likely to fluctuate in different stages of life and different individual contexts.

Epistemic Injustice

The forms of oppression mentioned above can also be seen as epistemic injustice. Fricker (2017) defines epistemic injustice as the unfair approaches of how knowledge is formed and valued. These approaches lead one to question the person's capacity to construct knowledge about themselves. This can take the form of silencing, ignoring, distorting meanings, dismissing lived experience and unfair power dynamics which marginalise people on multiple levels. Ho (2011) describes disabled people to be particularly susceptible to epistemic injustice due to their reliance on professionals' decisions, and their reduced power to challenge these norms. This power imbalance is frequently evidenced in the language that disabled people use to describe their interactions with services, which include terms like 'fight, 'battle', 'battleground', 'dictate', 'exhausted', 'survived' (Evans, Whitney-Mitchell, and Runswick-Cole, 2022). This is even more striking when one considers the large number of professionals that many disabled people must engage with. A participant in Norberg's (2022, p. 662) research stated that in one year, she had contact with over 200 professionals, repeatedly explaining her requirements but often feeling unheard, which negatively impacted her wellbeing. She stated: "I feel like a ball that is thrown around and never received".

Indeed, Katy, one of our authors, experienced this when she underwent a mental health crisis in 2020 and was passed around between almost 40 professionals in the span of eight weeks. Few providers could provide the physical access she needed, and even fewer were able to truly listen to her experiences as a disabled abuse survivor. Katy's suicidal feelings were dangerously dismissed when professionals wrongly assumed that she would be unable to take her life due to being disabled; inaccurately imposing their assumptions about disabled life onto her, instead of listening to her reality. This is despite disabled people in the UK being over four times more likely to die by suicide than non-disabled people (Disability Rights UK, 2023). Moreover, research on mental health experiences frequently excludes anyone who has pre-existing conditions, which further silences the voices of disabled people and limits how mainstream mental health knowledge can then be applied to disabled people's lives (Spandler, Anderson, and Sapey, 2015).

Both authors have frequently heard therapists say the phrase "I don't see disability". Whilst they undoubtedly mean this to be positive, underneath this is an inherent assumption that disability is 'bad', and the disabled person will be pleased that the therapist can look past this. In our experience, this is inaccurate and potentially harmful. It ties into epistemic injustice in that it ignores and silences the lived reality of disabled people. Katy says most of her therapy experiences have not been centred on disability. However, she goes on to say that disability is an important factor in her life and to ignore this would be failing to see her lived experiences and the whole person that she is.

Higher Prevalence of Trauma

Often, disability or the impairment is seen as the root of the disabled person's problems (Reeve, 2014b). But when we are trauma informed, we realise that trauma is often at the root of most people's challenges, be they disabled or non-disabled. As mentioned before, trauma is very prevalent in the lives of disabled people (Jones et al., 2012) and takes on many forms. We often think about accidents as trauma but forget that a medical diagnosis can cause a similar level of trauma, as can discrimination, exclusion and hate crimes (Disability Hate Crime, 2019). Often ignored is the daily accumulation of psycho-emotional disablism: experiences where you feel silenced, not heard, or not seen for who you are but rather viewed as a projection of what someone else fantasises about you (Reeve, 2014; Watermeyer and Swartz, 2016).

We often forget to consider that even medical interventions aimed at healing can cause trauma because of the involvement of anaesthetics, poor bedside manners by consultants, children being separated from caregivers, being restrained, or having painful or embarrassing procedures involving needing to be naked in front of health professionals. Reeve (2006) suggests that this amounts to accepted institutional abuse which leaves disabled people feeling vulnerable, exposed, and humiliated. Coombs exemplifies this:

> I dissociate in medical settings because I don't feel I am of much importance in the room. My body is, but particularly when I was growing up, my thoughts, feelings and opinions on what was happening to me, or being done to me, were almost never sought…and in those circumstances it's easier to

> mentally go elsewhere than engage with that sense of feeling otherness and wrongness.
>
> (Coombs, 2019, p. 172)

Katy echoes Coomb's words as someone who has had medical involvement since birth. She is also a survivor of childhood sexual abuse and believes these two experiences are inherently linked through the expectations of compliance and boundary violations she experienced in medical settings, which were later re-enacted in the abuse (Evans, 2021). Those of us who are trauma-informed understand that trauma has the potential to lead to opportunities: the development of new skills and abilities or chances to change our direction in life (Smart and Smart, 2006).

> According to several Buddhist and Taoist traditions, sex, meditation, death, and trauma share a common potential. These are the great portals – catalysts for… surrender and awakening.
>
> (Levine, 2005, p. 79)

Without trauma-informed approaches in therapy, it is difficult to support disabled people with lasting change and the skills to counter the daily stress and micro-traumas that occur almost constantly in the lives of disabled people.

The Critical Need for Disability-Affirmative Therapy

Isolation

Disabled people are often both practically and psychologically isolated, which has impacts on the therapy experience. For example, they may struggle to attend in-person appointments due to transport or support issues, pain, or fatigue. Many therapy services have very rigid cancellation policies, which make consistent attendance challenging for some clients. They may also be practically isolated because they have lost important people around them due to disability or have limited access to social and recreational venues that offer opportunities to socialise.

On a more unobservable level, disabled people are more isolated because they are usually surrounded by non-disabled people. This means that they do not see themselves reflected at home or in society (Gill, 2001). The disability they do see in society and the media is often portrayed negatively or is conceptualised as something to overcome, much like a superhero is expected to do in mainstream cinema.

During therapy however, psychological isolation is an important experience to consider. Much therapy training is about encouraging independence and eliciting related information from our clients. However, some disabled clients experiencing psychological isolation have been unable to share all parts of themselves with those around them because of how others have responded to them. They experience a kind of self-imposed silencing or bumping up against a "glass ceiling" in their relationships with others. Consequently, they may be very reluctant to show a non-disabled therapist what is beyond this glass ceiling.

Lack of Access to Services

Therapy services can be inaccessible in two ways: They can be physically inaccessible, for wheelchair users for example, or they can be inaccessible because the therapist is unable to work with them in an affirming way due to their own personal biases. Both areas need to be addressed for truly accessible therapy provision.

Like Ashley's situation, described above in Section "Introduction", Katy, one of the authors of this chapter and a disabled person herself, recently spent almost two years seeking a private therapist to work with in the UK. During this process, she encountered many therapists who had no wheelchair access, were unwilling to make any adjustments, and who lacked an accurate understanding of disability. In total, she contacted almost 200 therapists. The rejections she experienced reflected the trauma for which she was seeking therapy, resulting in further perpetuation of her trauma. This highlights Hunt's (2023) observation that therapy can harm disabled people through its inaccessibility and lack of socio-political understanding. At many points, Katy considered giving up, in order to protect her mental health. When the very act of seeking therapy can traumatise disabled clients, things urgently need to change.

In terms of physical access, we often think of ramps and accessible toilets, but there are many other factors to consider. For example, people who have assistive speech devices or personal assistants and need time to set up, those with service animals, those who need an interpreter or hearing loop must also be considered. Additionally, less obvious accommodations such as lighting and noise are also critical factors in affirmative care. Physical access also includes attention to session frequency, cadence, and length. For many disabled people, these factors need to be altered to cater to their energy and cognitive availabilities.

When a therapy space is inaccessible, telephone or online therapy is often offered as a reasonable adjustment. However, it is worth mentioning that for many people, this may not be suitable either. For example, for those with visual, speech, or hearing impairments, or those who have experienced trauma, (of which this is a high percentage), telehealth may not be the most appropriate form of treatment. At Spokz People, we estimate around 70% of our clients have experienced major or complex trauma. In these cases, it may be necessary to hire an alternative venue, explore working outside, hire an interpreter, or offer home visits. There are also unpaid voice to text interpretation services that may be suitable if the client and therapist mutually agree that therapy would be effective this way. Some video software also offers speech captioning, which may be useful. Even with accessible services and reasonable adjustments, many disabled people face assumptions, silencing, and harmful comments, leading to therapy termination and worsening mental health. These well-intentioned therapist responses often stem from a lack of training and awareness about living as a disabled person in a hostile, excluding environment.

Common questions disabled clients are asked in therapy often revolve around how to live well with continually relinquishing power and how to live when there is little control or independence, especially when you are assigned to a stigmatised minority. As therapists, we need to have given these questions some thought for ourselves, to provide DAT to our clients.

> We need therapists …who are used to confronting the depth of despair with their clients, whilst keeping their eyes on the possibilities ahead. We can never fake authenticity or existential courage. We can only help people to go as far as we have gone ourselves in our own lives.
>
> (Emmy Van Deurzen, Therapy Today, June 2020, p. 29)

Working Affirmatively: Strategies to Practice Disability Affirmative Therapy

Language and Communication

Currently, there is a lot of conflict surrounding discourse on identity, language, and terminology used among minority groups. This is challenging to navigate as therapists because it increases our fear of 'getting it wrong'. However, working affirmatively means being intentional about the language that we use when discussing disability and putting aside our fear of 'getting it wrong'. Therapists must enquire what terms the disabled person would prefer to use during sessions. In the same way, we might ask how a client's name is pronounced; we can ask what disability language a client prefers.

Discussing terminology is also helpful because we can observe how clients describe themselves. For example, if they use derogatory language (e.g. cripple) we can explore whether this is a view of themselves stemming from internalised oppression or shame, or whether they are taking back and turning around previously offensive words (e.g. the term 'queer' for the LGBTQ+ community or the term 'Crip' for the disabled community).

When it comes to communication, certain impairments such as those related to hearing, visual and speech, may impact the ability to communicate with the client. Many therapists understandably feel awkward and embarrassed if they do not understand the client. However, it is important to remember that a client with such an impairment is probably used to repeating themselves. A useful strategy is to have an open discussion regarding communication with the client before therapy commences. For example, sometimes we (authors) have agreed to allow a personal assistant to sit in during the first few sessions to support therapist's understanding of client communication.

Owning Discomfort

When people attend our training, they come in expecting to be given tips around how to work with their Deaf client or how to adapt their sessions for someone with a visual impairment/s. However, the core of our training focuses on building therapists' personal awareness. It places emphasis on recognising that whether you are a disabled or a non-disabled therapist, we all have a relationship with disability in some way. Disability can work in mysterious, complex, and unconscious ways, and is the only minority group to which we can all unexpectedly end up belonging to overnight.

Perhaps even reading this, you may experience an internal reaction to us saying that you at some point in your own life will be disabled, if you are not already. This response is common and understandable. Our work as therapists lies in addressing how to prevent our response from negatively impacting our therapeutic work. This centres around owning our discomfort and shame for any negative feelings that this internal response may entail. There is also tremendous opportunity within this process. Whether you are a disabled or non-disabled therapist, disability as a discourse offers us a choice to stop denying the truths that we are immortal, in control, and independent. We can use our personal therapy as well as supervision to explore these themes, and our own lives can be personally enriched because of what our clients bring in, challenging us to explore possibilities for truly affirmative care.

Allowing Space for Anger

As discussed earlier, so often disabled people are not allowed to be angry. Valerie Sinason (1992) discusses the "handicap smile" that she observed around disabled people with learning-related limitations. She coined this term to describe a smile she often saw which she believed was masking how disabled people were truly feeling; scared, angry, and/or upset. She writes that their true feelings were not allowed to be expressed. Generally, disabled people are expected to be grateful for any reasonable adjustments or inclusion they are offered. If unwanted assistance is given, and the disabled person responds angrily, they are often viewed as being unreasonable. A significant amount of healing can happen if anger is named and validated in the therapy room. One of the limitations of Cognitive Behaviour Therapy and related approaches is that clients often report that they are told to 'relax' or challenge ways of thinking, when a disabled person's thoughts are not the primary concern, disablement and inaccessibility are. Progress is not achievable unless clients have been given space to voice and process their experiences of years of silenced anger.

Disability Spread

This section describes the idea of 'disability spread'. It helps clinicians determine what parts of the presenting issue we can assign to an individual's impairment, and how much to assign to someone's response to disablement. There is a tendency to either assign all symptoms to the impairments (e.g., health professionals saying, "of course you are depressed, you are disabled", thereby missing secondary health diagnosis) or to completely deny its presence. The challenge that we face as therapists is to allow space for both. In conceptualisation, we need to consider the role of family systems and recognise that a disabled person's impairment may be a convenient scapegoat for other issues already present within the family (Haydon-Laurelut, 2011). It is essential to create space for clients to determine the extent to which their impairment contributes to the presenting issues.

Third Parties

As mentioned earlier, third parties are often involved in disabled people's lives, and during the initial phases of treatment, therapists must discuss with the client if and how to involve the third party in sessions. For example, a client may need a support worker before or during sessions to set up equipment or relay information. A client may have an interpreter or a service animal who needs to be present during the session. Sometimes a client may live in a care facility and there may be intrusions from care home staff. Discussions must be had around what is a suitable space for conducting therapy, even if not conventional. For example, although generally, a bedroom would be seen by most therapies as an unsuitable space to conduct therapy, it may provide more privacy than a group lounge for some disabled clients who do not have the privilege of full privacy.

Third-party relationships can be complex, and clients may feel ambivalent about them, even when these parties must be involved in therapy. However, with thoughtful and timely conversations, these dynamics can support effective therapeutic outcomes. For example, in the case of service animals, discussing their role in therapy with the client can reveal ways that these animals can enhance clients' engagement in therapy. Some clients experience comfort through their animal's sensitivity to their emotional state and may view the animal's presence as an important source of support during therapy sessions.

In one instance, Mel, a co-author of this chapter, used clicker training to help a client's assistance dog respond more effectively to the client's emotional cues.

Touch

It is difficult to address the nuances of the importance of touch for disabled people in just one chapter. What is important to highlight is that, generally in traditional therapy training, touching clients is often discouraged. However, when working with disabled clients, it may be necessary to incorporate touch for therapeutic and practical purposes. Practically, clients may need assistance to wipe tears or move their bodies. If therapists are not used to this, they may feel awkward about providing this type of assistance. For a disabled person who needs a support worker for daily living, they are used to this flexibility in boundaries.

It is also important to consider clients' cultural backgrounds and past experiences with regards to touch. A disabled client may have had past experiences of being touched in a harmful way medically, particularly in childhood, while being restrained during procedures. There is also higher prevalence of sexual abuse in childhood; how does a child differentiate between a doctor hurting them for a medical procedure, and an abuser? Consequently, disabled children and young adults are often targets of sexual exploitation (Pearce, 2019). Depending on their developmental history and impairments, some clients may only have experienced touch from care providers. They may use mobility aids, which prevent them from getting physically close to loved ones. Additionally, many non-disabled individuals often feel uncomfortable around disabled people and may avoid gestures like handshakes or hugs, which only reinforces social distance and exclusion. With appropriate discussions around consent during the initial phase of therapy, along with supervision and training, therapeutic touch can be used intentionally to counteract the harmful effects of past touch experiences.

Reasonable Adjustments: How Can We Be Proactive?

Many countries have equality legislation which *should* protect disabled people from experiences of inaccessibility and discrimination. In the UK, we have the Equality Act of 2010, which is applicable to all services offered to the public, including therapy. Within this act, service providers are required to make 'reasonable adjustments' to enable disabled people to access the service. This might include adjusting the session length, booking a wheelchair accessible room, or using online methods of conducting therapy.

However, what qualifies as a "reasonable adjustment" remains contested. The legal provision for such adjustments can, in practice, sanction spatial segregation such as requiring disabled individuals to use back entrances, fostering feelings of inferiority and second-class citizenship. Ironically, while intended to remove structural barriers, these measures can create new psycho-emotional obstacles. When adjustments are experienced as degrading or humiliating, they are effectively unusable, leaving the disabled person excluded from full participation in public spaces or activities (Reeve, 2014).

Katy (author) has previously written about the emotional impact that inaccessible therapy spaces and attitudes have had on her. Despite the Equality Act legislation, 70% of the therapists in her directory searches did not have wheelchair access (Evans, 2021). Notably, the Equality Act includes an 'anticipatory duty', which requires service providers to proactively consider and address access needs, rather than waiting for a disabled person to request accommodations. This means that accessibility should be regularly reviewed and improved in advance, ensuring that barriers are removed before they are encountered.

Therapists strive to value people in the work they do with them. Therefore, therapists also have a moral duty to ensure no one is excluded from their service. As disabled activist Mia Mingus (2018) writes, access can convey deeper meanings of value, visibility, and acceptance. Many clients within our practice report that proactivity from professionals and services is greatly healing and empowering. It has the potential to reduce a lot of the emotional labour and iatrogenic harm they experience. Are these not the very foundations on which effective therapeutic practice is based?

Assessments and Formulations

We have described the systematic ways that our society excludes and discriminates disabled people. In therapy practices, assessment procedures place all the power in the hands of an assessor. This assessor often has no lived experience of disability and yet decides what somebody's health should entail. As a result, the assessment process can reinforce systemic inequalities and deny disabled individuals' meaningful agency over their own care. Since it is so frequently requested (or demanded), intrusive paperwork is another common occurrence in the lives of disabled people. One participant in Norberg's (2022) study expressed the frustration and discomfort of having to explain her life to 200 professionals in just one year during this intake process.

Effective assessments help us understand client concerns and determine our ability to support them. Timing for paperwork is key here and should be considered, whether it is completed after sessions, or collaboratively during them. If done in-session, therapists must be mindful that clients are paying for that time. Historically, paperwork about disabled individuals is often completed without their input, leading to errors that are hard to correct. Involving clients in reviewing and editing paperwork empowers them and supports their autonomy.

Client formulations are typically developed privately but sharing them can be especially valuable when working with disabled clients. As clients process trauma, discrimination, and impairment-related experiences, formulations may evolve. Olkin (2017) offers a comprehensive guide to disability-affirmative assessment practices, recommending an exploration of disability status, developmental history, use of disability models, connection to disability culture, and internalised societal messages. For those new to this work, her book is a key resource to support affirming, context-rich formulations. This is important to learn, since to work in a disability affirmative way is to minimise the chance of repeated trauma within our therapeutic procedures.

Challenging Boundaries

We have discussed the concept of boundaries in the context of DAT earlier in this chapter, but mention it again in this section, since it is one of the major obstacles to providing effective therapy for disabled clients. Though an important component of therapists' training centres the enforcement of effective and safe boundaries with clients, there is minimal discussion on how boundaries need to be flexed for certain clients. As mentioned above, boundaries are often blurred if you need physical assistance frequently. Watermeyer (2013) devotes an entire chapter on describing how boundaries are frequently ignored and overstepped when you are disabled. Due to fairly rigid boundaries being a central part of traditional therapy training, it is understandable to experience discomfort around flexing boundaries, alongside the fear of 'getting it wrong'.

Sometimes therapists create personal boundaries that are used defensively, in a way to protect their own feelings of discomfort. In DAT, it may be necessary to step outside our traditional roles when a client needs assistance in ways that still lie within therapist's scope of competence and practice. For example, sometimes Mel (author) has been an advocate for and has written supporting letters to enable therapy to progress. She states, "I have worked outside in parks, in vehicles, bedrooms, care homes and had longer and shorter sessions bimonthly to several times a week". Allowing disabled clients to determine how and when they have their sessions can be empowering when they are rarely given that choice in their relationships with other health and welfare professionals. As we mentioned earlier when discussing epistemic injustice, stepping outside of our traditionally professional roles enables us to sit alongside a client rather than adding to the power differential that already exists within the clinical relationship. More information about working flexibly and holistically can be found in Halacre and Jalil (2017). Many therapists do not want to take on the complexity that sometimes comes with working with a client who has experienced multiple traumas through disablement. But if we as a profession, with access to supervision and personal therapy, do not open our hearts and support people to heal, who will?

Transference

Regardless of your therapeutic orientation, and whether you use the term 'transference' in your practice, most of us are familiar with the concept. Simply put, transference takes place when therapists project personal issues onto clients. If we have internal fears about our degrading bodies, illness, decline and/or death, they may be triggered by what clients bring into therapy, or even merely by what they visually represent in the room. Disability can often bring human myths and aspects of human life into awareness that many of us often strive to deny. For example, as a non-disabled therapist, one might feel anger toward the disabling world, recognising that they, too, are part of the very systems that have contributed to the client's marginalisation. Being aware of any related transference can reduce the risk of harming clients, enabling authentic DAT practices.

Utilising Supervision Differently

When describing her experience with supervision, Mel (author) shares,

> I was very lucky with my first supervisor. He very quickly assessed that I needed to change my way of working, if I wanted to be effective with the clientele that I was working with. He was not knowledgeable about disability,

> but what he did do was encourage me to step outside my comfort zone and try different strategies and approaches to see what would work best. This wisdom was vital in my development as a disability- affirmative therapist.

Within supervision spaces, it is important to reflect on several key considerations and factors, including:

1. Our own fears and anxieties about disability, the fragility of life, illness, degradation, and death, and how this may influence our clinical work.
2. How we can utilise our own experiences of trauma, exclusion, and difference to connect and relate to our clients.
3. How to offer a different approach to 'fixing' or rescuing. The themes and stories related to finding a fix, cure and "treating" a disabled person are prevalent in Western society and must be challenged.
4. Supervision is helpful in discussing 'disability spread'; how to help the client explore what is and isn't related to their impairments.
5. It is important to create a plan around how to address common areas of avoidance such as internalised ableism. Although disability is becoming more present in therapy training, Paluck (2006) suggests that short-term diversity training may in fact reinforce stereotypes and differences. With that in mind, it is far better to look at a sustainable approach and longer-term training to reduce any chance of unconscious biases. Supervision and training offer us safe spaces to process our inherent biases, thereby improving effectiveness (Kemp and Mallinckrodt, 1996).
6. Self-disclosure (or "use-of self) can often be practiced in impactful ways with disabled clients. It can help in strengthening the therapeutic relationship when we disclose our own experiences of exclusion and difference. If you are a disabled therapist, and feel comfortable doing so, it can be helpful to disclose some of your experiences to demonstrate similarities and helpful differences.

Conclusion

This chapter has explored some common barriers that disabled people experience in therapy and demonstrates how DAT practices can be deeply beneficial. Providing therapy services that are not only physically accessible but are also attitudinally affirming is our collective responsibility. We have chosen to conclude our chapter with the words of disabled activist Mia Mingus who defines disability justice as an act of love:

> When I say 'liberatory access', I mean access that is more than simply having a ramp, or being scent free, or providing captions. Access for the sake of access or inclusion is not necessarily liberatory, but access done in the service of love, justice, connection, and community is liberatory and has the power to transform.
>
> (Mingus, 2018)

We hope this chapter and the handbook as a whole has inspired you to join us as an advocate for change, working collectively to transform therapy services into truly inclusive, affirming spaces.

References

Barnes, C. (1991). *Disabled people in Britain and discrimination: A case for anti-discrimination legislation.* Hurst & Co Ltd. in association with the British Council of Organisations of Disabled People.

Barnes, C. (2012). Understanding the social model of disability: Past, present and future. In N. Watson, A. Roulstone, & C. Thomas (Eds.), *Routledge handbook of disability studies* (pp. 12–29). London, England: Routledge. https://doi.org/10.4324/9780203144114

BBC News. (2019, October 9). *Disability hate crime: Number of reports rising*. https://www.bbc.co.uk/news/uk-wales-54433753

British Psychological Society. (2017). *Practice guidelines* (3rd ed.). https://www.bps.org.uk/guideline/bps-practice-guidelines-2017-0

Clifford, E. (2020). *The war on disabled people: Capitalism, welfare and the making of a human catastrophe*. Zed Books Ltd.

Coombs, C. (2019). Disability, depression and the language of disorder. In J. Watson (Ed.), *Drop the disorder: Challenging the culture of psychiatric diagnosis* (pp. 168–173). PCCS Books Ltd.

Crow, L. (1996). Including all of our lives. In J. Morris (Ed.), *Encounters with strangers: Feminism and disability* (pp. 206–226). The Women's Press.

Devore, W., & Schlesinger, E. G. (1999). *Ethnic-sensitive social work practice* (5th ed.). Allyn and Bacon.

Dilemma: Disabled access. (2019, September). *Therapy Today, 30*(7), 44.

Disability Rights UK. (2023). *Disabled people far more likely to die by suicide than non-disabled people.* https://www.disabilityrightsuk.org/news/disabled-people-far-more-likely-die-suicide-non-disabled-people

Equality Act 2010, c.15. https://www.legislation.gov.uk/ukpga/2010/15/contents

Evans, K. (2021, December 3). *I was never taught to say no*. Spokz People. https://spokzpeople.org.uk/2021/12/03/i-was-never-taught-to-say-no/

Evans, K. (2021, December 3). *When getting into the room is the first hurdle: Lack of wheelchair access in therapy services.* Spokz People. https://spokzpeople.org.uk/2021/12/03/when-getting-into-the-room-is-the-first-hurdle-lack-of-wheelchair-access-in-therapy-services/

Evans, K., Whitney-Mitchell, S., & Liddiard, K. (2022). Desiring life and living with death. In K. Liddiard, S. Whitney, L. Watts, K. Evans, E. Vogelmann, R. Spurr, K. Runswick-Cole, & D. Goodley (Eds.), *Living life to the fullest: Disability, youth and voice* (pp. 125–146). Emerald.

Evans, K., Whitney-Mitchell, S., & Runswick-Cole, K. (2022). Labour in the lives of disabled young people. In K. Liddiard, S. Whitney, L. Watts, K. Evans, E. Vogelmann, R. Spurr, K. Runswick-Cole, & D. Goodley (Eds.), *Living life to the fullest: Disability, youth and voice* (pp. 99–114). Emerald.

Fish, D. E. (1986). Disabled persons and death anxiety in counselor trainees. *Journal of Rehabilitation, 52*, 53–55.

Fricker, M. (2017). Evolving concepts of epistemic injustice. In I. J. Kidd, J. Medina, & G. Pohlhaus Jr. (Eds.), *Routledge handbook of epistemic injustice* (pp. 53–60). Routledge.

Gill, C. J. (2001). Divided understanding: The social experience of disability. In G. L. Albrecht, K. D. Seelman, & M. Bury (Eds.), *Handbook of disability studies* (pp. 351–372). Sage.

Halacre, M., & Jalil, R. (2017). Holistic therapy with disabled adults from a social and individual perspective: A service evaluation feasibility study. *Counselling and Psychotherapy Research, 17*(4), 320–329. https://doi.org/10.1002/capr.12137

Haydon-Laurelut, M. (2011). Disablement, systemic therapy and people with learning disabilities. *Context, 7*, 7–11.
Ho, A. (2011). Trusting experts and epistemic humility in disability. *International Journal of Feminist Approaches to Bioethics, 4*(2), 102–123.
Hunt, J. (2023). On the need for structurally competent counselling and psychotherapy: Neoliberal ideology, disability and the psy disciplines. *Counselling and Psychotherapy Research, 23*(3), 598–602. https://doi.org/10.1002/capr.12649
Jones, L., Bellis, M. A., Wood, S., Hughes, K., McCoy, E., Eckley, L., Bates, G., Mikton, C., Shakespeare, T., & Officer, A. (2012). Prevalence and risk of violence against children with disabilities: A systematic review and meta-analysis of observational studies. *The Lancet, 380*(9845), 899–907.
Kemp, N. T., & Mallinckrodt, B. (1996). Impact of professional training on case conceptualization of clients with a disability. *Professional Psychology: Research and Practice, 27*(4), 378–385. https://doi.org/10.1037/0735-7028.27.4.378
Levine, P. A. (2005). *Healing trauma: A pioneering program for restoring the wisdom of your body*. Sounds True.
Liddiard, K. (2018). *The intimate lives of disabled people*. Routledge.
Lonsdale, S. (1990). *Women and disability: The experience of physical disability among women*. Macmillan Education.
Mackelprang, R. W., & Salsgiver, R. O. (2016). *Disability: A diversity model approach in human service practice* (3rd ed.). Lyceum Books.
Marini, I., & Stebnicki, M. A. (Eds.). (2012). *The psychological and social impact of illness and disability* (6th ed.). Springer Publishing Company.
Mason, M. (1992). Internalised oppression. In R. Rieser & M. Mason (Eds.), *Disability equality in the classroom: A human rights issue* (2nd ed., pp. 27–28). Disability Equality in Education.
McLeod, J. (1998). *An introduction to counselling* (2nd ed.). Open University Press.
Mingus, M. (2018, November 3). *"Disability justice" is simply another term for love*. Leaving Evidence. https://leavingevidence.wordpress.com/2018/11/03/disability-justice-is-simply-another-term-for-love/
Murphy, D. (Ed.). (2017). *Counselling psychology: A textbook for study and practice*. BPS John Wiley.
Norberg, I. (2022). Austerity as bureaucratic violence: Understanding the impact of (neoliberal) austerity on disabled people in Sweden. *Sociology, 56*(4), 655–672. https://doi.org/10.1177/00380385211051210
Oliver, J. (1995). Counselling disabled people: A counsellor's perspective. *Disability and Society, 10*(3), 261–280.
Olkin, R. (1999). *What psychotherapists should know about disability*. Guilford Press.
Olkin, R. (2017). *Disability-affirmative therapy: A case formulation template for clients with disabilities*. Oxford University Press.
Paluck, E. L. (2006). Diversity training and intergroup contact: A call to action research. *Journal of Social Issues, 62*(3), 577–595. https://doi.org/10.1111/j.1540-4560.2006.00474.x
Parritt, S. (2012). Disability. In C. Feltham & I. Horton (Eds.), *Handbook of counselling & psychotherapy* (3rd ed., pp. 586–589). Sage.
Pearce, J. (2019). *Child sexual exploitation: Why theory matters*. Policy Press.
Reeve, D. (2002). Oppression within the counselling room. *Counselling and Psychotherapy Research, 2*(1), 11–19. https://doi.org/10.1080/14733140212331384948
Reeve, D. (2004). Counselling and disabled people: A help or a hindrance? In S. French (Ed.), *Disability and psychology: Critical introductions and reflections* (pp. 94–107). Palgrave Macmillan.

Reeve, D. (2006). Towards a psychology of disability: The emotional effects of living in a disabling society. In D. Goodley & R. Lawthom (Eds.), *Disability and psychology: Critical introductions and reflections* (pp. 94–107). Palgrave Macmillan.
Reeve, D. (2014a). Counselling and disabled people: Help or hindrance? In J. Swain, S. French, C. Barnes, & C. Thomas (Eds.), *Disabling barriers – Enabling environments* (3rd ed., pp. 255–261). Sage.
Reeve, D. (2014b). Psycho-emotional disablism and internalised oppression. In J. Swain, S. French, C. Barnes, & C. Thomas (Eds.), *Disabling barriers – Enabling environments* (3rd ed., pp. 92–98). Sage.
Ryan, F. (2019). *Crippled: Austerity and the demonization of disabled people*. Verso Books.
Sinason, V. (1992). *Mental handicap and the human condition: New approaches from the Tavistock*. Free Association Books.
Smart, J. F., & Smart, D. W. (2006). Models of disability: Implications for the counselling profession. *Journal of Counseling and Development, 84*(1), 29–40.
Spandler, H., & Anderson, J. (2015). Unreasonable adjustments? Applying disability policy to madness and distress. In H. Spandler, J. Anderson, & B. Sapey (Eds.), *Madness, distress and the politics of disablement* (pp. 13–26). Policy Press.
Thomas, C. (1999). *Female forms: Experiencing and understanding disability*. Open University Press.
Thomas, C. (2004). Rescuing a social relational understanding of disability. *Scandinavian Journal of Disability Research, 6*(1), 22–36. https://doi.org/10.1080/15017410409512637
Thomas, C. (2012). Theorising disability and chronic illness: Where next for perspectives in medical sociology? *Social Theory & Health, 10*(3), 209–228. https://doi.org/10.1057/sth.2012.7
Van Deurzen, E. (2020, June). The big interview: Surviving and thriving in a global existential crisis. *Therapy Today, 31*(5), 29.
Watermeyer, B. (2012). Disability and countertransference in group psychotherapy: Connecting social oppression with the clinical frame. *International Journal of Group Psychotherapy, 62*, 393–417.
Watermeyer, B. (2013). *Towards a contextual psychology of disablism*. Routledge.
Watermeyer, B. & Swartz, L. (2016). Disablism, identity and self: Discrimination as a traumatic assault on subjectivity. *Journal of Community and Applied Social Psychology, 26*(3), 268–276. https://doi.org/10.1002/casp.2266
Weinberg, N. (1978). Preschool children's perceptions of orthopaedic disability. *Rehabilitation Counseling Bulletin, 21*, 183–189.
Wendell, S. (1996). *The rejected body: Feminist philosophical reflections on disability*. Routledge.
Withers, S. (1996). The experience of counselling. In G. Hales (Ed.), *Beyond disability: Towards an enabling society*. Sage.
Wright, B. A. (1960). *Physical disability: A psychological approach*. New York, NY: Harper & Row.

Bibliography

Oliver, M., & Barnes, C. (2012). *The new politics of disablement*. Palgrave Macmillan.
Swain, J., French, S., Barnes, C., & Thomas, C. (Eds.). (2004). *Disabling barriers – Enabling environments* (2nd ed., pp. 243–248). Sage.

10

THE CRITICAL ROLE OF MARRIAGE AND FAMILY THERAPISTS IN DISABILITY DISCOURSES

Kami L. Gallus, Jennifer L. Jones, Garrett M. Jones, and Natalie M. Richardson

Introduction

The goal of this chapter is to engage therapists and therapists-in-training in a clear, structured exploration of disability, expanding their awareness of disability discourse within systemic therapy. Throughout this chapter, the authors (KG, JJ, and GJ), describe our experiences as a marriage and family therapist (MFT), a mother and developmental disabilities scholar, and a self-advocate. We focus on outlining the steps necessary to expand diversity and equity in systemic family therapy, theory, and practice. Specifically, in this chapter, we will explain the shifts between two primary models of disability. We will then address how these shifts reflect changes in the conceptualization of disabled individuals regarding relationships, mental health, and mental health care. This chapter concludes by offering recommendations for integrating disability studies-informed approaches into systemic therapy research and theory. Throughout this chapter, we refer to the American Psychological Association (2023) language guide for identity-first language, with one exception where we intentionally use person-first language in recognition of the preference of the third author.

Our Lived Experiences

I'm Not the Therapist for You: An MFT's Perspective

I (KG) was well into my career as an MFT – fully licensed, a state and American Association for Marriage and Family Therapy (AAMFT) Approved supervisor,

DOI: 10.4324/9781003362586-17

and part of the core-faculty within a Commission on Accreditation for Marriage and Family Therapy Education (COAMFTE) accredited program – when I was confronted by a critical blind spot in my training within the field of systemic therapy. In the course of a rather mundane, daily conversation, my colleague and friend asked if I could provide any recommendations for therapists who could work with her adult son. This request would come to mark a turning point in my scholarship. My colleague shared that finding a therapist for her son who was experiencing symptoms of anxiety had been challenging. She explained that she had contacted numerous therapists over the years only to hear at the end of the intake phone call or in-person session that the therapist didn't feel comfortable or equipped to work with her son since Garrett has intellectual and developmental disabilities. "I'm not the therapist for you" were words I was trained and had trained numerous therapists to use only rarely and cautiously. This was especially true in response to diverse populations when effective collaboration and appropriate supervision could help serve a strongly underserved population. This is of course not the case if the clinician was certain that the appropriate treatment was outside their scope of competence. Yet, this unspoken message, of frequently being turned away by therapists, was heard repeatedly by my colleague and her family. I have since wrestled for more than a decade with this incongruence plaguing the field of systemic therapy as well as the broader mental health field (Parker & Gallus, 2021). How had the profession I loved and a field advanced by therapists and social scientists I respected, come to seemingly abandon the mental health needs of so many disabled individuals? Where are all the systemic therapists, members of a field that deeply value inclusion and multiculturalism, in the discourse regarding disability?

Disability as Diversity: Where Are the Systemic Therapists?

Disability is a natural component of human diversity. With 15% of people globally and approximately one in four (27%) adults in the United States experiencing disability, disabled individuals make up the world's largest minority group (Centers for Disease Control and Prevention, 2019; World Health Organization, 2019). Disabled individuals are included among protected classes (e.g., race, gender, age, and sexual orientation) and legally covered under anti-discrimination laws in the United States (Americans with Disabilities Act of 1990. Part 1, 1990). However, disability is unique in that it covers a broad range of characteristics. Disability can take many different forms including, but not limited to, sensory (e.g., hearing, visual), physical (e.g., ambulatory or mobility-related), and cognitive (e.g., intellectual; CDC, 2019).

While disabled people have been protected from discrimination by laws for over three decades, the shift beyond simply prohibiting discrimination to ensuring accessibility and equity in mental health care has been slow (Krahn et al., 2015). Disparities in the mental health of disabled individuals have been observed for centuries (Kinne et al., 2004; Lollar, 2002; Simeonsson & Leskinen, 1999).

Disabled adults report higher rates of mental distress and are at a higher risk for mental disorders than adults without disabilities (Cree et al., 2020; Okoro et al., 2021). For disabled individuals, mental health needs often introduce additional challenges in daily life, further impacting a sense of belonging and resilience for an already marginalized and stigmatized population. Despite experiencing consistently higher prevalence rates of mental health diagnoses, disabled individuals also experience significant barriers to accessing mental health care, constituting what Krahn and colleagues (Krahn et al., 2006) termed a "cascade of disparities" (p. 71). The common barriers disabled people face in accessing mental health care include the availability and affordability of care (Douma et al., 2006; M. W. Krauss et al., 2003). As a result of ongoing inequities in mental health, the holistic, biopsychosocial-spiritual well-being of many disabled individuals, as well as their family members, is often overlooked, and therefore, left unaddressed.

Inclusion Includes Disability: A Call to Action

As professionals, systemic therapists are defined by an enduring dedication to nondiscrimination and a respect for diversity. The Code of Ethics for the American Association for Marriage and Family Therapy (AAMFT, 2015) clearly states the professional expectations for nondiscrimination in Standard 1.1: "Marriage and family therapists provide professional assistance to persons without discrimination on the basis of race, age, ethnicity, socioeconomic status, disability, gender, health status, religion, national origin, sexual orientation, gender identity or relationship status." The AAMFT Code of Ethics further outlines two diversity-affirming values that guide the field in "acceptance, appreciation, and inclusion of a diverse membership" and "diversity, equity and excellence in clinical practice, research, education and administration."

Hardy (2016) suggested that the value of diversity in systemic therapy is about *who* the field includes, while the value of equity is about *how* they are treated. For disabled individuals, the field has much work to do. Like other health professions, they are not widely represented in the field of systemic therapy. Besides, many disabled individuals struggle to find mental health professionals willing and/or able to work alongside them in a way that is safe and effective to their mental health treatment. Despite some professionals in human service fields having personal experience or advanced training, most still feel ill-equipped to work with disabled individuals and their families (Werner & Stawski, 2012). The perpetuation of inequitable mental health care is clearly inconsistent with the ethical standards and values of the field of systemic family therapy (American Association for Marriage and Family Therapy, 2015). This stimulates questions about the neglect and exclusion of disability from sociocultural discourses in the field. It also directs attention to the critical issue that a field which inherently prioritizes diversity, equity, and inclusion may still be producing therapists who are ill-equipped to work alongside members of the largest minority group in the country.

Systems Theory: The Difference That Makes a Difference

As systems thinkers, MFTs are distinctly equipped to collaborate with diverse systems to effectively manage and cope with stressors faced across the lifespan (Carr, 2020). At the heart of a systems orientation is an emphasis on relationships. As Bateson (1988) suggested, this subtle but powerful shift in perspective from individual conceptualizations to a relational one when working with clients in psychotherapy generates *a difference that makes a difference*. Much of the work of family therapists is informed by considering one's broader context. Assessing family history and relational patterns is deemed necessary for effective treatment and positive outcomes (D'Aniello et al., 2016; McDowell et al., 2022). Therefore, every disabled individual is also connected in a systemic way to a network of formal and informal supports. These external but highly influential systems must be identified, assessed, and considered when addressing the mental health needs of the population. By uncovering new information about the roles of family and community relationships, systemic therapists can strive to empower and enhance the lives of individuals often systematically excluded from full participation in their communities.

Disability as Diversity: The Overlooked Sociocultural Competency

Systemic therapists are well-situated to play a critical role in disability discourse and provide effective services for individuals and families. However, work must be done to expand cultural competency and humility to encompass the lived experiences and intersectionality of disabled individuals and their families. Resources and trainings are needed that develop therapists' knowledge and skills to competently and confidently work with disabled individuals and their families. Despite the push within the field for systemic therapists to be socio-culturally attuned clinicians that hold competencies in working with diverse clientele and systems (D'Aniello et al., 2016; McDowell et al., 2022), there is a dearth of resources focused on effectively supporting disabled individuals. By neglecting elements of disability in diversity training, we further pathologize the experiences associated with disability. It is imperative that disability be acknowledged as an important diversity construct and an intentional part of diversity training.

Disability Discourse: A Tale of Two Models

Effectively engaging in disability discourse and training requires systemic therapists to consider how certain conceptualizations of disability exacerbate disparities in mental health care for disabled people. Disability operates as a unique identity context that distinguishes an individual within society. Yet, overtime, the meaning of the term *disability* has evolved – impacting the language people use to describe disabled individuals and influencing expectations and interactions. As systemic therapists expand the clinical conceptualization of diversity to better serve disabled individuals, professionals in the field must look beyond the terminology of disability to better understand the underlying theoretical perspectives that influence the social understanding and lived experience of disabled individuals and their families.

Over the past 50 years, the two most prominent models influencing disability discourse have been the medical model and the social model (Haegele & Hodge, 2016). Up until the 1970s, disability was predominantly viewed and constructed from a medical model. At the center of the medical model lies the idea that there is such a thing as normality and normative functioning. The person is viewed as a separate system, and disability is viewed as a disruption to normative individual and family functioning. This deficit-based, pathologizing perspective primarily views disability as a physiological deficit and deems nondisabled people as the standard of normality. Such conceptualizations view disability as a chronic medical condition that "is less than" and "needs fixing." As a result, the medical model has led to the expectation that interventions must be long-term, focused on helping the individual to "adapt" to their disability (Olkin & Pledger, 2003), thus requiring separate settings (e.g., institutions, separate schools and classes) and specialized professionals.

The field of disability studies, fueled by the disability rights movement (Patterson, 2018), emerged in the 1980s (Goodley, 2016). Disability studies offered a counter to the deficit-oriented, individualistic focus of the medical model of disability by advancing the social model. The social model views disability through a strength-based perspective and calls out the environmental, attitudinal, and systemic barriers that undermine the rights, access, and empowerment of disabled people (Oliver, 2013). From the social model perspective, the disadvantage of "disability" is not rooted in differences in how the brain or body works. Rather, it is societal barriers external to the individual, whether structural, programmatic, policy, or attitudinal, that are most debilitating for disabled people. When we view disability through this socio-ecological lens, it is the environmental and societal barriers that are most problematic for individuals and their families, not the differences in how one's brain or body works. A social model encourages a perspective of disability as a diversity construct that shifts our focus from increasing personal competence, to understanding and providing the supports individuals need across a variety of environments. As a result, the social model contends that effective supports for disabled individuals cannot be "prescribed" solely from a fixed diagnostic label, rather the nature and extent of support needed to participate in family and community life are ever evolving across contexts. Support needs are highly individualized, fluid, continuous, and ever-changing across time and context. The ultimate goal of a system is to "enhance opportunities for disabled people to better access and enjoy the people, places and activities they value" (Shogren et al., 2017, p. 28). Understanding disabled people from a social model perspective focuses professional efforts on modifying the context either through changes in the system or environment they are part of, or in the implementation of personalized supports.

Our Lived Experiences

Caught in a Double Bind: *A Mother's Perspective*

While I (JJ) did not always have the knowledge or language to describe the experience, I can now reflect on the last 30 years and recognize numerous times when I felt the rub of our family's understanding of disability against that of most healthcare professionals. We accepted and celebrated disability as a natural part of human diversity, while many of the professionals in my son Garrett's life and often, members of our community, viewed Garrett's disability as an individual deficit that society assumed resulted in both individual and family problems. Like all families, we experienced stressors and challenges. However, it often felt as though others blamed Garrett for whatever stressors our family experienced (e.g., financial, relational), because it was assumed that his disability was *the* liability for our family. These assumptions create a double bind, because as long as the understanding of disability is as a fixed trait that cannot be "cured," where is the hope? Professionals were often the barrier to Garrett being able to live a self-determined life and experience belonging.

One poignant example of this was when Garrett's high school special education teacher let us know that Garrett would no longer be allowed to sit with his wrestling friends at lunch because the other students in his special education class all sat at a separate table and felt left out. I was astounded. How was it that Garrett having a group of friends who embraced him was seen as the problem, rather than the historical and systemic segregation and discrimination experienced by his classmates? What our family needed, and thankfully occasionally experienced, was both professionals and a community who were willing to provide supports without pathologizing Garrett or our family system. We needed therapists who believed that Garrett was an asset, not a liability, to our family system and who used their professional expertise to address the normative stressors and challenges we experienced. This could have led to Garrett and the rest of our family living the life we desired. As Carter (2021) so beautifully reminds us, the desire to be included by your community, to have meaningful relationships, and to share life with people you love and that love you is not a "special need." Rather, the need to belong is deeply human.

Challenging the Dominant Discourse in Systemic Therapy and the Perpetuation of Ableism

Historically, systemic therapy, and the broader field of mental health, has been structured to support dominant norms and values that pathologize disability (Asch, 1988; Fine & Asch, 1988). Some scholars in the field contend that ableism has permeated the mental health field since its inception (Asch, 1988; Bogart & Dunn, 2019) and continues to have far reaching effects on how disabled persons access and acquire mental health care today. The term *ableism* refers to social oppression and dehumanization that results from the construction of disabled persons as marginalized and largely invisible to others (Campbell, 2001; Chouinard, 1999). Despite broad agreement that attunement to client's sociocultural experience is foundational to effective clinical practice (McGoldrick et al., 2020), to date, little, if any attention has been given to expanding diversity perspectives within systemic therapy to include sociocultural attunement to disability. Disabled people represent invisible others in the field. There are no standard genogram symbols representing the various forms of disability, and, when included, the term *disability* is relegated to a long list of potential vertical stressors that should be assessed for negative impacts when working with families (McGoldrick et al., 2020). Little to no clinical discussions explain or elaborate on the experience of disability beyond the diagnostic label. Students with marginalized identities, including disabilities, have expressed dissatisfaction with the narrowed conceptualization of diversity within required diversity curricula within COAMFTE accredited master's programs (Yzaguirre et al., 2022). Students indicated coursework primarily focused on race and ethnicity while placing less emphasis on other important aspects of identity such as sexual identity, religion, and disability status. Even within the systemic therapy literature focused on diversity, disability is all too often unnamed or exiled to the "etc." in the list of intersecting identities (see D'Aniello et al., 2016; Hardy & Bobes, 2016; McDowell et al., 2022). Clinical case examples rarely, if ever, introduce disabled clients (see McGoldrick et al., 2020; Reiter, 2014), and when disability is addressed, it is often limited to considering the physical characteristics of clients.

Increased awareness of the two distinct theoretical perspectives of disabilities, medical and social, helps systemic therapists better understand the current limitations to mental health services and identify new ways of improving access to mental health care for their disabled clients, while also enhancing opportunities and support for therapists-in-training and disabled therapists. Yet, in considering the two models of disability, Shakespeare and colleagues (Shakespeare et al., 2009) cautioned professionals that the dichotomy between the medical and social models of disability can be overstated – offering clinicians a both/and approach to integration consistent with systemic thinking. More contemporary models of disability, such as the human rights model of disability, offer additional perspectives on disability as a civil rights issue that must be recognized and understood. Overall, systemic therapists must be aware of the causes, consequences, and effective treatments of various disabilities that have been advanced by the medical model, while also being aware of incorrect assumptions about disability that result from stigmatized views about disabled people common within society.

For example, the ongoing practice of predominantly attributing symptoms and behaviors to an individual's disability – a phenomenon referred to as *diagnostic overshadowing* (Pickard & Akinsola, 2010) – often limits the exploration of the possibility of mental health symptoms, thus perpetuating the myth that individuals with disability are incapable of developing psychopathology and consequently reinforcing their exclusion from mental health care (Pickard & Akinsola, 2010; Reiss & Szyszko, 1983). Disabled people can and do experience significant mental health diagnoses, as well as the same life difficulties and challenges that commonly lead clients to seek out mental health care. Seeing difficulties or challenges purely as individual problems can ignore systemic issues that contribute to negative mental health outcomes and drive inequities. In fact, the understanding that people can be dually diagnosed with intellectual disability and mental health disorders is relatively recent. Up until the last 50 years, professionals across fields widely assumed that people with intellectual disability could not also have a mental health disorder (Reiss et al., 1982; Sovner & Hurley, 1983; Werges, 2007). Historically, when internalizing or externalizing behaviors (e.g., physical assault, self-injurious behavior) were noted, such behaviors were attributed to limitations in cognition and communication rather than the possible presence of mental health symptoms (Gardner & Cole, 1990; Szymanski & Grossman, 1984). Levitan and Reiss (1983), suggested that diagnostic overshadowing may be due to clinicians' tendency to attribute symptoms simply to the most noticeable factor of the client's presentation, which is generally apparent disability.

Likewise, negative assumptions exist toward disabled people when it comes to relationships. As a result of social norms and prejudices, it is often assumed that disabled people do not, or should not date, marry, or desire intimate relationships. However, research shows that disabled people both want and benefit from relationships (Bates et al., 2017; Retznik et al., 2022). Myths and stereotypes also exist regarding the sexual lives of disabled individuals. Disabled people are often assumed to be eternal children, asexual, or unable to inhibit their sexual desires. Numerous stereotypes and misconceptions exist about disabled people as parents, often questioning their ability to have and effectively parent children. Literature on parenting with a disability has often been limited by theoretical perspectives that pathologize disabled parents and presupposes negative outcomes for their children (Krauss & Olkin, 2020; Preston, 2010).

Disability Culture and Disability Pride: *Nothing About Us Without Us*

The disability community is demanding decisional control over health care and the access to effective mental health clinicians and interventions designed to address their needs. The emergence of the field of disability studies and the social model of disabilities brought attention to new understandings and conceptualizations of disability culture and disability pride. Disability culture rejects disability as a symbol of shame or pity, instead promoting solidarity and positive identity development. Disability pride acknowledges and embraces disability as a positive personal attribute and a source of pride, rather than a deficiency and source of shame. Understanding this creates the opportunity to differentiate one's perceptions and values about disability from the prevailing perceptions and values of an ableist society (Van der Klift & Kunc, 2019). Enhanced awareness of disability culture moves one away from the view that disability is an individual problem that requires individual solutions, to embrace the shared, collective experience of disability by reading and hearing the stories of other disabled people.

Our Lived Experiences

I Really Want to Find Another "Talking Doctor": A Self-Advocate Perspective

When I talked to a therapist, it helped me to feel better. It was something to look forward to. A therapist is very good because we talked about personal stuff – stuff that I wouldn't want to talk to my family or friends about. Therapists are very helpful I think. They help me feel comfortable and help with my stress. My therapist helped me learn to take deep breaths and helped me take a red squishy ball that you put in my hand – you squeeze it really tight and it helps you get all your stress and anxious out. We talked some and we also played games. When I talked to him, he would listen. "I think my advice to clinicians would be to always treat people with kindness and respect." I don't really think what I wanted to talk to my therapist about is really any different than any other person – decisions about my life and lifestyle, how to worry less, and about stress. I don't think my therapist ever talked to me about my disability. I think it would have helped. Even though I have a disability, it feels like people don't always know I have a disability and that would make it hard. Sometimes people can't understand my speech and that is also frustrating. I didn't like one therapist when I had to do stuff like homework. She had me do "tools" and always had a lot of papers. She didn't understand me. She didn't understand my story. I really want to find another talking doctor.

A Disability Studies-Informed Approach to Systemic Therapy

Systemic therapists are being called to work alongside the disability community to eliminate barriers to mental health care that reinforce health and relational disparities. To break down barriers to mental health care, the field needs to implement a multipronged approach-one that unites clinicians working with disabled clients, academic researchers, and disabled community members. To do this in a way that honors the experiential knowledge of disabled people, it is critical for the systemic therapy field to incorporate what Magasi (2008) referred to as a disability studies-informed approach. Magasi's approach focuses on how disability studies perspectives can be infused into, and ultimately strengthen human services training and practice.

For years, I (JJ) had a quote from Beart, Hardy, and Buchan (2005) on the dry erase board in my office that guided much of our (JJ + KG) scholarship over the past decade. Beart and colleagues stated that for individuals without disability, an understanding of disability lies at the level of discourse, rather than that of experience. They challenged researchers to acknowledge their limited perspective and to "try to understand at the level of experience by listening carefully to the people who live this identity every day" (Beart et al., 2005, p .55). This is not only a challenge for the researcher but also for all professionals who work alongside disabled individuals and their families.

Call to Action: Integrating Disability Studies into Systemic Therapy Research and Theory

There is an immediate need for evidence-based, systemic-focused interventions that supports the mental health care needs of disabled individuals. In partnership with the disability community, systemic therapists can play an important role in developing interventions to support the health and well-being of individuals with disability and the family systems they are part of. As echoed in the motto "nothing about us without us," disabled persons must be consulted and actively involved in all research, services, and supports affecting them. Use of community-based participatory research partnerships is one way to integrate disability studies principles into the systemic therapy research agenda (McDonald & Stack, 2016). In collaboration with disabled individuals, systemic therapists must work to identify common relational processes across the life cycle that combat relational stigma and stereotypes commonly held. Systemic therapists must work to better understand the core challenges and strengths for individuals and families and assess family-level relational processes. As Wampler and Patterson (Wampler & Patterson, 2020) pointed out, a rich description of the environment and the interaction between parts of the system was the accelerator for the development of systemic therapy. By embracing disability as diversity, greater value should be placed on expanding opportunities for therapists to understand the ordinary needs of disabled clients and their families.

Every Case Is a Systems Case

For systemic therapists, every case is a systems case (Wampler & Patterson, 2020) that takes a holistic perspective to health care and is concerned with the overall, long-term well-being of individuals and their families. The ability to acknowledge the system and its influence is a cornerstone of systemic thinking. Systemic therapists broaden the traditional emphasis on the individual to attend to the nature and role of individuals within primary relationship networks, such as marriage and the family. Shifting the focus from disability as a "problem," systemic therapists must look beyond the label to see the person and the system that they are a part of. For systemic therapy to be inclusive, it must go beyond being merely non-discriminatory. This includes the practice of more actively engaging in therapy, making consistent strides to be affirmative, and the promotion of a disability studies-informed approach.

For systemic therapists to effectively contribute to disability discourse, the field must work to define and use family- and system-level terms. The field must work to develop and expand system-level interventions that acknowledge and respect disability as a personal identity whose value is defined by the individual. Not only is it important for academic programs to incorporate trainings specific to the historical and systemic experiences of individuals impacted by disability, it is equally important that systemic therapists better understand the intersectionality of disability and other components of social location. For example, disability is often perceived as the primary component of the identity of disabled individuals. This assumption overlooks the fact that clients and their families are also impacted by other elements of identity and social location (i.e., race, gender, sexuality, ethnicity, nationality, religion/spirituality, and socioeconomic status). The intersectionality of disability with other experiences of inequity impacts the meaning related to disability for many families and often defines how an individual or the family is perceived or accepted/rejected by their own cultural or societal group. Additionally, it is important for systemic therapists to consider how the procedures they are already using in their practices can be adapted to meet the unique needs of disabled clients and their families.

Self-of-the-Therapist: Understand Your Values and Beliefs

The mental model that systemic therapists carry into their work with disabled individuals and families greatly impacts the treatment process. It is important for systemic therapists to identify and acknowledge their personal values, beliefs, biases, and assumptions regarding disability. As professionals, each of us has a working mental model of disability that defines our understanding of disability, determines the terminology we use, and ultimately provides the basis upon which we devise strategies for providing supports and services. All professionals must be aware of the mental model they bring to the therapeutic relationship and understand how such biases and assumptions impact the therapeutic relationship and process. Systemic therapists must check their prejudices and preconceptions, including believing the common myth that having a family member with a disability is a liability to couple and family relationships. On the contrary, research suggests that while families face unique stressors, having a family member with disability can positively impact relationships and individual and family quality of life (Blacher et al., 2013). Strategies applied when working with families of disabled individuals must include recognition of the unique strengths, resources, and experiences of each family member, including the disabled individual.

As part of the process of expanding understandings regarding disability, systemic therapists must be prepared to explore and challenge their own biases related to disability. Acknowledging how our own experiences and values influence our biases as clinicians is a crucial step in developing cultural humility. Potential self-of-the-therapist questions may include:

- What is my understanding of disability?
- What experiences do I have in interacting/working with disabled individuals?
- What do I know and not know about the systemic influences of disability?
- What have I observed in my own interactions with disabled persons and how is it different from my interactions with non-disabled individuals?
- What are my concerns with working alongside someone with an intellectual, sensory, and/or physical disability?
- What do I know or believe about the etiology or cause of intellectual disability?
- What are my beliefs or biases related to ability, relationships, work and education, communication, parenting, and so on for disabled people?
- What do I believe about the possibility for growth and change for disabled people in a clinical setting?

Supervisors in training programs must be prepared to prompt and engage in these conversations with therapists. This requires that supervisors who may not have experience working with this population also educate themselves and work through their own biases to build their own competencies.

Say the Word

Attention to nuances around language is critical to providing inclusive care. When working with disabled clients and their families, systemic therapists must also acknowledge their own comfort level or lack thereof with the language of disability. It is important that professionals work in collaboration with individuals and families to establish preferred language when discussing disability. While clients may need support when using terminology that is specific and empowers them to access the supports and services needed, therapists should be aware that internalized ableism might lead to the inappropriate use of self-identification for clients. Thus, professionals should approach such conversations with empathy and compassion, using a one-down position.

It is not uncommon for individuals, families, and professionals to use broad, imprecise terms (e.g., special needs) or incorrect terms that do not accurately identify the individual's current condition (e.g., using the term developmental delay for children or adults over the age of eight or learning disability for an individual with an intellectual disability). Professionals who are not adequately equipped with the appropriate terms and language as specified within the disability field cannot comfortably introduce the appropriate clinical language to individuals and families with whom they work. Clinicians should educate themselves on the most current and specific terminology within the field in order to avoid mislabeling individuals and misinforming families. The most recent Publication Manual of the American

Psychological Association, Seventh Edition (American Psychological Association, 2020) includes extensive revisions to bias-free language, including language and terms to use regarding disability. The manual requires authors to avoid perpetuating demeaning attitudes and provide specific guidelines for language that is affirming and inclusive. The Seventh edition also provides helpful and specific guidelines including the relevance of mentioning disability in academic writing as well as negative and condescending terminology to avoid.

While it is imperative that clinicians use bias free language, many individuals and family members are not aware of the changes and thus will not readily adopt disability terminology or change their use of outdated terminology. It is important to respect their choices, while simultaneously modeling best practices. I (JJ) am never going to correct the 75-year-old mom who has 55 years of lived experience in advocating and caring for her daughter with Down syndrome. When that mom uses words like "mental retardation" or even "idiot, imbecile or moron," I understand those were once clinical terms that professionals used to describe her daughter. The role and responsibility of clinicians is not to correct this mother, but instead to model best practice and terms – and, when appropriate, explain the power of language in the lives of disabled people.

Joining the Disability Discourse

To fully realize the stated values of acceptance, appreciation, and inclusion of diverse populations in the field of systemic therapy, we must first acknowledge that the field has not been value-neutral in the ongoing perpetuation of health disparities among disabled people. Moving forward, the field must be devoted to facilitating discourses and practices that bring the experiences of disabled people to light. We can begin by challenging biases and expanding current thinking about disability in systemic therapy. Fully embracing the "both-and" perspective of systems theory and thinking (Burnham, 1999), MFTs are uniquely positioned to expand disability discourse. They can move beyond the limitations of the medical and social models to promote new understandings of disability – ones that center not only the body or society but also the relational and systemic contexts in which disability is experienced.

References

American Association for Marriage and Family Therapy. (2015). *Code of Ethics.* https://www.aamft.org/Legal_Ethics/Code_of_Ethics.aspx

American Psychological Association. (2020). *Publication Manual of the American Psychological Association.* American Psychological Association.

American Psychological Association. (2024, December 20). *Inclusive language guide* (2nd ed.) [Webpage]. American Psychological Association. https://www.apa.org/about/apa/equity-diversity-inclusion/language-guidelines

Americans with Disabilities Act of 1990. Part 1: Public Laws: Hearing on 336, Senate 101 (1990). https://www.govinfo.gov/app/details/STATUTE-104/STATUTE-104-Pg327

Asch, A. (1988). Disability: Its Place in the Psychology Curriculum. In P. A. Bronstein & K. Quina (Eds.), *Teaching a Psychology of People: Resources for Gender and Sociocultural Awareness* (pp. 156–167). American Psychological Association. https://doi.org/10.1037/10066-019

Bates, C., Terry, L., & Popple, K. (2017). Partner Selection for People with Intellectual Disabilities. *Journal of Applied Research in Intellectual Disabilities, 30*(4), 602–611. https://doi.org/10.1111/jar.12254

Bateson, G. (1988). *Mind and Nature: A Necessary Unity*. Bantam Books.

Beart, S., Hardy, G., & Buchan, L. (2005). How People with Intellectual Disabilities View Their Social Identity: A Review of the Literature. *Journal of Applied Research in Intellectual Disabilities, 18*(1), 47–56. https://doi.org/10.1111/j.1468-3148.2004.00218.x

Blacher, J., Baker, B. L., & Kaladjian, A. (2013). Syndrome Specificity and Mother–Child Interactions: Examining Positive and Negative Parenting across Contexts and Time. *Journal of Autism and Developmental Disorders, 43*(4), 761–774. https://doi.org/10.1007/s10803-012-1605-x

Bogart, K. R., & Dunn, D. S. (2019). Ableism Special Issue Introduction. *Journal of Social Issues, 75*(3), 650–664. https://doi.org/10.1111/josi.12354

Burnham, J. (1999). Approach, Method, Technique: Making Distinctions and Creating Connections. *Human Systems: The Journal of Therapy, Consultation and Training, 10*(1), 3–26.

Campbell, F. A. K. (2001). Inciting Legal Fictions—Disability's Date with Ontology and the Abieist Body of the Law. *Griffith Law Review, 10*, 42.

Carr, A. (2020). Evidence for the Efficacy and Effectiveness of Systemic Family Therapy. In *The Handbook of Systemic Family Therapy* (pp. 119–146). John Wiley & Sons, Ltd. https://doi.org/10.1002/9781119438519.ch6

Carter, E. W. (2021). Dimensions of Belonging for Individuals with Intellectual and Developmental Disabilities. In J. L. Jones & K. L. Gallus (Eds.), *Belonging and Resilience in Individuals with Developmental Disabilities: Community and Family Engagement* (pp. 13–34). Springer International Publishing. https://doi.org/10.1007/978-3-030-81277-5_2

Centers for Disease Control and Prevention. (2019). *Disability Impacts All of Us.*

Chouinard, V. (1999). Disabled Women's Explorations of Ableist Spaces. In *Embodied Geographies* (pp. 141–156). Routledge.

Cree, R. A., Okoro, C. A., Zack, M. M., & Carbone, E. (2020). Frequent Mental Distress among Adults, by Disability Status, Disability Type, and Selected Characteristics—United States, 2018. *Morbidity and Mortality Weekly Report, 69*(36), 1238–1243. https://doi.org/10.15585/mmwr.mm6936a2

D'Aniello, C., Nguyen, H. N., & Piercy, F. P. (2016). Cultural Sensitivity as an MFT Common Factor. *The American Journal of Family Therapy, 44*(5), 234–244. https://doi.org/10.1080/01926187.2016.1223565

Douma, J. C. H., Dekker, M. C., & Koot, H. M. (2006). Supporting Parents of Youths with Intellectual Disabilities and Psychopathology. *Journal of Intellectual Disability Research, 50*(8), 570–581. https://doi.org/10.1111/j.1365-2788.2006.00825.x

Fine, M., & Asch, A. (1988). Disability beyond Stigma: Social Interaction, Discrimination and Activism. *Journal of Social Issues, 44*, 3–21.

Gardner, W. I., & Cole, C. L. (1990). Aggression and Related Conduct Difficulties. In J. L. Matson (Ed.), *Handbook of Behavior Modification with the Mentally Retarded* (pp. 225–251). Springer US. https://doi.org/10.1007/978-1-4899-2501-5_9

Goodley, D. (2016). *Disability Studies: An Interdisciplinary Introduction*. Sage.

Haegele, J. A., & Hodge, S. (2016). Disability Discourse: Overview and Critiques of the Medical and Social Models. *Quest, 68*(2), 193–206. https://doi.org/10.1080/00336297.2016.1143849

Hardy, K. V. (2016). Toward the Development of a Multicultural Relational Perspective in Training and Supervision. In *Culturally Sensitive Supervision and Training*. Routledge.

Hardy, K. V., & Bobes, T. (2016). *Culturally Sensitive Supervision and Training: Diverse Perspectives and Practical Applications*. Routledge.

Kinne, S., Patrick, D. L., & Doyle, D. L. (2004). Prevalence of Secondary Conditions among People with Disabilities. *American Journal of Public Health, 94*(3), 443–445. https://doi.org/10.2105/AJPH.94.3.443

Krahn, G. L., Hammond, L., & Turner, A. (2006). A Cascade of Disparities: Health and Health Care Access for People with Intellectual Disabilities. *Mental Retardation and Developmental Disabilities Research Reviews, 12*(1), 70–82. https://doi.org/10.1002/mrdd.20098

Krahn, G. L., Walker, D. K., & Correa-De-Araujo, R. (2015). Persons with Disabilities as an Unrecognized Health Disparity Population. *American Journal of Public Health, 105*(Suppl 2), S198–S206. https://doi.org/10.2105/AJPH.2014.302182

Krauss, M. W., Gulley, S., Sciegaj, M., & Wells, N. (2003). Access to Specialty Medical Care for Children with Mental Retardation, Autism, and Other Special Health Care Needs. *Mental Retardation, 41*(5), 329–339. https://doi.org/10.1352/0047-6765(2003)41<329:ATSMCF>2.0.CO;2

Krauss, L., & Olkin, R. (2020). Exploratory Research with Young Adult Children of Parents with Disabilities. *Stigma and Health, 5*, 2–10. https://doi.org/10.1037/sah0000169

Levitan, G. W., & Reiss, S. (1983). Generality of Diagnostic Overshadowing across Disciplines. *Applied Research in Mental Retardation, 4*(1), 59–64. https://doi.org/10.1016/S0270-3092(83)80018-6

Lollar, D. J. (2002). Public Health and Disability: Emerging Opportunities. *Public Health Reports (Washington, D.C.: 1974), 117*(2), 131–136. https://pubmed.ncbi.nlm.nih.gov/12356997/ . DOI: 10.1093/phr/117.2.131

Magasi, S. (2008). Infusing Disability Studies into the Rehabilitation Sciences. *Topics in Stroke Rehabilitation, 15*(3), 283–287. https://doi.org/10.1310/tsr1503-283

McDonald, K. E., & Stack, E. (2016). You Say You Want a Revolution: An Empirical Study of Community-based Participatory Research with People with Developmental Disabilities. *Disability and Health Journal, 9*(2), 201–207. https://doi.org/10.1016/j.dhjo.2015.12.006

McDowell, T., Knudson-Martin, C., & Bermudez, J. M. (2022). *Socioculturally Attuned Family Therapy: Guidelines for Equitable Theory and Practice*. Taylor & Francis.

McGoldrick, M., Gerson, R., & Petry, S. (2020). *Genograms: Assessment and Treatment.* W. W. Norton & Company.

Okoro, C. A., Strine, T. W., McKnight-Eily, L., Verlenden, J., & Hollis, N. D. (2021). Indicators of Poor Mental Health and Stressors during the COVID-19 Pandemic, by Disability Status: A Cross-sectional Analysis. *Disability and Health Journal, 14*(4), 101110. https://doi.org/10.1016/j.dhjo.2021.101110

Oliver, M. (2013). The Social Model of Disability: Thirty Years On. *Disability & Society, 28*(7), 1024–1026. https://doi.org/10.1080/09687599.2013.818773

Olkin, R., & Pledger, C. (2003). Can Disability Studies and Psychology Join Hands? *American Psychologist, 58*, 296–304. https://doi.org/10.1037/0003-066X.58.4.296

Parker, M. L., & Gallus, K. L. (2021, May/June). Disabilities and the Family: Where are the Marriage, Couple, and Family Therapists? *Family Therapy Magazine, 20*(3), 40–43. https://ftm.aamft.org/disabilities-and-the-family-where-are-the-marriage-couple-and-family-therapists/

Patterson, L. (2018). The Disability Rights Movement in the United States. In M. Rembis, C. Kudlick, & K. E. Nielsen (Eds.), *The Oxford Handbook of Disability History*. Oxford University Press. https://doi.org/10.1093/oxfordhb/9780190234959.013.26

Pickard, M., & Akinsola, T. (2010). *The Association Between Psychopathology and Intellectual Disability*. Psychology Press New York.
Preston, D. L. (2010). Finding Difference: Nemo and Friends Opening the Door to Disability Theory. *The English Journal, 100*(2), 56–60.
Reiss, S., Levitan, G. W., & Szyszko, J. (1982). Emotional Disturbance and Mental Retardation: Diagnostic Overshadowing. *American Journal of Mental Deficiency, 86*, 567–574.
Reiss, S., & Szyszko, J. (1983). Diagnostic Overshadowing and Professional Experience with Mentally Retarded Persons. *American Journal of Mental Deficiency, 87*, 396–402.
Reiter, M. D. (2014). *Case Conceptualization in Family Therapy*. Pearson.
Retznik, L., Wienholz, S., Höltermann, A., Conrad, I., & Riedel-Heller, S. G. (2022). Young People with Intellectual Disability and Their Experiences with Intimate Relationships: A Follow-up Analysis of Parents' and Caregivers' Perspectives. *Sexuality and Disability, 40*(2), 299–314. https://doi.org/10.1007/s11195-021-09721-z
Shakespeare, T., Iezzoni, L. I., & Groce, N. E. (2009). Disability and the Training of Health Professionals. *The Lancet, 374*(9704), 1815–1816. https://doi.org/10.1016/S0140-6736(09)62050-X
Shogren, K. A., Singh, N. N., & Wehmeyer, M. L. (Eds.). (2017). *Handbook of Positive Psychology in Intellectual and Developmental Disabilities: Translating Research into Practice* (1st ed.). Springer. https://doi.org/10.1007/978-3-319-59066-0
Simeonsson, R. J., & Leskinen, M. (1999). Disability, Secondary Conditions and Quality of Life: Conceptual Issues. *Issues in Disability & Health: The Role of Secondary Conditions & Quality of Life* (pp. 51–72).
Sovner, R., & Hurley, A. D. (1983). Do the Mentally Retarded Suffer from Affective Illness? *Archives of General Psychiatry, 40*(1), 61–67. https://doi.org/10.1001/archpsyc.1983.01790010063008
Szymanski, L., & Grossman, H. (1984). Dual Implications of" Dual Diagnosis": Guest Editorial. *Mental Retardation, 22*(4), 155.
Van der Klift, E., & Kunc, N. (2019). Segregation versus Solidarity: Rethinking the Uncritical Commitment to Inclusion. In *Promoting Social Inclusion* (Vol. 13, pp. 17–24). Emerald Publishing Limited. https://doi.org/10.1108/S1479-363620190000013002
Wampler, K. S., & Patterson, J. E. (2020). The Importance of Family and the Role of Systemic Family Therapy. In *The Handbook of Systemic Family Therapy* (pp. 1–32). John Wiley & Sons, Ltd. https://doi.org/10.1002/9781119438519.ch1
Werges, D. (2007). The Other Dual Diagnosis: Intellectual Disability. *The NADD Bulletin, 10*, 95–101.
Werner, S., & Stawski, M. (2012). Mental Health: Knowledge, Attitudes and Training of Professionals on Dual Diagnosis of Intellectual Disability and Psychiatric Disorder. *Journal of Intellectual Disability Research: JIDR, 56*(3), 291–304. https://doi.org/10.1111/j.1365-2788.2011.01429.x
World Health Organization. (2019). *World Report on Disability Summary*. https://www.who.int/publications-detail-redirect/WHO-NMH-VIP-11.01
Yzaguirre, M. M., PettyJohn, M. E., Tseng, C.-F., Asiimwe, R., Fang, M., & Blow, A. J. (2022). Marriage and Family Therapy Masters Students' Diversity Course Experiences. *Journal of Feminist Family Therapy, 34*(1–2), 15–37. https://doi.org/10.1080/08952833.2022.2052534

11

COUPLES THERAPY WITH DISABLED PARTNERS

Integrating Disability into Relational Practice

Rebecca Kammes, Madeline Barger and Debra L. Miller

Introduction

Recent data (2021) from the Centers for Disease Control and Prevention demonstrates that among disabled adults, approximately 44.5% are married or in unmarried long-term couples, 16.8% have divorced, 7.6% are widowed, and only 31.1% were never married or coupled. For cognitively or developmentally disabled adults, 41.1% are married or in non-married long-term relationships, 18.2% have divorced, 7.6% are widowed, and 33.1% were never married or coupled. With increases in numbers and visibility of couples living with disability, it is critical for marriage and family therapists to feel confident and be competent in working with disability in the context of couple's therapy. Many couples living with disability describe a desire to engage with a couple's therapist but consistently struggle to find a provider who understands how to work with disability effectively (Smith et al., 2021). Disabled individuals also feel strongly that knowledge on disability and the ability to adapt therapeutic methods to their needs are critical to effective treatment (Evans & Randle-Phillips, 2020). Though we offer some key insights and strategies into working with disabled couples in this chapter, it is crucial to recognize that these interventions are not universally applicable, and they will need to be adapted, depending on the couple's specific dis/ability experience.

Unique Characteristics of Couples Living with Disability

While many experiences of couples where one or both partners are disabled may mirror those of non-disabled couples, therapists must also recognize the distinct dynamics that can emerge in the context of disability. Working with couples where

DOI: 10.4324/9781003362586-18

physical disabilities, intellectual or developmental disabilities, or neurodivergence are present may require different considerations and adaptations. Neurodiversity, a non-medical framework, refers to natural variations in cognitive functioning and describes individuals whose brains engage with the world in ways that may differ from dominant neurotypical norms. This identity often intersects with societal barriers, including social exclusion and systemic misunderstanding, rather than arising from inherent deficits. Although neurodivergence itself is not a diagnosis, individuals who identify as neurodivergent may also navigate medical concerns or mental health diagnoses. It is essential for therapists to understand how different types of disability uniquely shape relational experiences-and to attend to the ways in which access, communication, and systemic ableism influence relational functioning, rather than focusing narrowly on levels of impairment.

Literature review searches related to disability and couples therapy commonly encompass articles related to couples living with physical disabilities, chronic conditions, and autism. Anecdotally, these are the types of couples living with disability that are most likely to engage in therapy, perhaps due to the greater visibility of these disabilities and the relative normalization or acceptance of these identities within dominant discourse (Morell-Mengual et al., 2017; Parchomiuk, 2012). Therapists may also encounter couples in which only one member of the couple is disabled. In these instances, it can be helpful to think of these relationships as "intercultural relationships" in terms of helping partners cope with and process their differences (Smith et al., 2021). With couples living with cognitive disability or neurodivergence, there may be differences in the methods and pace at which each individual processes information and communicates (Mitran, 2022). In those instances, therapy may be about "translating between two different brains." The therapist may work to help partners better understand one another's needs and communication styles to create shared meaning. However, it is important to note that many disabled individuals partner with other disabled individuals. These couples often share similar types of disability (e.g., both partners identifying as neurodivergent or living with a cognitive disability) and navigate similar systemic barriers together, reflecting a preference for shared understanding and mutual support within the relationship (Dammeyer et al., 2022). Regardless of whether one or both members of the couple are disabled, it is crucial for therapists to avoid making comparisons to able-bodied couples or framing non-disabled partnerships as the normative ideal.

Another critical aspect of couples living with disability is the impact of social exclusion. Some disabled individuals may face limited opportunities for social participation, including friendships and romantic relationships, not because of internal deficits but due to structural ableism and lack of access to inclusive spaces (Fulford & Cobigo, 2018; Gil-Llario et al., 2018; Turner & Crane, 2016). Many report a strong desire for intimate connection, yet encounter systemic barriers, including inadequate sexual and relationship education – both formal and informal. These gaps can result in challenges around coupling, and in some cases, vulnerability to exploitation, abuse, or mismatched partnerships (Black & Kammes, 2019). Social services often prioritize employment or independent living over social connection and intimacy, leaving relational and educational needs unmet until they become crisis points. As a result, some disabled individuals may begin dating later in life or may not receive the support necessary to pursue relationships in the ways they desire (Clarke & McKay, 2014; Janus, 2009; Nosek et al., 2001; Savage & McConnell, 2016).

Another factor worth noting is that some individuals may attend therapy alone to address relational issues. This may be particularly common among autistic individuals or when a disability is acquired later in life (Nowland et al., 2017). In these situations, it is important for the therapist to understand how disability identity, access, and communication patterns-rather than levels of functioning-may be shaping each partner's engagement with therapy. Therapists may also work with individuals who are not currently in a relationship but seek support around dating, relationship education, or building capacity for future intimacy.

Finally, language plays a central role in therapy with disabled clients and couples. Within disability communities, language is deeply tied to identity, community membership, and cultural pride. Clinicians must be mindful of the terms they use, recognizing that language carries implicit messages and can either affirm or marginalize. Using affirming, identity-respecting language is foundational to building trust and reducing stigma in therapeutic settings.

Recommendations for Affirmative Language-Use

1 Know and use your clients' preferred terminology.

  a Do they prefer person-first language (e.g., "individual with autism") or identity-first language (e.g., "autistic individual")?
  b Clarify and respect if preferences differ between members of the couple.
  c Understand that clients have likely experienced ableism, internalized ableism, and microaggressions related to their identities and/or their pursuit of sexual or romantic relationships. These experiences may influence how they relate to language and self-expression in therapy.

2 Take time to collaboratively define and establish shared meaning for any ambiguous, technical, or unfamiliar terms.
3 Be mindful of differences in expressive and receptive communication, including reading comprehension or language processing.

  a Verify understanding of terms and concepts in a way that is collaborative, respectful, and avoids assumptions about cognitive capacity or infantilizing clients.

4 Phrase statements as questions whenever possible.

  a Clients may have encountered patronizing, dismissive, or controlling behaviors from professionals or systems, and a questioning stance can demonstrate humility and foster autonomy and respect

Critical Disability-Related Considerations in Couples Therapy

Disability Diagnosis/Label

It is valuable to note that for couples where disability is present, the diagnosis or disability identity may play a meaningful role in the relationship. However, it is essential not to make assumptions about the nature or degree of its impact on the couple dynamic or presenting concerns. Therapists must practice curiosity and create space for open, client-led conversations about whether and how the disability is experienced as relevant to the therapeutic work. Rather than focusing on impairment or "functioning," clinicians should explore how clients understand their own experiences and identities, and how those meanings influence the relationship.

While conventional measures of functioning – such as intellectual abilities, social communication, or daily living skills – are often used in clinical contexts, these should not serve as proxies for capacity, insight, or relational value. Clients' understanding of their disability and its meaning may differ depending on whether it was acquired early in life or later on. In all cases, it is important to ask how individuals relate to their diagnosis and how it shapes their sense of self. Therapists should not assume a diagnosis to be either a strength or a limitation; instead, they should invite clients to articulate the significance of their disability in their own terms.

Clinicians should also explore how disability narratives, especially those shaped by early life experiences, labels, or imposed roles, may have become internalized and influence present-day identity, relational expectations, and emotional well-being. These early messages can affect how clients view themselves as romantic or sexual partners and how they perceive the dynamics of intimacy and support. Notably, beliefs about disability within relationships may vary across gender identities and societal role expectations (Brosnan & Gavin, 2021; Fitzgerald & Withers, 2013; Mimoun et al., 2024; Zhang et al., 2024). While research on couples navigating physical disability has received more attention (Brown & Ciciurkaite, 2021), similar explorations are still emerging for other types of disabilities. Disability may also shape couples' future desires and expectations, influenced not only by internal factors (such as embodied experiences or energy levels) but also by systemic variables, such as access to services or structural inequities. Caregiving roles, reciprocity, and relational interdependence may take on unique forms in disabled couples' lives. For example, in some partnerships, one individual may take on a caregiving role. Rather than assuming this to be inherently problematic, therapists should explore what this dynamic means for the couple, how it is experienced by each partner, and whether it aligns with their relational values (Neuman, 2020).

Clinical Vignette #1

To demonstrate common differences in experiences, let us compare the experiences of Mary and Claudia. Both are cisgender females in their mid-20s who are physically disabled and also identify as having cognitive differences. Mary uses a wheelchair and has frequent periods of immobility in her arms, while Claudia walks with a cane and must take frequent physical breaks. Both have a partner they cohabitate with who often helps them with daily tasks and engages in caregiving roles to varying degrees. However, for Mary, her partner views this as "part of the package," and their engagement in couples therapy was focused on sex therapy and increasing intimacy. For Claudia, her partner often expressed frustration about the extent of his household responsibilities, and their involvement in couples therapy was directly related to these caretaking dynamics.

Although both women had comparable experiences, the differences in how they experienced their disability within their relationships were shaped largely by their partners' perspectives and interpretations of disability. These variations in perception-not the disability itself-play a crucial role in shaping relational dynamics. Knowing this difference and discussing it openly can help guide therapy in a more meaningful and affirming direction.

The Role of the Family

Family members, especially parents, tend to be more involved in the relationships of couples living with disability, depending on the cultural positionality of the members and the developmental age of the partners within the couple (Chrastina & Večeřová, 2018; Kammes et al., 2023; Lunsky et al., 2017). This involvement can include serving as advocates for their adult children, providing relational coaching, and engaging in day-to-day support within the relationship – such as accompanying them on dates or assisting with caregiving tasks (Kammes et al., 2023; Rushbrooke et al., 2014). Given that most environments are not designed with disabled people or couples in mind, especially those who are neurodivergent, many individuals identify parents as essential sources of support and relational learning (Bertilsdotter Rosqvist, 2014). As such, family members are often included in therapy with predictable frequency.

In traditional couples therapy, the involvement of parents or other family members might be interpreted as triangulation or overreach. However, in the context of disability, their role is more often that of supporter, mediator, or access facilitator. Clinicians should reframe family involvement accordingly, understanding that these roles can offer stability, knowledge, and needed support (Neuman, 2020). The inclusion of family members should be led by the adult disabled client, in collaboration with a therapist who is grounded in systemic care and respectful of autonomy.

Some disabled individuals may also use their parents' relationship as a relational blueprint-modeling expectations for partnership, intimacy, shared responsibilities, or leisure based on observed dynamics in their family of origin. This may reflect a concrete and familiar reference point, shaped by the quality and tone of the parental relationship they witnessed growing up. Family rules and restrictions can also have a greater and more direct impact on couples living with disability. In some cases, family members or parents may retain legal guardianship or conservatorship over their disabled adult child. The scope and limitations of this guardianship vary by state, and therapists should be informed about relevant laws in their region. Certain forms of guardianship may give the guardian significant control over daily decisions, including those related to romantic and sexual relationships. In these circumstances, clinicians may need to include guardians in select discussions – not to override the couple's autonomy, but to advocate alongside them for their rights, desires, and relational goals, and to collaboratively clarify boundaries, expectations, or legal limitations.

For couples with intellectual or developmental disabilities in particular, adult services systems or family structures may impose restrictive rules around dating and intimacy. Research shows that such prohibitions – while often well-intended – can lead to secrecy, suppressed questions, and increased risk for exploitation or abuse, particularly when individuals fear punishment for discussing relationships (Azzopardi-Lane & Callus, 2015; Black & Kammes, 2019; English et al., 2018; Kammes et al., 2023). The role of family acceptance, support, and education emerges as especially important in fostering relational well-being for disabled couples, given the common need for ongoing family involvement in various areas of daily life (Brown & McCann, 2018).

Finally, therapists must remain attentive to the cultural identity and positionality of the individuals within the couple. Families from different cultural backgrounds, and the clients themselves, may hold a wide range of beliefs around topics such as legal marriage, cohabitation, independent living, and sexual intimacy. These expectations can shape both the couple's relationship and their interaction with extended family systems, especially when legal or caregiving roles intersect with cultural norms.

Cohabitation

Cohabitation may also be a significant topic for clinicians to explore with couples. There may be substantial systemic barriers to marriage and parenting for couples living with disability. Many disabled couples lose access to essential services if they legally marry and are reclassified as a dual-income household (Kammes et al., 2023). Additionally, due to medical concerns, a history of reproductive control, including forced sterilization, and the persistent influence of others' biased perceptions regarding their capacity to parent, many disabled couples may be unable-or may choose not to have children (Aunos et al., 2017). Because of these policy-driven and social challenges that make legal marriage more complex, cohabitation can become a significant milestone and meaningful commitment within the relationship.

However, for some couples, cohabitation may not be feasible-whether by personal choice, due to support needs, cultural values, or logistical constraints. For couples with intellectual or developmental disabilities, cohabiting in shared family homes or supported living arrangements is a common scenario. In couples where one or both partners have physical disabilities and require regular support, choosing to live with family members may be a strategic and affirming way to access additional assistance. This may also reflect the partner's desire to balance interdependence with care, without reinforcing dynamics of burden. Limited income and lack of access to affordable, accessible housing and financial resources can also pose substantial barriers to cohabitation for disabled couples.

For those couples who do choose to cohabitate, adapting to new routines can be a significant transition and requires a mutual commitment to navigating the shifts that arise. Many disabled individuals develop structured daily routines that support independence and wellbeing-particularly during transitions into adulthood. Merging or adjusting these routines to align with a partner's lifestyle may call for intentional planning, open communication, flexibility, and time.

For couples living together in structured care settings or family homes, privacy and relational autonomy may be more difficult to access. These couples may experience challenges related to intimacy, alone time, and engaging in everyday relational activities such as going out on dates (Brown & McCann, 2018). Clinicians can support couples in identifying creative, affirming strategies to maintain connection and intimacy, even within these environmental constraints.

Relationships within an Online Context

Disabled individuals are forming romantic and sexual relationships online or through other forms of electronic communication more frequently than ever before (Byers & Nichols, 2019). One aspect of this form of dating is that some relationships, particularly long-distance ones, may take place entirely online. Many disabled adults, especially neurodivergent and autistic adults, report that engaging with others online is more accessible and less anxiety-inducing than in-person interaction (Barros, 2020; Roth & Gillis, 2015). Due to the asynchronous nature of most online communication, these adults can set their own pace, reduce sensory and social pressures, and engage more authentically. Many clients report feeling that they can be more genuine and build deeper connections in these spaces.

However, with online communication, there is also an increased risk of abuse and exploitation, so safety planning and digital boundaries should be proactively explored. Romance scams and financial exploitation are unfortunately common experiences in online dating, particularly for disabled individuals (Buhagiar & Azzopardi Lane, 2022; Cross et al., 2018). It is important for clinicians to support clients in building awareness and protective strategies before these concerns arise.

Online communication also plays a vital role for many couples who have in-person relationships, whether or not they originally met online. For disabled individuals who experience limitations related to mobility or access, physical proximity may not always be possible. In these situations, digital connection becomes an essential part of the relationship. Audio or video calls may serve as substitutes for in-person dates, and texting or direct messaging may hold the same emotional and relational significance as face-to-face conversations. Clinicians should affirm these forms of connection as valid and meaningful expressions of intimacy.

Examining Different Relationship Stages

Relationship Education/Development

Disabled individuals face both environmental pressure and mythology. They live with the pressure to conform to ableist and neurotypical norms surrounding how relationships are initiated, learned about, and maintained. They also confront pervasive myths about their capacity to form and sustain romantic partnerships. These myths often include assumptions that disabled individuals lack the skills, independence, or desirability necessary to be viable partners-particularly in relationships with non-disabled or neurotypical individuals. Such narratives are both inaccurate and harmful. Disabled individuals are fully capable of learning, communicating, connecting, and engaging in intimate relationships, often in ways that are deeply meaningful and uniquely reflective of their lived experience. These forms of connection and coupling are no less valid or valuable than those of their non-disabled peers.

As a result of both societal pressure and enduring myths, opportunities for learning about relationships are often inadequate, inappropriate, or not tailored to meet diverse learning needs. This creates significant gaps in relationship-related knowledge and confidence. Therefore, early and individualized psychoeducation should be considered an essential component of the relational development process for some disabled client – not as a remediation effort, but as a support for autonomy, agency, and self-determined partnership. Psychoeducation about coupling and intimacy should be rooted in evidence-based practice, adapted to clients' communication and cognitive needs, and centered around the client's goals and preferences. This early work may involve exploring what the client hopes for in a partner, what they value in a relationship, and what they wish to contribute to a partnership.

Initiating Relationships

In the United States, dating is often the primary activity associated with the early stages of a romantic relationship. Most couples engage in some form of "getting to know you" interactions before pursuing a deeper commitment. For disabled individuals, these experiences are frequently desired, yet navigating them may require additional support. This is not due to a lack of desire or capacity, but because dating scripts are rarely taught in accessible, inclusive, or affirming ways. Some clients may benefit from guidance on dating-related skills and expectations. Depending on the client's communication style and support needs, therapists might ask questions like: "What does a date look like to you? How can you tell if this is a date or a platonic meet-up? What are your hopes for this interaction? How do you ask for and receive consent for physical or emotional intimacy?"

As noted previously, many disabled individuals begin dating and forming romantic relationships later in life. This may lead some to assign greater importance to early dating experiences and to progress through relationship milestones more quickly than is typical. These patterns are not pathological-they reflect context, access, and life experience. Some couples may not have regular access to traditional dating opportunities due to barriers such as inaccessible transportation or daily care routines. In such cases, online or virtual dates may serve as accessible and affirming alternatives. Unfortunately, many disabled couples experience discrimination while dating in public, including microaggressions and infantilizing comments. These experiences can come from strangers, service providers, or even family and friends, and may leave a lasting impact on the couple's sense of self and identity within their relationship. Therapists should validate these experiences while also helping clients develop strategies for resilience, boundary-setting, and self-advocacy.

Clinical Vignette #2

Mark, a 33-year-old autistic, cisgender male, attended therapy to work on self-esteem issues. His presenting issue was directly related to his desire to engage in intimate relationships and the distress he experienced following multiple dating-related failures. Throughout his engagement in therapy, the therapist helped him explore his desires and any assumptions regarding relationships. These open conversations helped him identify himself as bisexual and recognize that he may be looking for a relationship that looks "different than what's typically portrayed in media." His therapist with him also engaged in open discussions regarding dating and relationship activities, to ensure he had appropriate knowledge and a space to ask direct questions.

Forming New Relationships

The early relationship phase will also include how to blend the lives of two or more people in coupling and intimacy. Naturally, practicing and engaging in disability-related conversations about identity, support needs, diagnosis, and decision-making should be part of the couple's conversation in new relationships. Individuals or couples may encounter a spectrum of experiences when navigating the new aspects of a diagnosis.

There are three elements to effectively navigating diagnostic disclosure in therapy:

1 Identify the primary client or disabled clients' perspective and experience of their disability. What does the disability mean to them in their day-to-day life, and how do they feel about the diagnosis? Identify key points that are strengths-based and solution-focused.

2 Move on to learn about the history of disclosure. Have they, and how have they, shared their diagnostic information in the past? How has disclosure been received in positive or negative ways, historically? Highlight areas wherein they have been validated and supported, and model this validation in-session, to initiate/strengthen the positive experience of disclosure.
3 Plan an instance of disclosure, providing adequate support and practice for engaging in said disclosure. Clinicians must keep in mind that disclosure is not only about sharing a diagnosis, as a partner may already be aware of a diagnosis, but also about sharing a need in the couple system and/or external environment, related to the impairment. Therefore, disclosure is often an ongoing process of mutual understanding and adaptation in a couple's system.

Additionally, a clinician should examine the client's personal goals for a relationship, both for individual clients and for couples. In these early stages, this should include at least three requests that the client has of a partner or relationship and three contributions the client will bring to the relationship. Some criteria that are cited as important that the clinician should keep in mind during these discussions include environmental accessibility, the personality and communication style of the other partner, companionship, physical attraction between members, and having similar expectations of the relationship (Bates et al., 2017). Creating concrete lists of "must-haves" and "dealbreakers" in new or developing couple relationships can clarify individual needs and boundaries, while also framing the relationship as a deliberate and affirming choice that supports overall well-being and quality of life.

Coaching the initiation of building and strengthening new couple relationships may also involve the clients' family members or caregivers. For some clients, the logistics of planning, meeting, and maintaining relationships may require caregiver support or consent. The conversation about caregiver support should center around the clients' needs and desires, both for what they want out of, and will provide in, a couple relationship. First, ensure that the client's needs and desires remain central. Second, discuss how the clients can advocate or cue the need for support, what the support will entail, and who will be responsible for engaging in the supportive role (e.g., caregiver, parent, guardian, clinician, teacher, therapist, etc.).

In the early stages of a relationship, a clinician must feel prepared to answer relationship-related questions that are specific to the clients' needs. This could mean logistical questions regarding day-to-day coupling, sexual or intimacy-based activities, and other elements of daily living and relationship functioning. A clinician does not need to be an expert in all or even many of these aspects, but rather be prepared to listen, collect information in written or visual format, retain information, and help to organize the information. For example, if a client asks how they might engage in sexual intercourse with their partner, the clinician can collaboratively explore the question with the client, offering detailed, clear, and respectful guidance. This includes ensuring appropriate boundaries, clarifying consent, and considering the involvement of any relevant support persons or caregivers. For instance, a caregiver might assist with obtaining birth control as part of a predictable routine that supports the client's planned sexual activity, if appropriate.

Regarding mental health and advocacy, the early stages of a couple relationship may be anxiety-provoking for some disabled individuals. The individual may need to engage in behaviors such as modifying their daily routines and commitments, as well as educating and advocating with others in their life to effectively prepare for, initiate, and sustain an early-stage relationship. Additionally, because of the workload involved in the initiation of the relationship, in its early phases, the client may report fear of loss of the relationship or the partner. This anxiety and fear are common concerns associated with establishing early routines and boundaries in new relationships with disabled clients. Establishing a communication plan, preparing for the potential end of a new relationship, and exploring ways to pursue future connections are all important steps in fostering resilience for each individual in the couple. Additionally, elevated feelings of fear, anxiety, and overwhelm may shape the early stages of the relationship, adding complexity to what is often considered a dopamine-filled honeymoon phase. Supporting clients by normalizing emotional responses, building concrete contingency plans, and reinforcing established coping strategies are essential components of support during this formative period.

Clinical Vignette #3

Abby and Claire, a lesbian couple both in their mid-30s, were attending couples therapy due to anxiety related to the increased involvement of family members in their relationship. Abby was autistic and had an accompanying OCD diagnosis. Claire was non-disabled. Two of the main concerns the women presented with were Abby's struggles to be flexible and engage in activities that Claire was interested in, as well as what Claire saw as the "overinvolvement" of Abby's parents in her life. Therapy consisted of utilizing role plays and direct instruction to aid in the development of communication skills and perspective-taking for Abby, as well as allowing space for her to describe to Claire why her parents' involvement was meaningful and supportive to her. Defining the boundaries of the couple relationship as well as the family relationship was important to the progress of this case.

Commitment and Integration

This phase includes the middle phases of relationships wherein the couple has some agreement, contract, or arrangement, spoken or understood, that signifies the uniqueness and commitment of the relationship. This can be relevant in both monogamous and polyamorous relationships. Often for couples, this is a phase wherein there is a discussion of moving in together, getting engaged, bringing one another to activities as an identified pair (or more than a pair in the case of polyamory). For couples living with disability, clinicians may need to help them consider multiple relationship and living arrangements, depending on the disability.

Whether living apart or together, couples living with disability report needing to navigate a wide variety of coupling arrangements during the middle phase. For example, couples may live in an assisted living or group home setting together or near one another. They may also have in-person, virtual, cohabitation, or near-cohabitation relationships to accommodate needs such as sensory preferences and mobility adaptations. They may be more likely to experience a greater involvement of family members and caregivers in their daily lives, along with a higher likelihood of living in group or shared residential settings. Couples will also need to navigate financial requirements associated with disability. One key area to address is Social Security income, particularly the limitations on household income for disabled individuals who rely on government funding to supplement or replace their employment.

Additional considerations include the guardianship status of couples living with disability. Some clients may have a legal guardian that may include parents, relatives, guardians assigned by the state, and/or businesses or organizations identified as impartial guardianship sponsors. The clinician must educate themselves on the local state laws related to specific guardianship and living arrangements. Many states allow partial and/or complete guardianship status for clients aged 18 and older. As an example, a client could have guardianship specific to financial decisions only or have a legal guardian who is responsible for all their legal decisions. Guardianship status as well as legal disability status and level/type of government funding may impact a couple's ability to legally marry. For instance, a couple may wish to be legally married but may not have the privilege to be married within a court of law in the United States because doing so may result in the loss of critical benefits and supports if they legally marry and become a two-income household.

When it comes to government funding, some disabled individuals may be receiving Social Security Disability Insurance (SSDI), which is not impacted by increases or decreases in household income overall. However, the majority of individuals with significant or lifelong disabilities receive Supplemental Security Income (SSI). This level of funding is directly impacted by household income, and when two individuals combine their income, even if both are only receiving SSI, they can exceed the income threshold and are often denied SSI. Because of these unfortunate barriers, many couples choose to engage in a commitment ceremony or other non-legal agreement or celebration as a demonstration of their love and commitment. Clinicians must normalize the diversity of middle-phase living arrangements and use solution-focused methods for navigating any related logistical challenges that the couple may face.

Challenges extending beyond decisions about where and how to live as markers of relationship significance may also include navigating instances of internalized ableism. The couple in the middle phase of the relationship may be navigating visibility, legitimacy, and validation issues from family. They may have challenges in meeting some emotional, physical, mental health, or neurologically related boundary needs. For example, an individual may deeply value living alone and having complete privacy, yet require daily support with dressing or hygiene routines. Addressing the gap between personal desires and lived realities is essential to help mitigate self-esteem challenges and reduce the risk of depression for both the individual and within the couple system.

In this middle phase, couples also explore their needs and desires from a sexuality and intimacy perspective as they may have in the early phases of the relationship. Couples living with disability may struggle with access to privacy or experience a constant need to self-advocate when they require privacy for intimate activities such as dates or sexual interactions. While early-phase couples deal with the unknown, middle-phase couples may carry chronic anxiety related to the relationship. They may also experience exhaustion, deflation, and depression from constantly explaining or attempting to legitimize an underrepresented category of relationships, where living, legal, and daily routine arrangements differ from mainstream norms. It is important to note for clinicians that it is not uncommon for couples with disabilities to move into this relationship phase of commitment and integration faster than expected. This is often due to anxieties regarding legitimizing the relationship, in conjunction with a strong, understandable desire to experience all forms of relationships and human connections, especially when comparing their timelines to peers or family members.

For example, some clients may consider themselves in a serious relationship after only one or two positive dates. They may also stay in relationships or move toward commitment in relationships that are unhealthy or simply not embodying a strong connection due to a desire to have the label of being in a relationship or holding concerns over not being able to find another partner. For many of these individuals, dating and finding relationships has been a historically challenging process, and may result in settling into unsatisfactory relationships. Relationship education may be necessary to help the couple note what relationship stage they are in. It is critical to prioritize clients' desires and goals while working collaboratively to help clients work through any logistical or practical concerns that may arise in meeting these relationship goals.

Clinical Vignette #4

Jane and Fred were a heterosexual, cisgender couple in their 40s. Both were cognitively disabled and lived in a group home. They had been dating for 23 years but continued to live separately. Their family members and group home staff were very involved in helping them go on dates, find opportunities to be alone, and remain consistently engaged in one another's family activities. Jane began individual therapy first to address issues of depression she was experiencing. Through this process, she was directed to couples therapy with Fred due to arguments they were having. It was quickly discovered that the root of their issue was that Jane's same-aged cousin was finally getting married, and both Jane and Fred were upset that they felt this was a relationship step they would not be able to take at this stage in their lives. Members of both Jane and Fred's family were invited to therapy to discuss some of these concerns and barriers. Through these discussions, Jane and Fred were able to plan a commitment ceremony and buy rings for one another. They were also able to establish expectations for their future that included Jane moving to a new group home within walking distance of Fred's and discussing ways to find more flexibility in their ability to spend time alone with one another.

Long-Term Couples

This phase includes couples who have been in committed relationships for a significant amount of time. Some disabled individuals may face issues maintaining long-term relationships due to some of the concerns previously mentioned in this chapter. This includes a mismatch in adaptive functioning, barriers to cohabitate or share finances, concerns with caretaking needs, issues with guardianship or family involvement, and larger issues related to inaccessible structures and policies. Some autistic or other cognitively delayed individuals may encounter issues in maintaining long-term relationships specifically due to their experience of communication concerns and struggles with emotional connectedness. One study found that men with autism diagnoses experience less marital stress as well as overall stress if they perceive their spouse as understanding, accepting, and supportive of their diagnosis and the relationship challenges that may accompany it (Renty & Roeyers, 2007); an important strength to build on in couple's therapy.

Long-term couples living with disability experience many of the same issues as couples consisting of able-bodied members. The primary difference may be that therapists might need to directly address how the disability may be playing a role in the concerns being brought to the therapy room by the clients. For example, many couples might come to therapy to discuss concerns related to miscommunication or disagreement around current or future events. For couples in which one or both is autistic, the therapist might need to directly address concerns with perspective taking and empathic understanding, depending on the client's unique challenges. Therapists may need to provide psychoeducation or individual therapy before the couple is able to work through the issue together. Many neurodivergent individuals as well as those with additional support needs related to cognitive functioning may sometimes appear to lack an emotional response, and this can cause distress, especially if their partner is not neurodivergent or is cognitively delayed. Another issue that presents itself often for long-term couples is related to caregiving. If one member of the couple has more care-related needs, they can fall into significant over-functioning/under-functioning patterns. Despite agreements that may have been made earlier in the couple's history, over time, the caregiver can experience significant caregiving distress (Ledbetter et al., 2020; Nah et al., 2022; Polenick et al., 2017; Tough et al., 2019). The caregiving needs may also change as the individuals age, and the couple may need to renegotiate responsibilities.

Another challenge that often occurs in the long-term couple phase is parenting. There is minimal support provided to disabled parents from a societal, policy, and legal perspective due to misconceptions and biases about their ability to parent well. Couples living with disability often must rely on support from service providers or family members for support with parenting and may sometimes request family members or others to help with caretaking for their children (Aunos et al., 2017; Neuman, 2022). Disabled parents are also more often involved in child custody litigations (Aunos et al., 2017). There may be assumptions from others that due to their disability, these parents may engage in neglectful or inappropriate parenting. These concerns (most often mistakenly so) arise due to a lack of disability-focused parenting education as well as concerns with disabled parents juggling their own caretaking needs with those of their child. These parents often face ongoing struggles and policy changes related to unfair regulations and laws stemming from these assumptions about their caring abilities (Albert & Powell, 2021). It is imperative that therapists validate these struggles, and support clients to mobilize appropriate resources.

Due to changes in diagnostic criteria and a general misunderstanding of different cognitive, social, and learning disabilities, some individuals may not receive a diagnosis until later in life. This is often seen in autistic adults and others with borderline adaptive skills who demonstrated remarkable resilience and adaptability, allowing them to "fly under the radar" during school and early adulthood (Cage et al., 2024; Ghanouni & Seaker, 2023; Leedham et al., 2020). These misdiagnoses may impact a couple in important ways. In these instances, the therapist may need to discuss with clients how disability fits into the treatment plan. They may recommend beginning treatment with assessment and education before moving to the initial presenting issue that the couple brought into therapy. Gaining a new understanding of cognitive and behavioral patterns can cause couples to view and attend to their issues in a different light. Also, when a diagnosis comes later in life for an already established couple, it may sometimes feel like they are "moving back a phase" as the couple needs to reestablish boundaries and renegotiate how they are going to engage as a couple. It is vital to keep in mind here that treatment planning must be a collaborative process, with client autonomy consistently prioritized.

Clinical Vignette #5

Sam was a 42-year-old cisgender woman who had been diagnosed with ADHD as a child. She had been married for 18 years to Tom, a 41-year-old cisgender man who had recently been diagnosed with autism. They had one five-year-old son. Sam began attending individual therapy due to feelings of depression and concerns around her own difficulty in managing her emotions. She stated that Tom's new autism diagnosis was directly correlated to this presenting issue. She felt that because he now had the diagnosis, it was his responsibility to change, and she no longer wanted to "tolerate" some of the behaviors she had been upset about throughout their marriage. This eventually led them to couples therapy, where they worked together to process the new diagnosis and what it means for each of them. They practiced communication skills, developed a plan for meeting each other's emotional and relational needs, determined expectations for the future, discussed expectations for parenting, and how they would speak about the diagnosis with their son in the future.

Aging/Older Disabled Couples

Medical advances, as well as an increase in overall quality of health care, have led to disabled individuals, especially those with physical, cognitive, or genetic disabilities, experiencing longer life expectancies than they have in the past (Byram, 2018; Susano Jacinto et al., 2023). This, in turn, leads to more couples living into the aging/older couple stage. The most significant concerns that couples living with disability may face in this stage are related to caregiving. As care-related needs change, responsibilities may shift and need to be renegotiated. For couples living with cognitive or neurological disability specifically, they may be disproportionately impacted by dementia in later life (Jacobs et al., 2023). It will be important to work with these couples regarding care-related responsibilities and explore how they can support one another while maintaining their own well-being. For couples living with physical disabilities, these needs may become more heightened and impactful with age.

If one member of the couple is in a caregiving role, they may benefit from additional support as both members of the couple age. Multiple impairments, chronic conditions, and comorbidities may worsen over time. This, in turn, can cause increased depression and anxiety among this population when not supported well (Polenick et al., 2020). This is especially true if both members of a couple are disabled and have heightened care-related needs. It will be important to strengthen external support systems and access to appropriate resources.

Facilitating Sexual Education and Intimacy for Couples Living with Disabilities

Disabled individuals experience a significant lack of general sex education, including intimate partner relationship education (Chrastina & Večeřová, 2020). Unfortunately, there still exists a stigma of disabled individuals as being either asexual and lacking sexual interests or being "perpetual offenders" who are perceived as unable to control their own sexual urges (Gil-Llario et al., 2018). Due to this problematic misconception, therapists working with couples living with disability may need to check their own biases and prejudices before providing couples therapy and sex therapy to clients where one or both members are disabled. When relevant, therapists can provide psychoeducation and help clients enhance their understanding of personal values and desires related to intimacy. The therapist may also need to challenge inappropriate or incorrect information that individuals have received from peers, family members, or the media regarding their right and ability to engage with sex and sexuality.

Some individuals with cognitive or social impairments may present with the view that there is "only one way to have sex." To combat this misconception, it is important for the therapist to discuss what sexual activity can look like between consenting partners, when clients express a need or desire for such information. When assessing for any potentially inappropriate sexual behaviors, it will be important to be mindful of therapists' personal biases around disabled sexuality. As with all couples, it will be important to discuss values and ensure both members of the couple are aligned on an understanding of safe sexual behaviors and expectations. If an impairment limits a client's ability to engage in certain sexual behaviors, this needs to be discussed, followed by a conversation about alternative sexual behaviors that can result in similar or enhanced sexual pleasure and intimacy.

Diversity in Sexuality

According to the Human Rights Campaign (2022), approximately 36% of disabled people also identify as LGBTQ+. Therefore, it is important to note that while information in this chapter applies to many couples living with disability, therapists will need to make unique accommodations for those who are also living at the intersection of LGBTQ+ couples, multiracial/multiethnic couples, and other cultural intersections.

Disabled individuals may also present with varied sexual interests, practices, and histories. They may have a desire for specific objects, body types/parts, and/or role play scenarios. Unique brains and unique experiences may lead to diverse sexual interests or a need to engage in and negotiate varied sexual practices (Hall, 2018; Kattari, 2014). As with all couples, intimacy may not always be erotic or sexual. For some disabled individuals with physical limitations or touch and sensory requirements, it will be important to discuss what type of intimacy they desire. There is also an important pattern of neurodivergent adults describing themselves as falling on the asexual spectrum (Bush et al., 2021; Ronis et al., 2021).

Foundational Interventions in Sex Therapy

Disabled people have been desexualized throughout history, and it is critical that therapists do not perpetuate this harmful pattern. Therapists must prioritize respect, privacy, confidentiality, and safety when talking about sex with their disabled clients. It is important for the therapist to help the couple voice any needs, normalize different experiences, and provide an opportunity for the couple to discuss communication and safety around desired experiences. Specific behaviors and activities will need to be openly discussed, along with helping the couple understand each other's needs and desires, and what different experiences mean for each member of the couple. Some individuals may have a preference for solo pleasure over coupled pleasure. It is important to note that for some couples who may also be experiencing physical disabilities or lack of private time as a couple, self-pleasure can be a positive avenue for healthy sexual development. Some individuals may also engage with sexuality in a more visual way and may use pornography as a learning tool as well as a part of their sexual experiences. It will be important to discuss the use of pornography between members of the couple and ensure they agree on how it will be included within the relationship. Some other sex therapy interventions are described below.

1 **Role Playing**

   a Many disabled individuals have strong visual abilities (unless they have an impairment/s related to vision) and it can help to structure and talk members through different scenes and scenarios, based on their preferences. It can also be helpful to provide scripts to ensure consent and expectations for both partners.
   b Use the SOL technique:
   c Stop judging – understand that with diversity in development comes diversity in experiences and desires.
   d Observe – allow the couple to discuss their experiences and concerns openly.
   e Listen – hear what the couple has to say and why these experiences are important to them.

2 Sensate-Focused

   a Review the treatment plan, focusing on potential sensory differences and how to keep both members of the couple safe and enjoying the experience. Sensory differences may be related to unique neurology and/or physical disability.
   b Be prepared to draw or use visuals.
   c Varied/diverse forms of education, including materials that are inclusive of learners with different abilities – such as varying needs with vision, hearing, and verbal speech – must be provided. Be prepared to learn about the educational history of client(s) and adapt teaching materials accordingly.
   d Consider a more task-analysis format, breaking down steps and actions into parts as appropriate for the couple.

Abuse and Exploitation

Disabled individuals experience high rates of abuse and exploitation (Dike et al., 2022; Gil-Llario et al., 2018; Harrell, 2012). While the perpetrators are most commonly caregivers or strangers, there are still high rates of intimate partner violence and abuse among disabled couples, and this is unfortunately expected to continue to be a significantly underreported experience (Bernert, 2011; Bernert & Ogletree, 2013; Ward et al., 2010). Disabled women are most commonly the victims of these experiences, and it may take them years to fully comprehend its impacts, since open discussions about abuse in this community remain limited. Previous instances of exploitation perpetrated by strangers, caretakers, or peers may impact their current romantic or sexual relationship. The therapist may need to work with the individual to treat any trauma-related impacts and provide language to support them in understanding how it impacts their current couple relationship, if at all.

For instances of domestic violence between disabled couples, commonly used therapeutic techniques can work, with some important adaptations. The first is to remember that psychoeducation may help the couple learn about unhealthy relationship dynamics. Language such as "healthy and unhealthy" should be used as opposed to "typical or non-typical," as many couples may believe unhealthy relationship patterns are typical or expected due to inaccurate knowledge they have gained from others. Caretaking may also play a role in the probability of abuse occurring. One partner may use their caregiving role as an opportunity to exert power and control over the other member of the couple. An abuser may also use the disability itself as part of their control and abuse, telling the disabled person that they cannot be trusted or are incapable of caring for themselves-even when untrue (Bonomi et al., 2018). It will be important for clinicians to understand how the disability and any caregiving dynamics contribute to the cycle of abuse, as well as what level of education might be needed for the couple or a member of the couple to maintain safety within the relationship. Clinicians should also provide appropriate resources related to shelters, law enforcement, or specialized mental health referrals, when appropriate and led by the client's safety needs and choices.

Specific Therapeutic Techniques

Adaptations to Current Therapeutic Skills for Clinicians

Before we begin to address therapeutic approaches in working with this population, it is important to note that due to the variability and vast diversity of how disabled couples may be presenting in therapy, the following recommendations will change based on each individual's type and level of impairment and the presenting concern. Therapists must maintain that the individual is the expert in their own lives: ask questions and continually check in to ensure accurate understanding of experiences.

1. Deliver information and engage in therapeutic activities using multiple modalities, including visual, written, and other forms of communication.
   a. Provide written lists of any homework.

   b Provide diagrams when appropriate to help clients access concepts with pictures rather than just written or verbal teaching materials.
   c Similarly, drawings, either done in real time by the clinician and/or with the client, can be another way to teach new concepts.
   d Include ASL (American Sign Language) interpreters when appropriate.

2 Some clients may process information better in written format.

   a It may be helpful to write down or summarize key points that were discussed during session to aid in information processing outside of session.

3 Adapt interventions, concepts, and conversations for different processing needs.

   a Developing shared metaphors between the couple can provide a stronger communication bridge.
   b Provide examples of concepts and ideas.

4 Mirror the speed of processing and the pace of therapy that your client needs.

   a Every client will have different expressive/receptive language needs. Some individuals may need additional time to read or engage in communication, depending on their impairment (Mitran, 2022).
   b Trauma experiences, including past abuse and exposure to discrimination, are more prevalent in this population (McNally et al., 2021). This may impact the overall pace of therapy.
   c In-depth and holistic assessments during the initial phases of therapy are essential. Invest time at the beginning of treatment to understand your clients' functioning level, processing speed, and preferred methods of communication.

5 Collaborate on clear goals with concrete and behavior-based outcomes.

   a Refrain from highly abstract concepts (unless appropriate for the client's cognitive style) and focus more on connecting interventions to a direct behavior or outcome, depending on the client's needs and preferences.

6 Focus on active listening skills.

   a Looking at your client when speaking to them is important for all clients, regardless of ability. Sometimes, eye contact may be difficult for some disabled people, so the focus may be on maintaining attention.
   b Utilize warm and authentic body language such as nodding and turning toward the person, when appropriate.
   c Utilize verbal cues such as words of agreement or asking follow-up questions.

7 Therapists may need to review and practice certain social skills, if needed and appropriate to the presenting issue and the couple's functioning.

   a Offer examples of active listening skills: e.g., "I hear you. You said you are upset that I didn't wash the dishes last night. I can see why you might be having that experience. I have my own different experience: I feel as if I am the only one who washes the dishes and you never take a turn, and I would like if we could split the chores more evenly."
   b Discuss the importance of active listening and turn-taking, redirecting the couple as necessary when interruptions or distractions occur.

8 Think about utilizing technology when appropriate.
9 Many disabled individuals feel more confident connecting online and utilizing online assessments or completing tasks at home (Mitran, 2022).
10 Be cautious when using techniques that align with one partner to "unbalance the system," as these interventions are not accessible to clients with certain cognitive or social impairments and may risk damaging the therapeutic relationship (Barnes & Summers, 2012).
11 Allowing space for one person to work through a personal issue or engage in personal education can be helpful (Neuman, 2020).

Direction and Homework

Many disabled people are coping with multiple barriers and obstacles to daily living. A therapist who is able to be directive (in a collaborative and non-hierarchical manner) can lift some burden and create a sense of hope for disabled clients. The therapist should work with the couple to normalize and externalize the presenting issue, providing stability in the relationship and helping the couple focus on solutions. In session, this may include using visuals and asking questions to ensure understanding. Next, the therapist may need to model behaviors or provide other forms of visual and auditory engagement. Role playing is also a very useful tool, which includes having the therapist demonstrate the interaction, then asking the clients to role play while the therapist observes. Interventions such as this support clients in practicing new behaviors and interactions outside the therapy room. Given that, it will be important for the therapist to define specific behaviors related to the specific concern that the couple is experiencing. Finally, the therapist should provide clear, behavioral homework to the couple to ensure engagement on the issue outside of the therapy room, offering structured opportunities for practice. Of course, it is vital that these homework assignments are inclusive, paying attention to the unique needs, challenges, and strengths of each client in the relationship.

Using the ABCs of Couple Interactions

The ABC model of interaction stands for antecedent, behavior, and consequence. This is an intervention frequently used with disabled individuals when working on

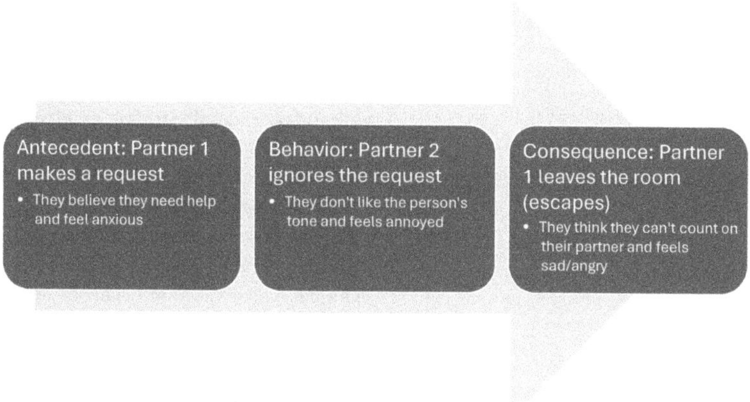

Figure 11.1 Example of an antecedent–behavior–consequence (ABC) pattern for one member of a couple.

individual behavior changes (Dyer, 2013). It can also be a helpful tool when working with couples. The model offers a clear and direct way of discussing behaviors and can be used alongside visuals and previously discussed interventions. Figure 11.1 illustrates how the ABC model can be applied in practice:

Adapting Systemic Couples Therapy Models for Disabled Clients

Systemic models of couples therapy provide a foundational framework for addressing relational dynamics, emotional processes, and intergenerational patterns. However, many of these models were developed without explicit attention to the lived experiences, access needs, or sociocultural positioning of disabled clients. To ensure clinical relevance and therapeutic effectiveness, systemic therapists must thoughtfully adapt core theoretical interventions in ways that affirm disability as a form of diversity rather than deficit. These adaptations must also be customized to the unique needs, identities, and interactional patterns of each client system, rather than applied prescriptively. Table 11.1 outlines illustrative modifications to several widely used models of couples therapy, offering practical guidance for integrating disability-affirmative practices while maintaining fidelity to each model's theoretical integrity.

Conclusion

In summary, couples navigating disability actively identify and express their relational needs. They also have the right to access safe and effective couples therapy, supported by tools and clinicians who are well-prepared to meet those needs with competence and care. Therapists must be sensitive to differences, avoid

Table 11.1 Examples of adaptations to common family therapy models

Emotion Focused Therapy	Incorporate drawings or other visual, auditory, or physical methods to the discussion, such as drawing out an illustration of the couple's cycle
Couples Cognitive Behavior Therapy	Adapt to the client's language, utilizing their labels, descriptors, and metaphors Utilize visuals to help describe concepts, including drawings, diagrams, audio-recorded explanations of concepts, or writing out summaries of discussions
Solution-Focused Therapy	Affirm their existing routines and break down tasks and goals into steps
Strategic Therapy	Find helpful replacement behaviors for arguing, that can be fun and draws on individual preferences
Intergenerational Therapy	Examine their family belief systems surrounding disability, independence, and expectations in adulthood and romantic relationships

comparisons with able-bodied couples, and use affirming, appropriate language to foster a supportive therapeutic environment (Table 11.1).

For couples living with disability, the impact of a disability diagnosis on the relationship should be explored with curiosity and openness, as each individual's understanding and acceptance of their disability can differ based on factors such as timing, societal reactions and narratives, stereotypes, and the nature of the impairment. Family members may play a significant role in the relationships of couples living with disability, offering support and guidance. However, their involvement in therapy should be collaborative and respectful of the disabled client's autonomy, while also accounting for cultural and legal contexts. It is important to consider how factors such as lived experience of disability, level of autonomy, and family involvement influence the couple across all stages of their relationship.

Another significant consideration is that disabled individuals often face a lack of comprehensive sex and relationship education. Therapists must accommodate the unique needs of couples at the intersection of disability, LGBTQ+ identities, and other cultural contexts, while creating space for safe and affirming discussions around sexual interests, intimacy preferences, and communication about desire. Therapists working with disabled couples should tailor their approach to each client's unique needs and preferences. They must use adaptive communication strategies, ensuring the pace and content of sessions align with the client's processing needs, while emphasizing concrete goals and strong active listening. Regular check-ins are essential to support accurate understanding. Therapists should avoid interventions that could undermine trust or accessibility and incorporate technology or individualized work when appropriate.

Ultimately, the most essential qualities in couples work with disabled clients include respect, empathy, and collaboration. These elements promote relational health by honoring each partner's voice, needs, and strengths.

Bibliography

Albert, S. M., & Powell, R. M. (2021). Supporting disabled parents and their families: Perspectives and recommendations from parents, attorneys, and child welfare professionals. *Journal of Public Child Welfare, 15*(5), 530–564. https://doi.org/10.1080/15548732.2020.1751771

Aunos, M., Feldman, M., Callow, E., LaLiberte, T., & Lightfoot, E. (2017). Parenting by people with intellectual disability. In M. L. Wehmeyer, I. Brown, M. Percy, K. A. Shogren, & W. L. A. Fung (Eds.), *A Comprehensive Guide to Intellectual and Developmental Disabilities* (2nd ed., pp. 679–694). Baltimore, MD: Paul H. Brooks Publishing Co.

Azzopardi-Lane, C., & Callus, A. (2015). Constructing sexual identities: People with intellectual disability talking about sexuality. *British Journal of Learning Disabilities*, *43*(1), 32–37. https://doi.org/10.1111/bld.12083

Barnes, J. C., & Summers, S. J. (2012). Using systemic and psychodynamic psychotherapy with a couple in a community learning disabilities context: A case study. *British Journal of Learning Disabilities, 40*(4), 259–265. https://doi.org/10.1111/j.1468-3156.2011.00704.x

Barros, D. M. (2020). Online dating, reproductive success and the rise autism spectrum disorder prevalence. *Medical Hypotheses*, *140*, 109679. https://doi.org/10.1016/j.mehy.2020.109679

Bates, C., Terry, L., & Popple, K. (2017). Partner selection for people with intellectual disabilities. *Journal of Applied Research in Intellectual Disabilities, 30*, 602–611. https://doi.org/10.1111/jar.12254

Bernert, D. J. (2011). Sexuality and disability in the lives of women with intellectual disabilities. *Sexuality and Disability, 29*, 129–141. https://doi.org/10.1007/s11195-010-9190-4

Bernert, D. J., & Ogletree, R. J. (2013). Women with intellectual disabilities talk about their perceptions of sex. *Journal of Intellectual Disability Research, 57*, 240–249. https://doi.org/10.1111/j.1365-2788.2011.01529.x

Bertilsdotter Rosqvist, H. (2014). Becoming an "autistic couple": Narratives of sexuality and couplehood within the Swedish autistic self-advocacy movement. *Sexuality and Disability, 32*(3), 351–363. https://doi.org/10.1007/s11195-013-9336-2

Black, R. S., & Kammes, R. R. (2019). Restrictions, power, companionship, and intimacy: A metasynthesis of people with intellectual disability speaking about sex and relationships. *Intellectual and Developmental Disabilities, 57*(3), 212–233. https://doi.org/10.1352/1934-9556-57.3.212

Blow, A., Seedall, R., Miller, D. L., Vaz, A., & Rousmaniere, T. G. (2022). *Deliberate Practice in Systemic Family Therapy.* Washington, DC: American Psychological Association. https://doi.org/10.1037/0000301-000

Bonomi, A., Nichols, E., Kammes, R., & Green, T. (2018). Sexual violence and intimate partner violence in college women with a mental health and/or behavior disability. *Journal of Women's Health, 27*(3), 359–368. https://doi.org/10.1089/jwh.2016.6279

Brosnan, M., & Gavin, J. (2021). The impact of stigma, autism label and wording on the perceived desirability of the online dating profiles of men on the autism spectrum. *Journal of Autism and Developmental Disorders*, *51*(11), 4077–4085. https://doi.org/10.1007/s10803-020-04830-8

Brown, R. L., & Ciciurkaite, G. (2021). The "Own" and the "Wise" Revisited: Physical Disability, Stigma, and Mental Health among Couples. *Journal of Health and Social Behavior, 62*(2), 170–182. https://doi.org/10.1177/0022146521998343

Brown, M., & McCann, E. (2018). Sexuality issues and the voices of adults with intellectual disabilities: A systematic review of the literature. *Research in Developmental Disabilities, 74,* 124–138. https://doi.org/101016/j.ridd.2018.01.009

Buhagiar, S., & Azzopardi Lane, C. (2022). Freedom from financial abuse: Persons with intellectual disability discuss protective strategies aimed at empowerment and supported decision-making. *Disability & Society, 37*(3), 361–385. https://doi.org/10.1080/09687599.2020.1833312

Bush, H. H., Williams, L. W., & Mendes, E. (2021). Brief report: Asexuality and young women on the autism spectrum. *Journal of Autism and Developmental Disorders, 51*(2), 725–733. https://doi.org/10.1007/s10803-020-04565-6

Byers, E. S., & Nichols, S. (2019). Prevalence and frequency of online sexual activity by adults with autism spectrum disorder. *Focus on Autism and Other Developmental Disabilities, 34*(3), 163–172. https://doi.org/10.1177/1088357618800061

Byram, E. (2018). Late-life challenges in caregiving for an adult child with a developmental disability. *Generations (San Francisco, Calif.), 42*(3), 9–14.

Cage, E., Botha, M., McDevitt, L., King, K. N., Biscoe, L., Tucker, K., & Pearson, A. (2024). Diagnosis as a new beginning not an end: A participatory photovoice study on navigating an autism diagnosis in adulthood. *Autism: The International Journal of Research and Practice, 28*(8), 2014–2027. https://doi.org/10.1177/13623613231220418

Centers for Disease Control and Prevention, National Center on Birth Defects and Developmental Disabilities, Division of Human Development and Disability. Disability and Health Data System (DHDS) Data [online]. [accessed Sep. 22, 2023]. https://dhds.cdc.gov

Chrastina, J., & Večeřová, H. (2018). Supporting sexuality in adults with intellectual disability: A short review. *Sexuality and Disability, 38*(2), 285–298. https://doi.org/10.1007/s11195-018-9546-8

Clarke, H., & McKay, S. (2014). Disability, partnership and parenting. *Disability & Society, 29*(4), 543–555. https://doi.org/10.1080/09687599.2013.831745

Cross, C., Dragiewicz, M., & Richards, K. (2018). Understanding romance fraud: Insights from domestic violence research. *British Journal of Criminology, 58*(6), 1303–1322. https://doi.org/10.1093/bjc/azy005

Dammeyer, J., Umino, A., & Chapman, M. (2022). Couple similarity with respect to physical and mental disabilities. *Scandinavian Journal of Public Health, 52*(1), 24–30. https://doi.org/10.1177/14034948221113652

Dike, J. E., DeLucia, E. A., Semones, O., Andrzejewski, T., & McDonnell, C. G. (2022). A systematic review of sexual violence among autistic individuals. *Review Journal of Autism and Developmental Disorders, 10*(3), 576–594. https://doi.org/10.1007/s40489-022-00310-0

Dyer, K. (2013). Antecedent-behavior-consequence (A-B-C) analysis. In F. R. Volkmar (Ed.), *Encyclopedia of Autism Spectrum Disorders*. New York: Springer. https://doi.org/10.1007/978-1-4419-1698-3_1003

English, B., Tickle, A., & dasNair, R. (2018). Views and experiences of people with intellectual disabilities regarding intimate relationships: A qualitative metasynthesis. *Sexuality and Disability, 36*(2), 149–173. https://doi.org/10.1007/s11195-017-9502-z

Evans, L., & Randle-Phillips, C. (2020). People with intellectual disabilities' experiences of psychological therapy: A systematic review and meta-ethnography. *Journal of Intellectual Disabilities, 24*(2), 233–252. https://doi.org/10.1177/1744629518784359

Fitzgerald, C., & Withers, P. (2013). "I don't know what a proper woman means": What women with intellectual disabilities think about sex, sexuality and themselves. *British Journal of Learning Disabilities, 41*(1), 5–12. https://doi.org/10.1111/j.1468-3156.2011.00715.x

Fulford, C., & Cobigo, V. (2018). Friendships and intimate relationships among people with intellectual disabilities: A thematic synthesis. *Journal of Applied Research in Intellectual Disabilities, 31*, 18–35. https://doi.org/10.1111/jar.12312

Ghanouni, P., & Seaker, L. (2023). What does receiving autism diagnosis in adulthood look like? Stakeholders' experiences and inputs. *International Journal of Mental Health Systems, 17*(1), 16. https://doi.org/10.1186/s13033-023-00587-6

Gil-Llario, M. D., Morell-Mengual, V., Ballester-Arnal, R., & Diaz-Rodriguez, I. (2018). The experience of sexuality in adults with intellectual disability. *Journal of Intellectual Disability Research, 62*(1), 72–80. https://doi.org/10.1111/jir.12455

Hall, M. (2018). Disability, discourse and desire: Analyzing online talk by people with disabilities. *Sexualities, 21*(3), 379–392. https://doi.org/10.1177/1363460716688675

Harrell, E. (2012). *Crime against People with Disabilities, 2009–2011—Statistical Tables* (NCJ 240299). Washington, DC: U.S. Department of Justice.

HRC Foundation. (2022, August 12). *Understanding Disability in the LGBTQ+ Community*. Human Rights Campaign. https://www.hrc.org/resources/understanding-disabled-lgbtq-people

Jacobs, P., Watchman, K., Wilkinson, H., & Hoyle, L. (2023). Couples with intellectual disability where one partner has dementia: A scoping review exploring relationships in the context of dementia and intellectual disability. *Ageing and Society, 44*(11), 1–40. https://doi.org/10.1017/S0144686X22001416

Janus, A. L. (2009). Disability and the transition to adulthood. *Social Forces, 88*(1), 99–120. https://doi.org/10.1353/sof.0.0248

Kammes, R. R., Douglas, S. N., & Black, R. S. (2023). Parental role in intimate relationships: Comparing adults with and without intellectual disabilities. *Journal of Intellectual & Developmental Disability, 48*(4), 397–408. https://doi.org/10.3109/13668250.2023.2198344

Kattari, S. K. (2014). Sexual experiences of adults with physical disabilities: Negotiating with sexual partners. *Sexuality and Disability, 32*(4), 499–513. https://doi.org/10.1007/s11195-014-9379-z

Ledbetter, A. M., Carr, K., & Lynn, G. (2020). When a romantic partner has a spinal cord injury: Caregiving tasks and resilience as moderators of support quality on psychosocial distress and relational closeness. *Journal of Social and Personal Relationships, 37*(8–9), 2551–2577. https://doi.org/10.1177/0265407520929761

Leedham, A., Thompson, A. R., Smith, R., & Freeth, M. (2020). 'I was exhausted trying to figure it out': The experiences of females receiving an autism diagnosis in middle to late adulthood. *Autism, 24*(1), 135–146. https://doi.org/10.1177/1362361319853442

Lunsky, Y., Robinson, S., Blinkhorn, A., & Ouellette-Kuntz, H. (2017). Parents of adult with intellectual and developmental disabilities (IDD) and compound caregiving responsibilities. *Journal of Child and Family Studies, 26*, 1374–1379. https://doi.org/10.1007/s10826-017-0656-1

McNally, P., Taggart, L., & Shevlin, M. (2021). Trauma experiences of people with an intellectual disability and their implications: A scoping review. *JARID. Journal of Applied Research in Intellectual Disabilities/Journal of Applied Research in Intellectual Disabilities, 34*(4), 927–949. https://doi.org/10.1111/jar.12872

Mimoun, E., Koslowsky, M., Margalit, D., & Ari, A. B. (2024). Impression formation following self-disclosure of an invisible (non-apparent) disability to a romantic partner. *Sexuality and Disability, 42*(2), 277–293. https://doi.org/10.1007/s11195-023-09829-4

Mitran, C. L. (2022). A new framework for examining impact of neurodiversity in couples in intimate Relationships. *The Family Journal: Counseling and Therapy for Couples and Families, 30*(3), 437–443. https://doi.org/10.1177/10664807211063194

Morell-Mengual, V., Gil-Llario, M. D., Díaz-Rodríguez, I., & Caballero-Gascón, L. (2017). Attitudes of parents, professionals and general population towards sexuality of people with physical and intellectual disabilities. *INFAD (Barcelona)*, *4*(1), 173–184. https://doi.org/10.17060/ijodaep.2017.n1.v4.1040

Nah, S., Martire, L. M., & Zhaoyang, R. (2022). Perceived gratitude, role overload, and mental health among spousal caregivers of older adults. *The Journals of Gerontology. Series B, Psychological Sciences and Social Sciences*, *77*(2), 295–299. https://doi.org/10.1093/geronb/gbab086

Neuman, R. (2020). Establishing and maintaining couple relationships as perceived by couples with intellectual disabilities: Implications for families, support staff, and policy change. *Journal of Policy and Practice in Intellectual Disabilities, 17*(2), 132–142. https://doi.org/10.1111/jppi.12329

Neuman, R. (2022). Supporting people with intellectual and developmental disabilities in their adult aspiration for sexual relationships and parenthood. *Sexuality Research & Social Policy, 19*(2), 599–609. https://doi.org/10.1007/s13178-021-00574-x

Nosek, M. A., Howland, C., Rintala, D. H., Young, M. E., & Chanpong, G. F. (2001). National study of women with physical disabilities: Final report. *Sexuality and Disability*, *19*(1), 5–39. https://doi.org/10.1023/A:1010716820677

Nowland, K. M., Roddy, M. K., & Doss, B. D. (2017). The online OurRelationship program for relationally distressed individuals: A pilot randomized controlled trial. *Couple and Family Psychology: Research and Practice, 6*(3), 189–204. https://doi.org/10.1037/cfp0000080

Parchomiuk, M. (2012). Specialists and sexuality of individuals with disability. *Sexuality and Disability*, *30*(4), 407–419. https://doi.org/10.1007/s11195-011-9249-x

Polenick, C. A., Birditt, K. S., Turkelson, A., & Kales, H. C. (2020). Individual-level and couple-level discordant chronic conditions: Longitudinal links to functional disability. *Annals of Behavioral Medicine, 54*(7), 455–469. https://doi.org/10.1093/abm/kaz061

Polenick, C. A., Leggett, A. N., & Kales, H. C. (2017). Medical care activities among spouses of older adults with functional disability: Implications for caregiving difficulties and gains. *The American Journal of Geriatric Psychiatry*, *25*(10), 1085–1093. https://doi.org/10.1016/j.jagp.2017.05.001

Renty, J., & Roeyers, H. (2007). Individual and marital adaptation in men with autism spectrum disorder and their spouses: The role of social support and coping strategies. *Journal of Autism and Developmental Disorders, 37*(7), 1247–1255. https://doi.org/10.1007/s10803-006-0268-x

Ronis, S. T., Byers, E. S., Brotto, L. A., & Nichols, S. (2021). Beyond the label: Asexual identity among individuals on the high-functioning autism spectrum. *Archives of Sexual Behavior*, *50*(8), 3831–3842. https://doi.org/10.1007/s10508-021-01969-y

Roth, M. E., & Gillis, J. M. (2015). "Convenience with the click of a mouse": A survey of adults with autism spectrum disorder on online dating. *Sexuality and Disability, 33*(1), 133–150. https://doi.org/10.1007/s11195-014-9392-2

Rushbrooke, E., Murray, C., & Townsend, S. (2014). The experiences of intimate relationships by people with intellectual disabilities: A qualitative study. *Journal of Applied Research in Intellectual Disabilities*, *27*(6), 531–541. https://doi.org/10.1111/jar.12091

Savage, A., & McConnell, D. (2016). The marital status of disabled women in Canada: A population-based analysis. *Scandinavian Journal of Disability Research SJDR, 18*(4), 295–303. https://doi.org/10.1080/15017419.2015.1081616

Smith, R., Netto, J., Gribble, N. C., & Falkmer, M. (2021). "At the end of the day, it's love': An exploration of relationships in neurodiverse couples. *Journal of Autism and Developmental Disorders, 51*(9), 3311–3321. https://doi.org/10.1007/s10803-020-04790-z

Susano Jacinto, M. Â., Matos, R., Branquinho Gomes, B., Caseiro, A., Antunes, R., Monteiro, D., Leitão Ferreira, J. P., & Carvalheiro Campos, M. J. (2023). Physical fitness variables, general health, dementia and quality of life in individuals with intellectual and developmental disabilities: A cross-sectional study. *Healthcare*, *19*(11), 2688. https://doi.org/10.3390/healthcare11192688

Tough, H., Brinkhof, M. W., Siegrist, J., & Fekete, C. (2019). Social inequalities in the burden of care: A dyadic analysis in the caregiving partners of persons with a physical disability. *International Journal for Equity in Health*, *19*(3), 1–12. https://doi.org/10.1186/s12939-019-1112-1

Turner, G. W., & Crane, B. (2016). Pleasure is paramount: Adults with intellectual disabilities discuss sensuality and intimacy. *Sexualities*, *19*(5–6), 677–697. https://doi.org/10.1177/1363460715620573

Ward, K. M., Bosek, R. L., & Trimble, E. L. (2010). Romantic relationships and interpersonal violence among adults with developmental disabilities. *Intellectual and Developmental Disabilities*, *48*(2), 89–98. https://doi.org/10.1352/1934-9556-48.2.89

Zhang, Z. (Meredith), Smith-Johnson, M., & Gorman, B. K. (2024). Who cares? Unpaid caregiving by sexual identity, gender, and partnership status among U.S. adults. *Demography*, *61*(1), 115–140. https://doi.org/10.1215/00703370-11145841

12

DISABILITY-AFFIRMATIVE FAMILY THERAPY (PART I)

Historical Foundations and Philosophical Assumptions

Manasi Shankar

Family Science, Systemic Therapy, and Disability: A Historical Overview

The field of Family Therapy is one of the most foundational and influential disciplines in the history of psychotherapy. The origins of the field trace back to the mid-20th century when mechanistic ways of thought and conceptualization were rampant. With the rise of Systems Theory in the 1950s and 1960s, a groundbreaking paradigm shift from the focus on the individual to the entire family system emerged (Signs, 2022). For the first time, this transition allowed for a more holistic interpretation of presenting issues. This shift was a welcome change from historically reductionistic approaches to case conceptualization. It facilitated a much-needed shift in treatment focus from the isolated individual to an understanding of the client as inseparable from the social contexts within which they exist. Early pioneers like Minuchin, Bowen, and Satir developed important models rooted in systemic thinking, reinforcing the foundational assumptions of the field, and emphasizing the value of moving away from individual pathology.

Since then, the field of Family Therapy has evolved tremendously, often representative of shifts within larger societal discourse. In the 21st century, the field recognizes and prioritizes the importance of case conceptualization through an Intersectional (Crenshaw, 1989), Biopsychosocial (Bronfenbrenner, 1979) and spiritual, trauma informed, multicultural, and justice-oriented framework. Advocacy and social justice are cornerstones of the field today, as many family therapists recognize and hold space for clients who hold identities that are oppressed and marginalized by various social structures. Today, we recognize the sociocultural

DOI: 10.4324/9781003362586-19

dimensions of our client's experiences, while drawing from their strengths and sense of community. One could argue then that the discipline of Marriage and Family Therapy is at the forefront of conversations surrounding social justice, inclusion, equity, and diversity.

At the same time that Family Therapy was shifting from a focus on individual pathology to systems thinking, the field of Disability Studies was also undergoing a meaningful transformation. Very gradually, and very importantly, disability conceptualizations were moving away from the individual, deficit-focused, and pathologizing ways of the medical model to a more contextual, nuanced representation through the formation of the social model (Oliver, 1983). The social model is founded on the premise that social structures significantly shape disability experiences. It shifts the "problem" away from the body-mind of the individual, moving the onus instead to the social structures that disable them. If we were to take a step back and examine the evolution of these two parallelly occurring movements, we would have expected them to align in a way that has the power to create transformational change. Unfortunately, the two disciplines evolved in isolation, missing the opportunity for truly collaborative care for disabled communities.

Disabled clients and their families have been underserved in therapy spaces since the conception of our discipline, despite our prioritization of equitable and fair mental health care (Chen et al., 2024; Wang et al., 2024). Extant research exists on how systemic therapists, including MFTs, have overlooked the disability community in their provision of care (Parker & Gallus, 2022). One potential reason is the idea that this writer defines as "disciplinary fragmentation"; the reality that the study of disability, unlike most others, spans a variety of fields, instead of being relevant to only one. The overmedicalization of disability made it *feel* less relevant to us as psychotherapists and MFTs.

In this chapter (a series of two parts), consistent with the philosophies on which this handbook is founded, identity-first language is utilized when describing disability experiences. When referring to the family, I use "disabled family members", even when only one member of the family may be directly impacted by disability. This language is consistent with family systems theory that understands all parts of the unit as being interrelated.

The Interplay between Disability and Family Functioning

The personal experiences of disabled individuals including diagnosis, adaptation, and communication have a significant impact on family functioning (Bertschi et al., 2021; Charles, 2020; Shojaee et al., 2018). When an impairment is diagnosed, particularly later in life, it can shift family roles, structures, and relationship dynamics. A single diagnosis can create ripple effects throughout the entire family system, influencing all members. Additionally, patterns of interaction within the family, as well as engagement with external systems such as healthcare and political structures, play a crucial role in shaping individual behavior (Rolland,

1994). Familial support is well-documented as a powerful factor in helping individuals with marginalized identities navigate their experiences optimally (Balsam et al., 2011; Hernandez & Wilson, 2022). However, many families with disabled members enter the world of disability without a psychosocial map leading to experiences that can feel isolating (Rolland, 2018). Without guidance, families may struggle to adapt, highlighting the need to understand and address the systemic and relational dimensions of disability.

It is vital to correct assumptions that might arise about the nature of the effects of disability on a family. Disability can have positive effects on the family systems and its members. It can foster greater levels of empathy, resilience, meaningful family bonds, appreciation for diversity, and a deeper sense of purpose (Trute et al., 2012). One mother who is raising a disabled daughter shared that she derives more excitement from the little joys that other parents may not even think to celebrate, bringing immense joy to the parenting experience (Lodewyks, 2009).

Dr. John Rolland was one of the first theorists to describe this reciprocal nature of disability experiences and family systems. Dr. Rolland's model, the Family Systems Illness model (FSI) offers a family systems-oriented, normative, and preventive approach to assessment and intervention for families coping with chronic or life-threatening conditions. The FSI model is "a family-focused, resilience-based, and prevention-oriented clinical model that fosters healthy psychosocial adaption of the family" (Rolland, 2018, p. 5). Applicable to both adult and childhood-onset illnesses and disabilities, including neurocognitive and genetic disorders, the FSI model presents a systemic perspective on how families adapt to disability, viewing this adaptation as an ongoing developmental process that families collaborate on. Though Dr. Rolland primarily focuses on illness experiences, many philosophies and practice components remain relevant to disability experiences.

Research on Autism Spectrum Disorders (ASD) has also made significant contributions to understanding how diagnoses impact family functioning, uncovering both challenges and positive outcomes. For example, research illustrates that caring for a child with ASD can lead to heightened stress and tension between parents, often resulting in conflicts and decreased marital satisfaction. The responsibilities associated with caring for a child with ASD can lead to greater dissatisfaction and disagreements between parents on how to handle care and necessary interventions (Amate & Rosa, 2024). However, Kishimoto et al. (2023) found that high levels of family adaptability and cohesion (FAC) are linked to lower parental stress in families with children affected by ASD. FAC, which encompasses a family's ability to adapt to stress and the emotional bonds among its members, plays a crucial role in navigating the challenges associated with ASD. Caregivers of disabled family members can also benefit from adaptive family functioning. Kim et al. (2020) discussed the importance of considering the quality of family functioning when developing a social support intervention program to improve the quality of life of caregivers of children with intellectual disabilities. These findings speak to the critical role that healthy family functioning plays on an adaptive and positive experience of living with a developmental disability such as ASD. With these findings, it becomes clear that supporting families in developing healthy and positive family adaptation processes may be one of the most critical components of care in the lives of disabled people.

Foundational Philosophies and Principles

Traditional Systemic Models

Traditional systemic models such as Structural Family Therapy (SFT) (Minuchin, 1974), Narrative Therapy (White & Epston, 1990), and Bowenian Family Therapy (Bowen, 1974) among others, address family dynamics, structures, communication patterns, and roles among other family processes. However, like many other disciplines, disability has unfortunately not been a key consideration in the adaptation of these foundational models, despite their strong potential for use in conceptualizations of disability-related presenting issues.

For example, the concept of "circular causality", which is a critical component of Family Systems Theory, can be utilized to effectively understand how the reaction of one family member (such as a sibling) to the acquisition of an impairment can influence the disabled member, creating a continuous loop of interaction that is reflective of the complex interplay between disability, individuals members, and the family unit. Similarly, Minuchin's SFT is one that I (this writer) utilize frequently to address the reorganization of family structures and hierarchies, power dynamics, and the clarification of boundaries on the onset of a diagnosis. I also utilize SFT to discuss the value of flexibility in these roles and rules, a construct that will be expanded upon in another chapter. Therapists can also draw inspiration from the concepts and interventions of Narrative Therapy, such as reframing narratives about the disability experience, helping clients to re-authoring their stories to one that is less limiting, and possibly more strengths-based. Families may find themselves trapped in the societal discourse that is tied to pathology, disempowerment, and exclusion. Helping clients construct reframed narratives that are focused more on empowerment can create hope, a deeper sense of purpose, and potentially stronger levels of cohesion and unity.

Therapists can also utilize elements of Bowenian Family Therapy (Bowen, 1978) to psycho-educate clients about important constructs such as "differentiation of self". Many disabled family members have to experiment with processes like dependence and caregiving, and helping disabled individuals maintain their sense of self while receiving care from family members could be transformative for the family system. Therapists could examine ways in which generational patterns of coping with disability manifest within the family system. We could also assess for any transmission of trauma and/or resilience factors related to disability experiences across generations. In conclusion, traditional MFT models are highly relevant to disability, but they must be adapted equitably and fairly to address the unique dynamics and needs of families navigating disability experiences.

Contemporary Approaches to Disability

During the 1980s and 1990s, the integration of justice, advocacy, and social change gradually gained momentum in the discipline of MFT. Today, there is a growing recognition of the importance of conceptualizing client experiences from a Postmodern, Feminist, social-justice framework. Feminist Theory, in particular, advocated for more equitable and fair therapy practices that acknowledge the role of social structures in framing family relationships (Anderson & Stewart, 2003). Similarly, Bronfenbrenner's Bioecological model also expanded our view of the presenting issue, paying close attention to the influence of varying systems on the individual. It would be remiss not to address the widespread influence of Crenshaw's concept of Intersectionality on understanding our clients' identities and experiences in a more holistic way (Crenshaw, 1989). The spread of these movements reflects the ongoing recognition of the interconnectedness between individual well-being, relational health, and societal structures. Integrating disability into these discussions is essential, as it offers a critical perspective on how multiple forms of oppression and identity intersect, shaping individuals' lived experiences. Disability interacts with other identities, including race, gender, immigration status, and socioeconomic status, affecting how individuals encounter societal barriers and access resources. By embedding disability within the framework of Intersectionality, we cultivate a more comprehensive and inclusive approach to addressing inequality, enhancing support for marginalized communities, and advancing social justice for all.

References

Amate, J., & Rosa, M. (2024). The effect of autism spectrum disorder on family mental health: Challenges, emotional impact, and coping strategies. *Brain Sciences, 14*(11), 1116. https://www.mdpi.com/2076-3425/14/11/1116

Anderson, C. M., & Stewart, D. (2003). *Feminist family therapy: Empowerment in social context*. Sage Publications.

Balsam, K. F., Molina, Y., Beadnell, B., Simoni, J. M., & Walters, K. L. (2011). Family, social support, and depression among Black and Latinx sexual minority men. *Cultural Diversity and Ethnic Minority Psychology, 17*(3), 301–309. https://doi.org/10.1037/a0023244

Bertschi, I. C., Meier, F., & Bodenmann, G. (2021). Disability as an interpersonal experience: A systematic review on dyadic challenges and dyadic coping when one partner has a chronic physical or sensory impairment. *Frontiers in Psychology, 12*, 624609. https://doi.org/10.3389/fpsyg.2021.624609

Bowen, M. (1978). *Family therapy in clinical practice*. Jason Aronso.

Bowen, M. (1974). Toward the differentiation of self in one's family of origin. In J. Framo (Ed.), *Family interaction: A dialogue between family researchers and family therapists* (pp. 111–173). Springer.

Bronfenbrenner, U. (1979). *The ecology of human development: Experiments by nature and design*. Harvard University Press.

Charles, M. L. (2020). Communication experiences of family caregivers of hospitalized adults with intellectual and developmental disabilities—A qualitative study. *Nursing Open*, *7*(6), 1725–1734. https://doi.org/10.1002/nop2.557

Chen, S.-W., Espin-Tello, S. M., Keleman, A. A., Bollinger, R. M., Snyder, M., Storey, K., Kaesler, M., Kinder, E., Lewis, G., Dashner, J., Devine, M., & Stark, S. L. (2024). Underrepresentation of working-age and older adults with disabilities in behavioral clinical trials in the US: A review of registered behavioral clinical trials. *Occupational Therapy Faculty Publications*, Paper 1. https://digitalcommons.wustl.edu/ot_facpubs/1/

Crenshaw, K. (1989). Demarginalizing the intersection of race and sex: A Black feminist critique of antidiscrimination doctrine, feminist theory, and antiracist politics. *University of Chicago Legal Forum*, *1989*(1), 139–167. Retrieved from https://chicagounbound.uchicago.edu/uclf/vol1989/iss1/8/

Hernandez, M., & Wilson, C. M. (2022). "Family before anyone else": A qualitative study on family, marginalization, and HIV among Hispanic or Latino/a/x Mexican sexual minority males. *International Journal of Environmental Research and Public Health, 19*(15), 8899. https://doi.org/10.3390/ijerph19158899

Kim, Y., Lee, H., & Park, J. (2020). Mediating effects of family functioning on the relationship between care burden and family quality of life of caregivers of children with intellectual disabilities in Mongolia. *Journal of Applied Research in Intellectual Disabilities, 33*(6), 1293–1302. https://doi.org/10.1111/jar.12814

Kishimoto, T., Liu, S., Zhang, L., & Li, S. (2023). How do autistic severity and family functioning influence parental stress in caregivers of children with autism spectrum disorder in China? The important role of parental self-efficacy. *Frontiers in Psychology, 14*, 956637. https://doi.org/10.3389/fpsyg.2023.956637

Lodewyks, J. (2009). *Parent and child perceptions of the positive effects that a child with a disability can have on the family* [Master's thesis, University of Manitoba]. https://mspace.lib.umanitoba.ca/xmlui/bitstream/handle/1993/3143/Lodewyks%20final%20thesis.pdf

Minuchin, S. (1974). *Families and family therapy*. Harvard University Press.

Oliver, M. (1983). *Social work with disabled people*. Macmillan.

Parker, R., & Gallus, K. (2022, May). *Disabilities and the family: Where are the marriage, couple, and family therapists?* Family Therapy Magazine. https://ftm.aamft.org/disabilities-and-the-family-where-are-the-marriage-couple-and-family-therapists/

Rolland, J. S. (1994). *Families, illness, and disability: An integrative treatment model.* Basic Books.

Rolland, J. S. (2018). *Helping couples and families navigate illness and disability: An integrated approach.* The Guilford Press.

Shojaee, S., Khakhaninejad, M. S., & Najafi, M. (2018). Family communication patterns of individuals with and without disabilities. *Health Psychology Research*, *6*(1), 7080. https://pmc.ncbi.nlm.nih.gov/articles/PMC6280074/

Signs, T. (2022). *Historical overview of family systems theory*. Family Therapy Magazine. Retrieved April 7, 2024, from https://ftm.aamft.org/historical-overview-of-family-systems-theory/

Trute, B., Benzies, K. M., & Worthington, C. (2012). Mother positivity and family adjustment in households with children with a serious disability. *Journal of Child and Family Studies, 21*(3), 411–417. https://doi.org/10.1007/s10826-011-9492-x

Wang, K., Ostrove, J., Manning, R., Fodero, S., Ash, S., Whang, J., Bogart, K. R., Cipollina, R., Nario-Redmond, Adler, J., & Lowe, S. (2024). Ableism in mental healthcare settings: A qualitative study among U.S. adults with disabilities. *SSM – Qualitative Research in Health*, *7*, 100498. https://doi.org/10.1016/j.ssmqr.2024.100498

White, M., & Epston, D. (1990). *Narrative means to therapeutic ends*. Norton & Company.

13

DISABILITY-AFFIRMATIVE FAMILY THERAPY (PART II)

Clinical Applications

Manasi Shankar

Introduction

Prior chapters have highlighted the concerning gap in the field of family therapy regarding disability, emphasizing the urgent need to integrate disability dialogue into discussions on diversity, equity, inclusion, and justice. We have also explored the responsibility that we, as Marriage and Family Therapists (MFTs), hold in providing comprehensive mental health care to disabled clients and their families. By this point, the reader has grasped the profound significance and transformative power of systemic therapy in fostering meaningful support for disabled clients and their families. Before delving into concrete strategies, it is essential to first outline the foundations of Disability-Affirmative Therapy (D-AT). Several core assumptions of this framework are interwoven throughout the approach that is presented in this chapter, and therapists would benefit from having a foundational understanding of these principles before beginning to work with disability in clinical settings.

Foundations of Disability-Affirmative Therapy

In her seminal work, *What Psychotherapists Should Know About Disability* (Olkin, 1999), Dr. Rhoda Olkin introduces Disability Affirmative Therapy (D-AT) as both a philosophical concept and a clinical practice. At its essence, D-AT emphasizes the importance of affirming and validating the lived experiences of disabled individuals within therapeutic spaces. The approach challenges traditional models that are steeped in ableist tendencies and proposes concrete strategies that are

DOI: 10.4324/9781003362586-20

more inclusive of disabled experiences and identities. Olkin's work, along with the broader propositions of D-AT, has profoundly shaped the development of this handbook. While D-AT is well-integrated into many disability-focused mental health spaces, the discipline of MFT has yet to fully embrace its potential.

Olkin categorizes the practice of D-AT into two main components that therapists must consider. One component is related to the "stance of the therapist" (p. 3). This "stance" involves therapists taking on an active role in embodying a constructivist view of disability, viewing disabled people's rights as an integral component of the civil rights discourse, and contributing actively toward dismantling archaic structures that are deeply ableist. Therapists must view disability as a social construct, wherein societies actively disable individuals, rather than pathologizing the client's experiences. This process is instrumental in contributing toward more attitudinally accessible family therapy experiences. Therapists must also adopt the World Health Organization's Bio-Psychosocial view of disability, recognizing the unity of mind, body, and society, and their influences on each other (World Health Organization, 2001).

The second component is related to assessment; nine specific areas that clinicians must explore in collaboration with the disabled family. The knowledge that is acquired from this assessment will offer key insights into case formulation. While this handbook does not provide an in-depth exploration of all nine areas, therapists can refer to "Disability-Affirmative Therapy: A Case Formulation Template for Clients with Disabilities" (Olkin, 2017) for a more comprehensive discussion. The objective of this chapter is to offer a broad overview, equipping therapists with foundational principles that can inspire the development a customized treatment plan.

The nine areas of D-AT (Olkin, 2017) that therapists must pay attention to during the initial phases of treatment are:

1 **The developmental history of the individual and family and how disability has affected this history**. This writer frequently utilizes genograms as a tool to bolster an assessment of history. Detailed and multi-faceted genograms can offer insights into the generational history of disability experiences.
2 **The current sequala of disability, with an emphasis on pain, fatigue, sleep, and falls**. This could include an exploration of chronic pain symptoms, any mobility limitations, cognitive impairments, or secondary health issues like fatigue or sleep disturbances that stem from symptom-management.
3 **Models of disability of the individual and their family members, as well as the therapist**. Misalignment between family members in the way they understand the construct of disability, can perpetuate feelings of misunderstanding and isolation for the disabled member. The model that the therapist embodies is impactful as well, often informing implicit and explicit interactional patterns in therapy. Psychoeducation of the varying models as well as a discussion of the importance of some alignment in models may be valuable

in helping disabled members progress toward feelings of validation, empathy, and cohesion.

4 **Disability in the context of other demographic and cultural variables**. MFTs are trained to conceptualize cases through an Intersectional lens. It is critical that therapists understand the multi-cultural experiences of clients, assessing for the potential impact of multiple layers of marginalization.
5 **The disability culture and community, and the client's knowledge and interface with this culture and community**. An integral component of the MFT's role is to connect clients with resources and communities of support. Disabled people often benefit from a sense of belonging that is characteristic of many local, national, and virtual disability-centered groups. It can be beneficial to ask clients about their interactions with disability communities (including ones online) and the broader culture.
6 **How disability is impacting the individual's (and family's) current social interactions**. Therapists will benefit from inquiring about the family's social interactions with extended family members, friends, school systems, religious communities, medical health structures, etc.
7 **The experiences of microaggressions and the person's (and family's) reactions to these aggressions.** Expressing curiosity, asking questions about lived experience, and centering these experiences in assessment can meaningfully enrich the therapeutic alliance. It also allows for the gathering of critical information regarding the impact of microaggressions and ableism on the family's experiences.
8 **The management of affective prescriptions (mourning, cheerfulness, bravery) and prohibitions (anger)**. Able-bodied people often hold presumptions about how a disabled person "should be" feeling and/or behaving. We prescribe affective responses that are reflective of how able-bodied people make sense of the experience of disability. It feels more "digestible" when let's say, a disabled person expresses sorrow, or even grief, because this emotion-based response is consistent with tragic views of disability that are rampant in the worlds around us. Similarly, anger might be interpreted as maladaptive, rather than a typical, even healthy response to disablism, and so we may "prohibit" it, even if unintentionally. As therapists, it is our responsibility to be mindful of, and correct both affective prescriptions and prohibitions that we may perpetuate. By practicing this, we contribute to the empowerment of disabled people, recognizing that they are the only ones with expertise on the "correct" way to feel.
9 **Current intimacy (sexuality, partnership relationships) and disability within the context of these relationships**. Disabled individuals have historically been desexualized (Chin, 2024), leading to harmful stereotypes and misconceptions about the intersection of disability and sexuality. These assumptions overlook the complexity and richness of disabled people's experiences of intimacy. It is essential for therapists to actively dismantle these biases rather than inadvertently reinforcing them. In the context of family therapy, therapists

will benefit from inquiring about sexuality and intimacy-related questions in private with the disabled member, to respect their privacy.

A Clinical Framework for Addressing Disability in Family Therapy

The interventions outlined by Olkin, as described above, serve as foundational tools that therapists can integrate into ongoing assessment practices when working with disabled clients. The following section presents a concrete, clinical framework that family therapists can utilize to deliver effective disability-affirmative family therapy. It includes practical strategies, tools, and interventions to support clients in meeting their therapeutic goals in a client-centered way. It is important to recognize that this framework is one clinical plan and does not attempt to be applicable to every family living with disability. Considering the vast diversity within the community, an attempt to generalize would be unrealistic and potentially even harmful. The framework includes the following phases: (a) self-of-the-therapist work, (b) defining the client system, (c) identifying the presenting issue/s, (d) case assessment and formulation, and (e) developing a treatment plan. Establishing and maintaining a strong therapeutic alliance with all members in a manner that prioritizes feelings of safety, advocacy, and collaboration is essential to effective treatment, and must be a component of every phase.

Self-of-the-Therapist Work

If you, the reader, have followed along through the different chapters of this handbook, you are aware of the frightening gap that exists in the field of family therapy, in relation to disability. You may have also established for yourself that the issues that disabled individuals and their families struggle with mostly originate from socially inaccessible structures, policies, and attitudes, rather than individual pathology. This departure from the pathologization of disabled individuals, combined with constructivist and social model perspectives, reframes disability as a societal issue, rather than an individual deficit. Although we, as intellectual, compassionate, and socially aware professionals may grasp these concepts on a theoretical level, many therapists (even disabled therapists) still grapple with internalized ableism, implicit biases, stereotypes, and deeply ingrained misconceptions. These biases often lead to unintended, yet harmful interactions with disability within therapy contexts (VanPuymbrouck et al., 2020).

The first step in treatment (and arguably the most important one) lies in a commitment to ongoing self-of-the-therapist work, which includes an awareness of biases and ableism-related tendencies. Ask yourself these questions when you encounter a disabled person approaching you for care: *what are my instinctive thoughts when I see a disabled client in my practice? Do I experience fear, anxiety, incompetence, pity, confidence? What do these initial thoughts and feelings say about my own model of disability? Are there any assumptions I am making here? Is my own family history with disability impacting the way I feel about this person?* These reflective questions provide a crucial foundation for examining biases; an important first step in cultivating an inclusive practice.

Therapists must also engage in ongoing training in D-AT, disability rights history, contemporary trends within disability discourse, and frequent professional development opportunities. Organizations like the American Association for Marital and Family Therapy (AAMFT) and National Council on Family Relations (NCFR) frequently host disability-focused trainings and webinars on related topics. Supervision can be an essential tool for therapists at different stages in their career, especially when addressing obstacles that are influenced by the therapist's personal experiences, thoughts, and attitudes. Clinical effectiveness will be significantly strengthened by learning directly from disabled experts in the field through supervision, trainings, or consultations. For able-bodied clinicians, we may never fully understand our clients' experiences or always know the most accurate way to respond, but that holds true for all clients, regardless of their ability status. What matters most is approaching each client with humility and respectful curiosity.

Defining the Client System

The second component of the framework emphasizes a clear determination of the primary client system and communicating this with all members. As systemic thinkers and those trained in traditional systemic models, we know that in the context of family therapy, the entire family makes up the client system. Often, this can include family members that are not physically present in therapy, extended family members, friends, guardians, fictive kin etc. Remaining attuned and sensitive to the family's cultural identities and belief systems will help clinicians expand their notions of what "family" entails. Clearly establishing the family as the client system during the early stages of treatment helps shift the focus from pathologizing the individual to understanding the family unit's overall functioning. This approach emphasizes relational dynamics rather than placing responsibility on a single person, fostering a more systemic and supportive framework for therapy. It is also aligned with the departure from the problematic medical model that attempts to "fix" the individual, which often leads to feelings of blame. When the entire family is the unit of care, cohesion is strengthened, and adaptive functioning becomes a shared responsibility.

Identification of Presenting Issue(s)

One of the most pertinent challenges that MFTs report in working with disabled clients is the fear of either minimizing the role of the impairment on the presenting issue, or overinflating it (Turns et al., 2018). This is an understandable concern considering MFTs care deeply about not causing further harm, while receiving little to no training on how best to do so. On a foundational level, *collaboration* and *curiosity* are key in overcoming this challenge. Collaborating with all family members in determining the presenting issue places the client as the expert, dismantling years of disempowerment that disabled people have experienced within healthcare systems. It also reduces any assumption-making on the part of the therapist regarding the role of the impairment on the presenting issue. Curiosity should arise not from ignorance but from an acknowledgment that the client is the expert in defining their presenting issues and that every experience of disability is unique. Additionally, research indicates that understanding individuals with lived experience of disability as the experts can improve the relevance and effectiveness of therapeutic interventions (Gupta et al., 2023).

Olkin (1999) addresses the importance of explicitly inquiring about disability and its role on the presenting issue. Even if the client does not raise the topic **and if the clinician believes it might be relevant to the case**, this is an important question to ask. Once clients describe what brings them to therapy, Olkin recommends asking "Are there any ways in which your disability is a part of this problem that you describe?" (p. 167). When we fail to ask these questions, we shift the burden onto clients to ease clinicians' discomfort in discussing disability. Similar to other client experiences that we frequently work with, clients may experience denial and/or a lack of insight on the impact of the impairment on the presenting issue. In these moments, prioritizing the client's pace and maintaining a strong therapeutic alliance is essential, allowing them to revisit the question when they feel ready.

In the context of family therapy specifically, all these elements of curiosity, collaboration, and respect for pace are applicable. I often use Gottman-inspired methods of communication (Gottman, 1999) during the initial phase of treatment, where while one "active speaker" is describing their understanding of the presenting issue, other family members serve as "active listeners". Each family member takes turns as the "active speaker", fostering a layered and holistic understanding of the presenting issue. The therapist then synthesizes these perspectives, framing and presenting them to the clients for validity and refinement. Some common presenting issues faced by disabled families can include: (a) difficulty in navigating external, inaccessible, systemic barriers such as medical systems, housing, state and federal-level policies, or school systems, (b) adjustment and coping with a new diagnosis, (c) caregiver stress and burnout, (d) communication challenges, (e) conflicts over generational attitudes toward disability, and (f) parent-child and/or sibling conflicts related to balancing care, feeling infantilized, or lacking agency in family decisions. These are just some common challenges, but it is critical to ensure that the identification of the presenting issue(s) remains primarily client-driven.

Case Assessment and Formulation

A thorough case assessment and formulation are critical elements of an effective treatment plan. An in-depth assessment leads to a formulation that accurately captures the challenges within the system, identifies contributors to maladaptive patterns, and highlights areas of family functioning that need attention in therapy. Understanding if and how the disability influences the presenting issue allows for a case conceptualization that is comprehensive and free from bias. Clinicians can think of assessment as collecting information about client history, health symptoms, behaviors, relationships, quality of interactions with people and systems, and overall functioning. Case formulation, on the other hand, is about interpreting this information to create a meaningful framework for therapy.

Assessment

Clinical assessment procedures include several important components, both individual and relational. Clinical interviews and standardized screening tools such as the PHQ-9 (Patient Health Questionnaire-9) and GAD-7 (Generalized Anxiety Disorder-7) are valuable in evaluating individual well-being, which is a crucial contributor to overall family functioning. Depending on the developmental age of members, individual clinical interviews can help therapists assess mental health concerns that may affect (or be affected by) family interactions. It can also help in uncovering family dynamics and patterns that might be contributing to the maintenance of the presenting issue. Often, exploring individual perspectives on family issues can also help with a more holistic conceptualization of the family's struggles.

With regard to the assessment of the family system, the primary goal is to gain a comprehensive understanding of the family's dynamics, strengths, and challenges, to be able to inform effective treatment interventions. It also helps in the process of aligning individual and family needs to establish meaningful treatment goals. Effective assessment practices must include a bio-psychosocial (Engel, 1977) (and spiritual), cultural assessment of the issues. It also must include an incorporation of a truly Intersectional lens that flows through every stage of treatment. Therapists could utilize a model like the Eco-Systemic Family Therapy model (ESFT) (Lindblad-Goldberg & Northey, 2013) to assess how the disability interacts with different layers of the system. Therapists can also use scales such as the Family Adaptability and Cohesion Evaluation Scales (FACES) (Olson, 2011), the McMaster Family Assessment Device (FAD) (Epstein, Baldwin, & Bishop, 1983), or the Parenting Stress Index (PSI) (Abidin, 2012) to better understand relational dynamics. Some disability-specific family assessment tools are also available. These include the Family Needs Survey (FNS) (Dunst et al., 1988) and the Impact on Family Scale (IOF) (Stein & Jessop, 2003) both of which evaluate the interaction of disability with family dynamics. The utilization of strengths-based tools is also important in shifting the therapeutic focus away from challenges to existing strengths and resources. Some examples include the Parenting Sense of Competence Scale (PSOC) (Gibaud-Wallston & Wandersman, 1978; Johnston & Mash, 1989), Family Strengths Inventory (Stinnett & DeFrain, 1985), and the Family Resilience Assessment Scale (FRAS) (Patterson, 2002; Sixbey, 2005).

Other structural tools can also assess the influence of external systems. A disability-focused genogram can help therapists track generational patterns related to disability experiences such as diagnoses, any deaths, generational attitudes and narratives toward disability, as well as any strengths and protective factors. If any long-standing cultural narratives regarding disability exist, the therapist can discuss this during the assessment phase as well. Therapists can also benefit from "time-lining" disability events to track how important transitions such as diagnosis, diagnosis-disclosure, coping, etc. have shaped the family's adaptation over time. Often, this opens the door to conversations about experiences of trauma that are rampant within the disability community (Sullivan & Knutson, 2000; Wang et al., 2024). Clinicians can also draw from Olkin's interventions outlined in a prior section of this chapter, for a full assessment. An effective assessment will result in an in-depth, holistic understanding of the presenting issue and the factors that impact it.

Formulation

Following a thorough assessment of the family's presenting issue, the information gathered must be synthesized to create a case formulation (or conceptualization) that can guide treatment. This includes but is not limited to:

1 **Revisiting the presenting issue(s) to include any new and pertinent information gathered**. At this stage, therapists must collaborate with the family to discuss conclusions regarding the assessment process.
2 **Highlighting family system dynamics (such as roles, rules, hierarchies, power) and the role of disability (if any) on these dynamics**. This is where relational processes such as enmeshment and parentification can be explored with the family. It is crucial to acknowledge that constructs like these are not always culturally informed or fairly researched. These concepts, along with the individual experiences related to them, are deeply shaped by cultural influences.
3 **Considering any disability-specific factors when relevant**. This includes any medical or functional limitations, prescribed drug usage, access to services and support systems, and quality of interactions with healthcare workers.
4 **Acknowledging the influence of sociocultural factors**. Therapists must consider any financial stressors, resource limitations, immigration-related stressors, and employment-related factors when formulating the case.

These formulations will facilitate the generation of a hypothesis about the patterns that contribute to the presenting issue. Therapists must arrive at this juncture in collaboration with the client. Based on the formulation, therapists can then work with clients to set goals that also account for individual member needs and well-being. It is also encouraged to outline treatment approaches that the therapist plans to use with the clients, to demonstrate collaborative care. When working with disability, this could also entail collaborating with other professionals such as those within school systems, advocates, law professionals, medical providers, and social workers.

Establishing Treatment

For disabled individuals, the term "treatment" in the context of care is a complex one and has been a source of harm to the community for decades. Historically (and aligned with archaic ideas regarding eugenics), "treatment" was equated to erasure, erasure not just of symptoms but of people. This age-old understanding of treatment, that stems from medical model conceptualizations, is what we are moving (far) away from. Instead, deeply aligned with systemic notions of treatment, within safe MFT spaces, treatment must entail the healing of interactional patterns that are dysfunctional and/or maladaptive that may or may not be impacted by impairment. Treatment must also incorporate a strengths-based approach whenever relevant. For this reason, therapy sessions must prioritize the optimization of functioning (ex, health, well-bring, and hardiness), rather than on the amelioration of negative symptoms (Olkin, 1999).

Integrating the lived experiences of disabled individuals into therapeutic frameworks can significantly enhance treatment outcomes and family adaptation. A recent study by Mona (2023) emphasizes the necessity of client-led psychotherapy when working with physically disabled clients, highlighting how affirming approaches can foster empowerment, while clinician-driven methods may cause harm. These foundational principles must be established before delving into specific treatment plans.

The sections below offer clinicians a blueprint to help structure treatment. Given the wide range of experiences within the community, this template is not intended to be universally applicable to all disabled families. Rather, it serves as a starting point that clinicians can adapt to meet the unique presenting issues and needs of their clients.

Family Resilience Approach

The term "resilience" has often been misused, especially when directed at marginalized communities that are in need of systemic support. Rather than acknowledging the structural barriers they face, resilience is sometimes framed as an individual responsibility, placing undue pressure on those who are already navigating significant challenges. Walsh defines resilience as "the ability to withstand and rebound from serious life challenges" (Walsh, 2016, p. 4). With regard to disability experiences, it is critical that we do not presumptuously equate disability to adversity. While many disabled individuals and family members may view their experiences as challenging, equating disability with adversity or trauma can be harmful and reductive. Many disabled people draw strength from their identity

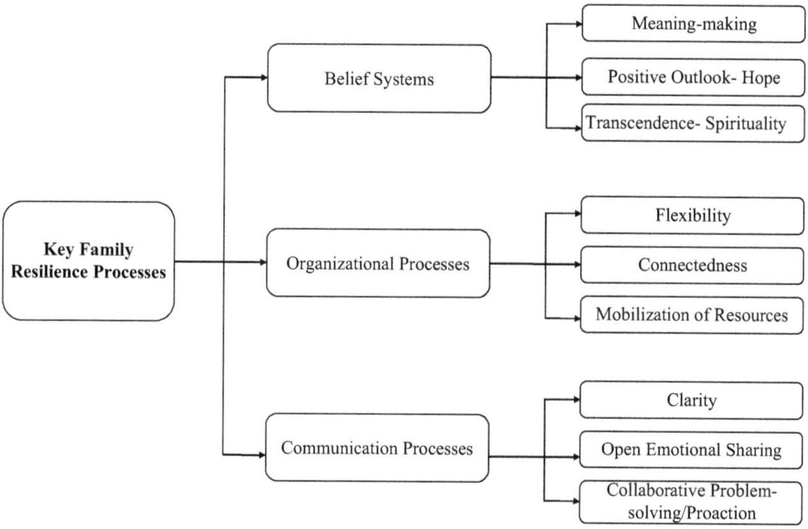

Figure 13.1 Walsh's Family Resilience Framework.

as a disabled person. They enjoy meaningful life experiences, not despite the disability, but because of it (Martz & Livneh, 2015; Sniatecki et al., 2021). For most people in the community, their experiences exist somewhere in between these two points of the spectrum, dynamically moving from one end to the other, based on context(s) and many times (I have found anecdotally), on perceived social and communal support. This section introduces an adaptation of Walsh's Family Resilience Framework tailored for family therapy with disabled individuals and their families. Figure 13.1 outlines the key family processes of resilience based on Walsh's model that can be utilized in the treatment phase, when adapted to work with disabled clients and families.

Belief Systems: Cultivating a Shared Meaning of Disability

Walsh describes *belief systems* as the "heart and soul" of all family functioning (Walsh, 2016, p. 39). Belief systems that individual members and the family hold about disability determine the meaning that they make of the experience. The way in which the family views challenges can make all the difference between coping and mastery, or dysfunction and despair (Walsh, 2016). Often belief systems that we hold are determined by larger societal discourses, cultural influences, intergenerational narratives, parental messaging, media influences (particularly social media), and politics. These beliefs, in turn, trigger emotional responses, inform behavior, attitudes, values, convictions, and ways of behaving. Walsh addresses the important difference between *constraining beliefs* that perpetuate problems and cause despair, and *affirming beliefs* that focus on acceptance, self-worth, and support. When we help family members to cultivate more affirming beliefs, we support them in rallying through crises. Throughout history, disabled individuals have been depicted as weak, incapable, and in need of "fixing". These harmful narratives have permeated societal belief systems, shaping the ways in which individuals perceive and interact with disability. In the context of belief systems, our objective is twofold: (1) assess, explore, and critically discuss the diverse beliefs and assumptions surrounding disability. A conversation about models of disability becomes relevant here. If one member identifies with the social model of disability, and another, the medical model, this could create important differences in the way they interact with the disability and with each other. Therapists could engage in psychoeducation about the different models, so that members have a deeper understanding of each model, and the way in which it impacts the disabled member. (2) Work toward developing alignment and a shared belief system within the family. In well-functioning families, members hold a congruent set of beliefs and are open to differing viewpoints (Walsh, 2016). This step is crucial in ensuring that the disabled family member feels understood, accepted, and less isolated.

Within this stage in treatment, therapists can conduct clinical interviews and talk with members about their *meaning-making* related to the acquisition of the impairment. Therapists could ask *That must have been hard for you to watch your daughter struggle when she was first diagnosed. In that moment, how did you make sense of what was happening.* Therapists can encourage individual members to tell stories about past experiences that may have impacted personal meaning-making. This creates a sense of understanding, empathy, and more clarity in behavioral motives. It also results in loyalty and trust where members can feel a sense of unity in navigating adverse situations.

A *positive outlook* is not the same as dismissive or forced optimism; rather, it emphasizes strength-based interactions, constructive hope, and meaningful support. Extant research demonstrates the power of a forward-looking perspective on working through challenges (Snyder et al., 2002). This process does not entail ignorance of past ruptures, present struggles, or future concerns, but a strengths-based approach in helping the family heal. Often, disabled people feel hopeless and discount their personal contributions to the family's well-being. This can be challenged by asking questions such as

> I understand that because of the fibromyalgia, your energy is limited. You cannot always help your partner with household chores that demand high levels of mobility. You seem to have a good way around numbers though. Are you able to use these skills to contribute towards financial planning?

This intervention shifts the focus from the impairment to accessibility, increasing feelings of inclusion and unity.

The final component of belief systems in Walsh's model is *transcendence and spirituality.* Walsh clearly addresses the distinction between religion and spirituality, the latter being less about intuitions and entities, and more about a connection with the meaning of life, values, purpose, and joy. Researchers have described how suffering invites us into the spiritual domain (Wright, 2009), and it is imperative that we accompany our clients on their spiritual journeys as they navigate the meaning of living with disability. By facilitating conversations about meaning and purpose, families can align on forging new meaning, purpose, and ways of healing. I once worked with a family living with a father who recently acquired a traumatic brain injury (TBI). One question that was discussed that truly shifted the course of healing was *In the midst of this life-altering transition, what personal values that you hold can we draw on to help you find purpose again?*. Walsh also highlights the power of "role models and heroes" in the journey toward transcendence (p. 61). Disabled activists with a strong social media presence, such as Alice Wong and Lauren Spencer, among numerous others, serve as important role models for many disabled people. Supporting clients in finding purpose and a sense of connection through the stories of these individuals can have profound impacts.

Organizational Processes: Adjusting Family Dynamics for Long-Term Adaptation

MFTs often work with a family's structural dynamics in treatment, particularly during periods of transition. Minuchin's Structural Family Therapy provides a framework aimed at reorganizing the family system, including facilitating shifts in family members' roles and positions when social contexts demand it (Minuchin, 1974). Similarly, Walsh discusses the importance of mobilizing and organizing resources (both internal and external) and reorganizing family structure to fit changing family conditions. When an individual acquires an impairment, their abilities and preferences, be it physical, emotional, psychological, behavioral, or relational may change. This evolution in a client's identity may result in a shift in the family's rules, roles, and/or patterns of relating with one another. One study by Becerra and Michael-Makri (2012) revealed the value in educating family members about healthy boundary-formation and shifts in boundaries, when working with Mexican and Mexican-American families who are raising a disabled child. Therefore, from a structural perspective, the objective of the therapist is to support clients through the process of healthy reorganization and adaptation, throughout the evolution of the disability experience.

"Like all human systems, families tend to resist change beyond a certain familiar range" (Walsh, 2016, p. 65). Fortunately, Walsh offers strategies to help families attain successful readaptation. The positive impact of *flexibility* in structures has been well-documented in family therapy research (Chung et al., 2014). Satir (1988) describes the adaptability of certain healthy families in challenging situations as a particularly healing force within the system. Especially during the initial phases of disability acquisition or diagnosis, flexibility in familial roles, rules, hierarchies, power dynamics, caretaking, expectations, and interactions with external systems such as extended family members become critical. For this author's doctoral dissertation, adult children who were raised by disabled parents were interviewed, to examine their experiences and perspectives (Shankar, 2021). Across these interviews, participants consistently emphasized the value of flexibility within their families, particularly in family roles and rules. Many participants contributed to household chores, with some also taking on caregiving responsibilities for their parents. Western views on child-rearing often regard emotional and instrumental parentification as inherently negative. However, adopting a culturally informed and nuanced perspective requires directly engaging with individuals to assess the impact of developmentally appropriate roles. Notably, what is deemed "appropriate" in one cultural context may be considered "inappropriate" in another. Without empirically sound, and inclusive research methods, claims regarding the long-term impacts of these experiences may be stemming from bias and may not be reflective of lived experiences.

Throughout this readaptation process, Wash describes the importance of *strong leadership*- establishing that the parents and other elders are the "architects" of this transformational process. This strong leadership can "protect, nurture, and guide" (p. 35) members through the readaptation process. Often, disabled parents, depending on the disability, may not be able to demonstrate this leadership in a traditional or overt manner. In these situations, another parent, or an elder may step in to take on this role. Throughout the chaos and disruption that the disorganization and reorganization process entail, therapists must normalize this reaction and gently support the family through re-stabilization.

A second process within organization in Walsh's framework is *family cohesion.* Extant research has established the power of familial support in the navigation of chronic illness and disability (Martz & Livneh, 2015). An important study by Li and Moore (2010) demonstrated that emotional support from family members and friends determined the quality of adjustment to a recently acquired disability. With respect to healthy functioning at the face of challenging times, families tend to do best when they are able to balance mutual support, closeness, and commitment with respect for individual needs, growth, and separateness. A strong sense of teamwork can facilitate resilience for families when they are navigating stressful times (Walsh, 2016). Some research has also demonstrated that potentially testing transitions such as a disability diagnosis, can further strengthen feelings of connectedness, loyalty, and teamwork among members (Sutherland et al., 2025). The role of the therapist then is to normalize any disruptions to feelings of cohesion during the initial phases, psycho-educate about the value of teamwork, and engage clients in interventions that will enhance feelings of closeness.

Sometimes, clients' feelings of closeness are tested by the need to reimagine and reconstruct previously established *family boundaries* (Walsh, 2016). Family boundaries are a critical point of discussion for many disabled families. Minuchin (1974) describes family boundaries as the specific roles of each family member and how they interact with one another. In the face of disability, these boundaries are tested, and must be re-established, based on the new social context of disability. "People's experiences change as their positions relative to one another are transformed". Minuchin describes this process as "movement in therapy" and therapists can support family members through this transformation (Minuchin, 1974, p. 117). A few years ago, I got the opportunity to work with a family where the mother was recently diagnosed with a spinal cord injury resulting in paralysis, due to a car accident. Her diagnosis disrupted family roles, forcing a redefinition of boundaries. The father struggled to step into the caregiving role, while the children grappled with their mother's changing presence. Therapy helped them restructure their roles, fostering adaptation and deeper connection, albeit in a new form.

In the context of disability, the importance of the final organizational process in Walsh's framework-*social and economic resources* cannot be overstated. For centuries, disabled people have experienced systemic isolation, inaccessibility to community resources, and inequitable legal frameworks, policies, and care provision. A lack of societal focus on supporting disabled families has led to extreme feelings of exclusion and loneliness for the community. In today's era of social media and increased social comparison, the fragmentation of social connections can significantly affect a disabled person's mental well-being and sense of belonging. Walsh explains that healthy families maintain clear, yet flexible boundaries, allowing members to mobilize external resources and engage with outside systems in a helpful manner.

Similar to the expectations that we as clinicians place on families to be flexible in their roles, it is vital that we are adaptive in our therapeutic role as well. Often, therapy with disabled members entails more roles than is traditionally expected, which must include advocacy. This could include connecting clients with housing resources, medical professionals, lawyers, testing and assessment centers, writing employment-related leave of absence letters that can be used for the Family and Medical Leave Act (FMLA), support for emotional support animals (ESA), service animals, and more. In sessions, we are building a "support team" for the family, consisting of multiple professionals working together to support the family in a holistic manner. This helps the family feel supported and strengthens the perceived sense of loyalty and teamwork that was described earlier.

Disabled individuals disproportionately face financial challenges, often due to systemic barriers that limit their access to fair employment opportunities. They are unemployed at higher rates, facing discrimination and inadequate workplace accommodations that restrict their economic independence (U.S. Bureau of Labor Statistics, 2024). Therefore, once a strong rapport has been established and members feel comfortable to do so, therapists and clients can engage in an open discussion regarding any financial stressors that might be hindering the family's healing. Offering sliding scale fees when possible is an effective way to increase the financial accessibility of therapy. Therapists can also support disabled individuals by connecting them with financial resources such as Social Security Disability Insurance (SSDI) and Supplemental Security Income (SSI), as well as programs like Federal Disability Benefits (FDB) that provide financial assistance and access to essential services.

Finally, helping the family to mobilize appropriate sociocultural resources such as extended family, fictive kin, appropriate disability communities, and support groups is crucial. Miller et al. (2009) emphasized the important role that health-care professionals can have in helping families navigate complex care systems. Of course, practicing culturally informed care is vital in the mobilization of appropriate resources. In many collectivistic cultures, grandparenting roles are often synonymous with parenting, and extended family members hold significant influence in family decision-making, shaping the course of treatment. In this way, therapy with disabled families inadvertently involves far more people than those physically present in the room.

Communication Processes: Facilitating Change Through Clear and Collaborative Dialogue

Communication involves the transmission of beliefs, information exchange, emotional expression, and problem-solving (Ryan et al., 2005). The final process within Walsh's framework is often considered one of the most difficult to navigate in family therapy, yet one of the most transformative. In the context of disability, open communication among family members (regardless of the format or modality) becomes particularly crucial, as experiences with disability often involve uncertainty in diagnosis, prognosis, and meaning-making. It is important to recognize that communication is not solely verbal. It also includes non-verbal messaging, modeling behavior, intergenerational and cultural messaging, body language, tone, pace, voice, and much more. In fact, many disabilities involve non-verbal communication methods, such as those used by individuals with autism, speech impairments, and those who belong to the Deaf and non-speaking communities.

With regard to therapy, the quality of communication that we model in our interactions with clients is also crucial. Since there is tremendous value for clients in receiving treatment in the most accessible language (de Bruin & Brugmans, 2006), several therapists learn and practice American Sign Language (ASL), have written documents in Braille, and utilize assistive technologies to communicate with their clients. The important study by de Bruin and Brugmans (2006) analyzed the unique and valuable relationship between the psychotherapist and the sign language interpreter who many therapists collaborate with to make therapy accessible.

Clarity in communication entails clear, consistent verbal and behavioral messaging (Walsh, 2016). The primary objective of clarity in communication is to foster a shared understanding of disability processes, similar to the family process of "belief systems". When communication is vague, it breeds confusion, anxiety, and in the case of disability, even fear. Another important finding in this writer's dissertation was the emphasis on open and clear communication. (Shankar, 2021).

Participants who were raised by disabled parents talked about a lack of clarity in parental diagnosis leading to intense feelings of confusion, fear, and "feeling left out". One participant who was raised by a mother with fibromyalgia shared "I wished they just told me. They kept saying 'mom is sick'. I had no idea what that meant. Like, was she going to die? I carried that fear everyday". Many parents engage in family secrecy surrounding the diagnosis, prognosis, and limitations, to "protect" their children. This lack of transparency can have detrimental effects on the child's own understanding of disability and can even lead to strained relationships. Walsh asserts how prolonged silence, secrecy, and distraction create barriers to true understanding and informed decision-making. (Walsh, 2016). When conversations are developmentally appropriate, open discussions about the disability can be incredibly valuable. These conversations can foster a sense of collaboration and teamwork, ultimately enhancing family cohesion and connectedness.

Walsh describes this process of talking openly about the distressing event as "sharing the bad news" (p. 84). In the context of disability, this can be interpreted instead as a "collaborative conversation", "important update", "diagnosis", "impairment" – all more strengths-based phrases, dependent on the unique needs of the family. When working with families with young children, therapists can meet with parent/s first to understand the diagnosis and the disabled member's experience with the impairment. The therapist can then coach parent/s on how to openly, respectfully, and kindly share this information with their child/children. The conversation with the child must lead to "open communication pathways", demonstrating that parents are always available to answer questions (to the best of their ability) whenever the child needs it. Often, disability may include components that are consistently unpredictable, and clarity and predictability become a privilege known only to some. In these instances, it is important to be honest with children (and partners) about the unpredictable nature of the disability. Parents can instead, emphasize the predictability and stability of the support systems and the skills and qualifications of care professionals who serve the family.

Extant research demonstrates the value of *open emotional sharing* between family members (Rimé et al., 1996). Open emotion-focused conversations within families play a crucial role in emotional development and connection. Discussions about sadness often involve reflection and resolution, fostering a sense of self in relation to others, while promoting healthy coping strategies. In contrast, conversations about anger primarily focus on the emotional experience itself, strengthening self-definition and personal identity (Fivush et al., 2003). Gentzler et al. also found that emotional-focused communication between parents and children strengthened the child's coping mechanisms (Gentzler et al., 2005). This can be particularly valuable during periods of adversity, when emotional vulnerability becomes a critical element in the healing process. When parents model healthy emotional expression and vulnerability, they communicate to their children that such behaviors are not only acceptable but encouraged. This sets a powerful precedent, fostering an environment where emotional openness is both supported and valued.

This chapter has addressed the importance of family members navigating disability experiences as a "team", with parents and/or elders as the "leaders" of this team. For the final component of her framework, Walsh describes the value of *collaborative problem-solving.* Aligned with the ideologies that underpin this handbook, it is crucial to recognize that the issue requiring collaborative problem-solving is not the impairment itself, but rather the "disablement" caused by inaccessible social structures, policies, infrastructure, healthcare systems, and societal discourse, along with their detrimental effects on the well-being of the family and individual members. Once family cohesion has been strengthened through a shared understanding of disability and stronger communication, therapists can support the family in navigating both the challenges and the strengths of disability as a team, where each member makes their contribution toward achieving these shared goals. As described earlier, these roles are dynamic, developmentally-appropriate, and openly communicated with room for flexibility as social contexts change.

Integrating shared belief systems, flexible organizational processes, and open communication into family therapy helps families build resilience and adapt to the effects of disability and disablement. Shared belief systems shape how families make meaning of their experiences, fostering hope, a sense of collective identity, and connection. Organizational processes including roles, rules, and flexibility provide the structure needed to maintain stability while adapting to change. Open communication creates space for emotional expression, validation, and collaborative problem-solving, strengthening family connectedness. When these processes are intentionally incorporated into therapy, families can better manage stress, support one another, and navigate disability in more optimal ways.

Case Example

This section presents a case vignette to illustrate the application of the treatment structure described above. It is only a summary and does not delve into specific interventions or clinical tools.

Case Vignette

The Park family, Korean immigrants who moved to the U.S. six years ago, have been facing increasing challenges since the father (Jun) was diagnosed with progressive Multiple Sclerosis (MS) a year ago. All other members are non-disabled. The mother (Bora) works long hours to provide for the family, while 13-year-old Mina has taken on a caregiving role, helping her father with daily tasks and supporting her younger sister, eight-year-old Soo. Soo struggles to comprehend the changes in her father's health and often feels neglected as the family focuses on his care. Financial pressures have also led to strain between the parents. Bora feels exhausted and Jun is experiencing guilt over his declining condition and its effects on the family. Despite their strong bond, the family finds it difficult to communicate openly about their emotional struggles and the evolving dynamics in their household, bringing them to us for family therapy.

1 **Self-of-the-therapist work**

- Reflect on and work through any implicit/explicit biases and/or stereotypes. The family holds several minoritized identities including being immigrants, East Asian in America, facing a financial crisis, and a recent disability diagnosis. Self-reflect on any prejudice as well as skill and competence levels, and refer out if appropriate.

2 **Defining the client system**

- In family therapy, the entire family is the unit of care. During the intake process, therapists can inquire about external support systems such as extended family and fictive kin, who may also need to be a part of the client system, if relevant.

3 **Identification of the presenting issue**

- Collaborate with family members to understand what brings them to therapy from a place of non-judgement. Ask respectful, open-ended questions about specific concerns and challenges. Keep in mind that the client is the expert here. Asking Jun about the meaning he makes of his recent diagnosis, Mina about her experiences helping with caretaking, Bora about the impact of the diagnosis on her psychosocial well-being are good places to start.
- Utilize Gottman-inspired communication interventions to create space for all members to share their perspective on the presenting issue, regardless of age. As long as the family member has a desire to share, and is developmentally able to, check in with each unit of the family. Be open to the idea of facilitating individual sessions with each member, if needed.
- Remain mindful of not overinflating the role of the impairment or minimizing it. Since the disability is relevant to the case, it is important to gently inquire about its impact on the presenting issue. As Olkin (1999) stated, when disability is in fact relevant to the case, it is vital that therapists do not shy away from openly discussing it.

4 **Case assessment and formulation**

- **Individual Well-Being Assessments**: Use standardized screening tools such as the PHQ-9 and GAD-7 to assess symptoms of depression and anxiety in each family member in a developmentally appropriate manner.
- **Clinical Interviews**: Conduct individual interviews with each family member, ensuring developmental appropriateness, to explore their personal experiences, coping strategies, and perceptions of family dynamics. This will help identify mental health concerns that may be influencing, or are influenced by family interactions.

- **Family System Assessment**: Utilize the McMaster FAD or FACES to evaluate the family's cohesion, adaptability, and communication patterns. These tools can highlight areas of strength and strain within the family structure.
- **Bio-Psychosocial-Spiritual and Cultural Considerations**: Conduct a culturally responsive assessment, acknowledging the family's Korean immigrant background, financial stressors, and potential cultural stigmas around disability and mental health. Exploring their beliefs about disability, intergenerational expectations, and available community supports is essential. Since the family has mentioned difficulties with emotional expression, respectfully explore cultural norms and beliefs regarding emotional vulnerability and openness.
- **Disability-Specific Assessment**: Use the FNS and the IOF to assess how Jun's MS diagnosis affects family functioning, roles, and emotional well-being. These tools can help identify unmet needs and guide interventions that enhance family support.
- **Strength-Based Tools**: Incorporate measures like the FRAS and the PSOC to identify existing family strengths, coping mechanisms, and sources of resilience.
- **Family system dynamics**: Traditional Korean values may be influencing caregiving expectations, with the mother assuming primary responsibility and Mina stepping into a caretaker role. A non-judgmental, culturally sensitive approach to discussing any impacts of these roles is imperative.
- **Disability-specific factors**: Jun's medical needs, access to health care, and interactions with providers may be impacting family stress. Navigating disability services and financial constraints may be adding further strain.
- **Sociocultural influences**: Acculturation and assimilation-related stress, grief and feelings of loss related to immigration, political climates, and limited resources may be shaping the family's experiences.
- **Hypothesis generation**: The combination of financial hardship, disability-related stress, and evolving family roles may be contributing to their distress. Given the family's strong emotional bond, therapists can utilize this as a foundation for developing strengths-based interventions.

5 Treatment

- **Belief Systems**: Explore the family's shared beliefs about disability, considering the cultural and intergenerational influences that shape their perspectives. Recognize the differences in how each member interprets the disability-one may see it as a tragedy, while another views it as a challenge to overcome together. The therapist's goal is to foster alignment in meaning-making while honoring each individual perspective.
- Collaborate with the client to cultivate a hopeful perspective, moving away from self-limiting and defeating thoughts. Encourage them to focus on their strengths, particularly the emotional closeness they share.

- Explore any spiritual or religious beliefs that may serve as sources of motivation, reinforcing hope and a positive outlook.
- **Family Organizational Patterns**: Provide psychoeducation about the importance of flexibility, normalizing the disruption in structure that the family is undergoing. Work in collaboration with all members to openly discuss roles, rules, and their dynamic nature. We only move forward from this stage when all members feel ready and open to adaptation.
- Therapists must assert the value of connectedness and mutual support in creating a strong sense of "teamwork" between family members. Both parents must serve as the "leaders" of this team. If Jun (father) has days where he cannot engage in physical tasks, he can still demonstrate this leadership through emotion-based check ins, household planning, and other chores that he is able to take on. Psycho-educate clients about the "spoon theory of disability" (Miserandino, 2003), where the family can utilize a "code word" when all of Jun's "spoons" have been depleted for the day and another member needs to step in.
- Build a support team in a detailed, strategic manner. This team is built to support not only Jun, but the entire family. This support team could include healthcare professionals, social workers, friends, neighbors, fictive kin, extended family, cultural communities, supportive school officials, and a list of financial resources. In this case, there are numerous external struggles that are beyond the control of the therapist, such as economic hardship. However, therapists can still pay attention to this and connect the family with appropriate resources.
- **Communication and Problem-solving**: Emphasize the value of clarity in communication. Help parents find developmentally-appropriate language to talk with both children about MS, the prognosis, symptoms, and its often-unpredictable nature. Discuss what strategies help when the pain flares up and how to support each other on challenging days. Remember to help parents foster "open communication pathways", so that children know that even when time lapses, they can always approach parents if questions related to disability come up in their own personal lives.
- Highlight the importance of open emotional expression, guiding parents and children in sharing their feelings in ways that remain respectful and aligned with cultural values.
- Once therapy establishes a sense of teamwork and strong family cohesion, challenges can be reframed as opportunities for collective problem-solving.
- As therapy progresses, the goal is for the family to feel more connected, develop a shared understanding of their experience, honor individual perspectives, and strengthen moments of collaboration, connection, hope, joy, and resilience.

Conclusion

This chapter has explored the critical intersection of family therapy and disability, emphasizing the systemic, disability-affirmative lens essential for effective treatment with families where disability is present. Olkin's philosophical assumptions provide the foundation for understanding disability as a social construct, highlighting the need for therapists to adopt an empathetic, anti-ableist stance in clinical practice. This perspective challenges traditional models by urging therapists to recognize and affirm the lived experiences of disabled individuals within their familial contexts. Moving from theory to practice, Walsh's Family Resilience Framework offers a nuanced approach to treatment. By focusing on the strengths and adaptive capacities of families, it provides concrete strategies for addressing the challenges of living with disability. Through this lens, therapy becomes not just about managing disability experiences but also about fostering resilience, empowerment, and cohesion within the family system.

Family therapists have the compassion, training, expertise, and systemic lens to create meaningful change in the lives of families navigating disability. As therapists committed to relational healing and justice, we must recognize that integrating disability-affirmative practices is not an optional expansion of our work-it is an overdue and necessary shift; it is a part of our ethical code. This work may be complex, but if we are to truly define ourselves as an inclusive field, we must not overlook the world's largest minority group.

References

Abidin, R. R. (2012). *Parenting Stress Index (PSI) manual* (4th ed.). Psychological Assessment Resources.

Becerra, M. D., & Michael-Makri, S. (2012). Applying structural family therapy with a Mexican-American family with children with disabilities: A case study of a single-parent mother. *Journal of Applied Rehabilitation Counseling, 43*(2), 17–22.

Chin, N. M. (2024). The structural desexualization of disability. *Columbia Law Review, 124*(1), 1–45. https://columbialawreview.org/content/the-structural-desexualization-of-disability/

Chung, B. D., Mikesell, L., & Miklowitz, D. J. (2014). Flexibility and structure may enhance implementation of family-focused therapy in community mental health settings. *Community Mental Health Journal, 50*(7), 787–791. https://doi.org/10.1007/s10597-014-9733-8

de Bruin, E., & Brugmans, P. (2006). The psychotherapist and the sign language interpreter. *Journal of Deaf Studies and Deaf Education, 11*(3), 360–367.

Dunst, C. J., Cooper, C. S., Weeldreyer, J. C., Snyder, K. D., & Chase, J. H. (1988). Family needs scale. In C. J. Dunst, C. M. Trivette, & A. G. Deal (Eds.), *Enabling and empowering families: Principles and guidelines for practice* (pp. 163–167). Brookline Books.

Engel, G. L. (1977). The need for a new medical model: A challenge for biomedicine. *Science, 196*(4286), 129–136. https://doi.org/10.1126/science.847460

Epstein, N. B., Baldwin, L. M., & Bishop, D. S. (1983). The McMaster family assessment device. *Journal of Marital and Family Therapy, 9*(2), 171–180. https://doi.org/10.1111/j.1752-0606.1983.tb01497.x

Fivush, R., Berlin, L. J., Sales, J. M., Mennuti-Washburn, J., & Cassidy, J. (2003). Functions of parent-child reminiscing about emotionally negative events. *Memory, 11*(2), 179–192. https://doi.org/10.1080/741938209

Gentzler, A. L., Contreras-Grau, J. M., Kerns, K. A., & Weimer, B. L. (2005). Parent–child emotional communication and children's coping in middle childhood. *Social Development, 14*(4), 591–612. https://doi.org/10.1111/j.1467-9507.2005.00319.x

Gibaud-Wallston, J., & Wandersman, L. P. (1978). *Development and utility of the parenting sense of competence scale*. Paper presented at the annual meeting of the American Psychological Association, Toronto.

Gottman, J. M. (1999). *The seven principles for making marriage work*. Crown Publishers.

Gupta, V., Eames, C., Golding, L., Greenhill, B., Qi, R., Allan, S., Bryant, A., & Fisher, P. (2023). Understanding the identity of lived experience researchers and providers: A conceptual framework and systematic narrative review. *Research Involvement and Engagement, 9*(1), 26. https://doi.org/10.1186/s40900-023-00439-0

Johnston, C., & Mash, E. J. (1989). A measure of parenting satisfaction and efficacy. *Journal of Clinical Child Psychology, 18*(2), 167–175.

Li, H., & Moore, S. M. (2010). The impact of family support on the quality of adjustment to disability. *Journal of Rehabilitation, 76*(3), 44–51.

Lindblad-Goldberg, M., & Northey, W., Jr. (2013). Ecosystemic structural family therapy: Theoretical and clinical foundations. *Contemporary Family Therapy, 35*, 147–160. https://doi.org/10.1007/s10591-012-9219-1

Martz, E., & Livneh, H. (2015). Psychosocial adaptation to disability within the context of positive psychology: Findings from the literature. *Journal of Occupational Rehabilitation, 26*(4), 4–12. https://doi.org/10.1007/s10926-015-9598-x

Miller, A. R., Condin, C. J., McKellin, W. H., Shaw, N., Klassen, A. F., & Sheps, S. (2009). Continuity of care for children with complex chronic health conditions: Parents' perspectives. *BMC Health Services Research, 9*, Article 242. https://doi.org/10.1186/1472-6963-9-242

Minuchin, S. (1974). *Families and family therapy*. Harvard University Press.

Miserandino, C. (2003). The spoon theory. *But You Don't Look Sick*. https://www.butyoudontlooksick.com/articles/written-by-christine/the-spoon-theory/

Mona, L. R. (2023). Psychotherapy with adults with physical disabilities: Recommendations for affirmative practice. *American Psychological Association*. https://www.apa.org/education-career/ce/psychotherapy-adults-physical-disabilities

Olkin, R. (1999). *What psychotherapists should know about disability*. Guilford Press.

Olkin, R. (2017). *Disability-affirmative therapy: A case formulation template for clients with disabilities*. Oxford University Press.

Olson, D. H. (2011). FACES IV and the circumplex model: Validation studies and applications. *Journal of Marital and Family Therapy, 37*(1), 64–80. https://doi.org/10.1111/j.1752-0606.2009.00175.x

Patterson, J. M. (2002). Understanding family resilience. *Journal of Clinical Child Psychology, 31*(2), 233–243.

Rimé, B., Dozier, S., Vandenplas, C., & Declercq, M. (1996). Social sharing of emotion in children. In N. Frijda (Ed.), *ISRE 96: Proceedings of the IXth Conference of the International Society for Research on Emotion* (pp. 161–163). Toronto, Canada: International Society for Research on Emotion.

Ryan, R. M., Deci, E. L., Grolnick, W. S., & La Guardia, J. G. (2005). The significance of autonomy and autonomy support in psychological development and psychopathology. In D. Cicchetti & D. J. Cohen (Eds.), *Developmental psychopathology: Theory and method* (2nd ed., Vol. 1, pp. 795–849). Wiley.

Satir, V. (1988). *The new peoplemaking*. Science and Behavior Books.

Shankar, M. (2021). *She is a formidable woman, a powerhouse of sorts: A transcendental phenomenology examining the experience of growing up with parental disability* (Unpublished doctoral dissertation). Virginia Polytechnic Institute and State University.

Sixbey, M. T. (2005). *Development of the family resilience assessment scale to identify family resilience constructs* (Doctoral dissertation). University of Florida.

Sniatecki, J. L., Ashton, J. R., Perry, H. B., & Snell, L. H. (2021). Positive aspects of disability among college students. *Journal of Research in Innovative Teaching & Learning, 14*(2), 150–161. https://doi.org/10.1108/JRIT-09-2019-0069

Snyder, C. R., Rand, K. L., & Sigmon, D. R. (2002). Hope theory: A member of the positive psychology family. *Clinical Psychology: Science and Practice, 9*(3), 249–275. https://doi.org/10.1093/clipsy.9.3.249

Stinnett, N., & DeFrain, J. (1985). Family strengths inventory. In N. Stinnett & J. DeFrain (Eds.), *Secrets of strong families* (pp. 25–36). Berkley Books.

Sullivan, P. M., & Knutson, J. F. (2000). Maltreatment and disabilities: A population-based epidemiological study. *Child Abuse & Neglect, 24*(10), 1257–1273. https://doi.org/10.1016/S0145-2134(00)00190-3

Sutherland, D., Flynn, S., Griffin, J., Thompson, P. A., & Hastings, R. P. (2025). Programme recipient and facilitator experiences of positive family connections for families of children with intellectual disabilities and/or who are autistic. *Journal of Applied Research in Intellectual Disabilities, 38*(1), 45–60. https://doi.org/10.1111/jar.13085

Turns, B. A., Springer, P. R., & Sibley, D. S. (2018). Removing the "mystery" in therapy: Transparency as a continuous intervention in family psychotherapy. *Journal of Family Psychotherapy, 29*(1), 1–19. https://doi.org/10.1080/08975353.2018.1488127

U.S. Bureau of Labor Statistics. (2024). Persons with a disability: Labor force characteristics—2024. https://www.bls.gov/news.release/pdf/disabl.pdf

VanPuymbrouck, L., Friedman, C., & Feldner, H. (2020). Explicit and implicit disability attitudes of healthcare providers. *CQL|The Council on Quality and Leadership.* https://www.c-q-l.org/wp-content/uploads/2020/03/CQL-2020-VanPuymbrouck-Friedman-Feldner-Health-Care-Providers-Disability-Attitudes.pdf

Walsh, F. (2016). *Strengthening family resilience* (3rd ed.). Guilford Press.

Wang, K., Lowe, S. R., Fodero, S., Whang, J., Ostrove, J. M., Manning III, R. B., Bogart, K. R., Cipollina, R., Adler, J. M., Nario-Redmond, M. R., & Cipollina, R. (2024). Ableism in mental healthcare settings: A qualitative study among U.S. adults with disabilities. *SSM - Qualitative Research in Health, 6*, 100498. https://doi.org/10.1016/j.ssmqr.2024.100498

World Health Organization. (2001). International classification of functioning, disability and health (ICF). *World Health Organization.* https://www.who.int/classifications/icf/en/

Wright, L. M. (2009). *Beliefs and illness: A model for healing.* 4th Floor Press.

Bibliography

Stuntzner, S. (2012). Resiliency and coping: The importance of framing. In D. A. LeBlanc (Ed.), *Cultivating change: The impact of positive psychology* (pp. 35–48). Nova Science Publishers.

14

CONSTRUCTING ACCESSIBLE THERAPY SPACES

Looking beyond Infrastructure

Toni Saia and Gabrielle Ficchi

Author Note: We intentionally use identity-first language to indicate disability as a sociopolitical construct and valid human identity. Additionally, given the wide audience, the word "professionals" will be used to encompass counselors, therapists, educators, trainees, students, and others in related mental health fields. Before we proceed with this chapter, it is vital to also share our positionality. We enter this conversation as proud disabled, female, wheelchair users, members of the disability community; the largest growing minoritized group in the United States, and as community members longing for accessible therapy spaces for all. This is an important distinction, given that disabled people aren't typically the authors of chapters within textbooks. Our expertise as disabled people, coupled with our clinical backgrounds as rehabilitation and mental health counselors, has provided us with both knowledge and lived experiences to connect with our readers in a meaningful way. It is our hope that this information will bridge the gap between the textbook and real-life application consistent with the phrase "nothing about us without us" (Charlton, 1998).

Introduction: Accessibility as Access Intimacy

This chapter aims to explore the numerous and varied dimensions of accessibility within therapy spaces. However, it is important for us to first describe how we define accessibility. We frame our lens of accessibility in alignment with "#AccesslsLove", created and led by three disabled women- Sandy Ho, Mia Mingus, and Alice Wong, who state, "accessibility is understood as an act of love, instead of a burden or an after-thought" (Ho et al., n.d., para.1). This framework moves us beyond compliance and the letter of law (American with Disabilities Act), which

DOI: 10.4324/9781003362586-21

has little to no enforcement measures in place, resulting in the burden falling on disabled people to fight for access. It allows us to think about access as an act of care, rather than an act of obligation or duty. Furthermore, we do not want to narrow the definition of accessibility to purely physical parameters such as ramps, curb cuts, captions, or braille (Thomas, 2020). Attitudinal access is much more nuanced than just physical access. Mingus (2011) coined the term "access intimacy" to name the freeing feeling when someone else understands and "gets" your accessibility needs. Mingus (2011, para. 9) says:

> It is a freeing, light, loving feeling. It brings the people who are a part of it closer; it builds and deepens connection. Sometimes access intimacy doesn't even mean that everything is 100% accessible. Sometimes it looks like both of you trying to create access as hard as you can with no avail in an ableist world. Sometimes it is someone just sitting and holding your hand while you both stare back at an inaccessible world.

As professionals, it is our responsibility to ensure that our clients feel safe and heard, which should be no different for disabled clients. Thus, we must proactively embrace strategies that address the holistic needs of disabled clients by creating accessible therapy spaces. We recognize that truly accessible spaces do not come to fruition overnight. Accessible spaces are built with intention, purpose, planning, trust, and a little bit of failing, because it is impossible to always get it right, especially as we mingle in a world that is not designed for disabled people. At this point, you're probably thinking either where do you begin, or where do you go from here; both valid thoughts. Before we move forward, we must define ableism. This will help frame the conversation that is about to ensue.

Professionals are often positioned in roles of power, which can inadvertently reinforce ableist reactions toward disabled people, such as fear, pity, shame, avoidance, or the belief that they are inherently dependent on providers. These biases can undermine the therapeutic relationship and hinder the development of a collaborative, empowering dynamic (Vash & Crewe, 2003). Therefore, in its most basic form, ableism is defined as the discrimination of disabled people (Slesaransky-Poe & García, 2014). This can take the form of microaggressions, attitudes, beliefs, and physical and attitudinal barriers that prevent disabled people from being active members of their community. Talia Lewis (2022) takes a more Intersectional approach and defines ableism as

> a system of assigning value to people's bodies and minds based on societally constructed ideas of normalcy, productivity, desirability, intelligence, excellence, and fitness. These constructed ideas are deeply rooted in eugenics, anti-Blackness, misogyny, colonialism, imperialism, and capitalism. This systemic oppression leads to people and society determining people's value based on their culture, age, language, appearance, religion, birth or living

place, "health/wellness", and/or their ability to satisfactorily re/produce, "excel" and "behave". You do not have to be disabled to experience ableism.

Ableism is also manifested when we ignore disability as an aspect of diversity. Although topics of multiculturalism and diversity have increased in counselor education, the same cannot be said for disability (Rivas, 2020; Rivas & Hill, 2018). Disability representation is lacking in counseling journals, syllabi, and student experiences. Researchers have identified that since 1990, only 1% of the articles published in general counseling journals have addressed disability (Emir Öksüz & Brubaker, 2020; Woo et al., 2016). In addition, a study by Priester and colleagues (2008) found disability to be addressed in only 25% of multicultural counseling course syllabi. Another study revealed that more than half the sample of counseling students reported that disability received less attention than other cultural identities in their coursework (Deroche et al., 2020). Such oversights of disability require reflection on the current landscape of counseling and counselor education; to question whether "there is something inherent in the way diversity is considered, that makes it impossible to recognize disability as a valid human identity" (Davis, 2011, p. 4).

There is growing concern regarding the insufficient attention given to disability content in counselor education programs and the preparedness of instructors to effectively teach such material. A survey of counselor educators in CACREP-accredited programs revealed that fewer than 30 participants were required to instruct disability-related courses in their programs. Moreover, over half acknowledged that too little time was devoted to disability concepts and expressed that their students were only somewhat prepared to work with disabled clients (Feather & Carlson, 2019). These educational gaps have real-world implications, translating directly into inadequacies in professional practice. For example, mental health professionals working with disabled clients rated their perceived competence highest in awareness, moderately in knowledge, and lowest in practical skills (Strike et al., 2004). The issue extends further, represented in a study focusing on disability professionals, which included those whose work involves disability or supports disabled people. A total of 77.2% explicitly preferred working with nondisabled people. Alarmingly, many participants displayed significant levels of ableism. A majority (37.8%) were categorized as symbolic ableists, exhibiting high explicit and implicit ableist attitudes, while approximately one-third (31.1%) were classified as aversive ableists, demonstrating low explicit but high implicit bias against disability (Friedman, 2023). These findings, spanning decades of research, underscore a persistent and systemic issue: the failure to prioritize and address the needs and lived experiences of disabled clients within both education and practice.

Creating accessible (remember our definition from above) therapy spaces is a necessity to help counter the ableism that disabled clients face daily. What follows is a list of themes and suggestions as you begin to or continue to create accessible therapy spaces. We attempted to refrain from disability-specific recommendations as that tends to reinforce the hierarchy that surrounds the disability experience. However, when appropriate, we provide specific examples. This should not be confused with disability etiquette which fails to recognize the nuance and depth of disability experience (Purlang, 2022). As Judy Heumann (often thought of as the mother of disability rights) (2021) once said:

> Change never happens at the pace we think it should. It happens over years of people joining together, strategizing, sharing, and pulling all the levers they possibly can. Gradually, excruciatingly slowly, things start to happen, and then suddenly, seemingly out of the blue, something will tip.
>
> (p. 183)

Prioritize Accessibility

To prioritize accessibility, you must plan for it. It should not be an afterthought that sends clear messages about who is valued in your space. This can include the physical location of your building as well as your office space. If there are elements outside of your control (i.e. accessible parking, building location, tight spaces), be transparent so that disabled clients can make informed choices. Flexibility is essential to being proactive. Flexibility in your approach, flexibility in your physical space (i.e. furniture with wheels so it is easily moveable for navigation) flexibility in what you expect to get done in the allotted time, and flexibility in the options you provide is critical to the process. During the COVID 19-pandemic, society embraced flexibility with work-from-home options, virtual participation, telehealth, etc. This is akin to the flexibility the disability community begged for years, but were denied. Thus, Saia et al. (2021) argues for the "new flexible;" rather than a return to normal that failed to include disabled people. Purlang (2021, para. 24) is urging people to view the pandemic as "a learning experience for everyone that will carry over into the post-pandemic world. Maybe it will finally add some urgency to the decades-long push to make life more accessible and sustainable for disabled people". As Meenakshi Das stated (in Ruiz-Grossman, 2021):

> I am a person with a speech disability, specifically a stutter. Working from home has been great for me since I can use the chat feature in online meetings to type and share my thoughts. … Before COVID-19, work from home was generally not popular, and disabled people had to try hard to get these accommodations. However, now that everyone needs that accommodation, it's considered alright and doable. It took a pandemic for people to realize how accommodations are low-cost and totally doable, and I hope it stays that way.
>
> (Ruiz-Grossman, 2021, para. 11)

Flexibility allows professionals to meet clients where they are on any given day. Disability is a fluid experience. Some days a client may be able to have an hour-long session without a break and some days that may not be an option. Miserandino (2003) who has lupus, developed the "Spoon Theory" to describe this idea of limited energy, using "spoons" as a unit of energy. Trust that disabled people understand their bodies and experiences best. Use this as an opportunity to check in with your client and to affirm flexibility instead of forcing them forward. Here are some reflection questions to support proactive planning as you embrace an accessible and flexible approach with disabled clients:

- Who is the activity initially designed for?
- Does the activity consider diverse learning styles?
- What kind of movement must a user perform to participate?
- What shapes, colors, text, and graphics must a user understand to participate?
- What sounds are required for a user to participate?
- How much time must a user spend to participate/engage in the activity?
- Are there multiple ways to participate in the activity?
- Does the activity fit with the time allotted?
- How can you adapt the physical space to ensure participation?

Increase Physical Access

To promote access intimacy, we must first understand that the Americans with Disabilities Act is the floor, not the ceiling in terms of access for disabled people. Settling for minimum standards halts society's progress forward. "The current state of the law allows for 'separate but equal,' but usually results in simply unequal" (Wentz et al., 2011, n.p.). Therapists must consider the physical accessibility of their space to ensure a welcoming and safe environment for disabled clients. Professionals should make sure (1) clients have adequate room to navigate the space, (2) there is clear signage with braille and tactile indicators, (3) information/flyers are not hung too high on the walls, (4) information and email communications are written in accessible fonts such as Verdana, (5) fluorescent lighting is scarce, (6) information is available in alternative formats, (7) to regularly check in with clients about how physical access can be improved and most importantly, and (8) respond efficiently when improvements are suggested and be transparent about your plan to increase access. While not exhaustive, these tangible practices focused on improving physical accessibility also play a crucial role in fostering attitudinal accessibility. Wherever you are in this journey to improve access, even a small change like changing your font (which is free of charge) sends a message about the prioritization of your practice as an inclusive clinician.

Ensure Communication Access

Communication is an important right, especially in clinical settings (Agaronnik et al., 2019). Disabled people use diverse methods of communication and self-expression, all of which are equally valid and deserving of recognition and respect. Professionals should also pay close attention to body movements as a form of communication. Inclusive communication strategies prioritize the use of clear, accessible language, while providing information in multiple formats such as visual, auditory, and tactile, to ensure accessibility for all clients. This approach aligns with the principles of Universal Design, which advocate for creating products and environments that are usable by as many people as possible, minimizing the need for adaptations (Mace, 1985). Professionals play a critical role in fostering an environment where diverse communication methods, such as augmentative and alternative communication (AAC) devices, sign language, or text-based interactions, are not merely accommodated but actively embraced. For example, learning basic phrases in sign language, familiarizing yourself with common AAC systems and most importantly, giving disabled people time and space to communicate. By implementing these suggestions, professionals demonstrate respect for their clients' experiences and build stronger therapeutic alliances (Beukelman & Light, 2020).

Embrace Disability Culture and Include Authentic Representation

Integrating disability culture into your therapeutic approach not only affirms the identities and experiences of disabled clients, but also fosters greater attitudinal accessibility to create a more welcoming environment (Saia, 2023). Disability culture highlights the immense value disabled people bring to our communities. Brown (2002) shared:

> Disabled people have forged a group identity. We share a common history of oppression and a common bond of resilience. We generate art, music, literature, and other expressions of our lives and our culture, infused from our experience of disability. Most importantly, we are proud of ourselves as disabled people. We claim our disabilities with pride as part of our identity. We are who we are: We are disabled people.
>
> (p. 49)

We share this powerful definition as an invitation for reflection on how to meaningfully incorporate disability culture into your practice. A starting point is to actively promote authentic representation of disability whether in the resources you use, the discussions you facilitate, or the spaces you create, ensuring that disabled voices and experiences are celebrated and centered. This does not mean that every client identifies with disability as a culture. However, as professionals, it is essential to be prepared to discuss disability culture and provide support to disabled clients as they explore and connect with their communities. We suggest starting with thinking about how your physical space (i.e. office, building, school) reflects the community you serve. Think about decorating your space with artwork by disabled people or hanging a disability pride flag (Saia, 2023). Intentionally seeking ways to authentically represent disabled people within your environment sends a powerful message that disability is a natural and valued part of life.

Incorporate the Independent Living Philosophy

The Independent Living (IL) Philosophy asserts that disabled individuals deserve the same civil rights, opportunities, and control over their lives as non-disabled people. (McDonald & Oxford, 1995). At its core, IL champions self-determination, empowerment, autonomy, and equal opportunities. These are the very principles that professionals must integrate into their practice to dismantle ableist biases and validate the lived experiences of disabled people. To uphold these principles, professionals must recognize disabled individuals as the foremost experts in their own lives. This involves respecting their needs, preferences, and right to make autonomous decisions (Feather & Carlson, 2019). Empowering clients to take charge of the therapeutic process, set meaningful and appropriate goals, and make informed choices is essential. Professionals, parents, and other stakeholders must actively respect and support the autonomy and judgment of disabled individuals, ensuring that therapy is a collaborative and empowering experience. In practice, therapists should regularly review and adapt goals to promote growth, while encouraging clients to exercise decision-making within sessions. Giving disabled clients control over how they want to use their time in therapy fosters a sense of agency and reinforces their ability to navigate their lives with confidence and independence. By centering these values, professionals can create an inclusive therapeutic environment that aligns with the foundational ideals of Independent Living.

Acknowledge and Respect Intersectionality

Crenshaw's (1989, 1991) groundbreaking essays laid the foundation for expanding Intersectionality into a framework that encompasses a wide variety of issues, social identities, structural power dynamics, and interconnected social systems. Thus, it is vital for professionals to recognize that disability is not an isolated identity. It intersects with other dimensions of a person's identity, such as race, gender, sexual orientation, age, socioeconomic status, and cultural background. These intersections can create unique challenges, amplify systemic barriers, and shape the experiences of disabled individuals in significant ways. For example, a Black disabled woman may face compounded discrimination based on ableism, racism, and sexism, which could influence how she accesses services and perceives support systems. Professionals must adopt a culturally responsive and an Intersectional approach that acknowledges these complexities. This means being attuned to how systemic oppression, privilege, and cultural values interact with disability in a client's life. Practically, respecting Intersectionality involves taking time to learn about and understand clients' cultural and social contexts. It requires professionals to ask thoughtful, open-ended questions about how clients' intersecting identities influence their lived experiences and what barriers they may face. Additionally, it involves incorporating culturally relevant practices and materials into sessions to enhance accessibility and honor diverse forms of communication and expression. For example, professionals working with disabled clients from low-income backgrounds should consider the financial constraints that may limit access to resources. Furthermore, professionals should also consider access to transportation when sharing resources and planning for appointments. When possible, offer virtual options as that can increase access. Ultimately, this requires professionals to support clients throughout the therapeutic process, celebrate their multifaceted identities, and engage in advocacy to ensure equitable experiences.

Understand the Diverse Experiences of Disability

Disabled people represent the largest growing minoritized group, with diverse experiences, needs, and aspirations that deserve intentional consideration in the therapeutic process. These needs encompass social, physical, emotional, and vocational aspects, all of which intersect in unique ways to shape their lives. Counselors must understand these intersections to provide holistic support. "Socially", disabled clients may encounter isolation and discrimination, often resulting in loneliness, diminished self-esteem, and strained interpersonal relationships (Shakespeare, 2016). "Physically", they may require accommodations such as ramps, accessible seating, or adaptive communication tools to ensure equal access to therapy spaces. "Emotionally", the societal stigma surrounding disability and personal challenges can contribute to heightened stress, anxiety, and depression, all of which require nuanced and empathetic intervention (Goodley, 2016). "Vocationally", navigating workplace barriers and advocating for rights under disability legislation are common challenges that many disabled individuals face, underscoring the need for tailored vocational counseling and support (Wehman, 2013). A major obstacle is the prevalence of ableist attitudes among professionals, which often manifest as infantilizing perspectives or a lack of empathy (Strike et al., 2004). Such biases can hinder the therapeutic relationship and limit the potential for fostering independence and empowerment among disabled clients. To address these barriers, counselors must commit to ongoing education, critical self-reflection, and adopt anti-ableist practices (Feather & Carlson, 2019). Creating an accessible and equitable therapeutic space extends beyond physical accommodations; it requires a paradigm shift toward equity and intentionality. This means acknowledging the diversity within the disability community, promoting autonomy, and embracing counseling approaches that prioritize client-centered and culturally responsive care. By addressing these systemic barriers, counselors can foster an inclusive environment that truly meets the needs of disabled clients, enabling them to thrive socially, emotionally, and professionally.

Attend Trainings and Engage in Self-Reflection

Continuous, ongoing training to expand and deepen one's understanding of accessibility is essential for fostering equity and challenging ableism (Shakespeare, 2016). However, this training must go beyond superficial efforts designed merely to "check a box". Professionals must intentionally seek out educational opportunities that are authentic, impactful, and centered on uplifting the expertise of disabled people. Training should be led by disabled individuals who bring lived experience and nuanced understanding to the conversation. Their insights can illuminate the systemic barriers disabled people face, and provide practical, real-world strategies for fostering accessibility (Hartley & Saia, 2022). By prioritizing training that uplifts and validates the experiences of disabled individuals, professionals can gain a more accurate, empathetic, and comprehensive understanding of accessibility.

Professionals should engage in self-reflection and challenge themselves to think creatively (beyond a one size-fits-all approach) about accessibility. Professionals must hold themselves accountable by applying the knowledge gained from these trainings in their regular practice. This includes reevaluating biases, implementing inclusive strategies, and advocating for systemic change within their organizations. Professionals must regularly examine their own biases and assumptions about disability, which are often shaped by societal norms and stereotypes. This self-awareness can be cultivated through reflective practices, peer discussions, and supervision, enabling professionals to identify and address unconscious biases that may influence their work (Brown, 2019).

Commit to Further Learning

Professionals have an ethical responsibility to continuously learn, grow, and actively engage in anti-ableist practices. It is essential not to assume that their training has adequately covered disability-related topics, as disability is often underrepresented or inadequately addressed in many educational and professional programs. To support further learning, we have shared resources for the resource guide at the end of this handbook. All our recommendations center and uplift the experiences of disabled people.

Conclusion

The core message of this chapter is that, to construct accessible therapy spaces, professionals must expand their understanding of both accessibility and disability. Every aspect of the therapeutic process should center on empowering and amplifying the voices and experiences of disabled people, ensuring their access needs, identities, and autonomy are prioritized and celebrated. We, as the authors, hope that this chapter motivates you to take action to best support disabled clients, regardless of where you are on the journey of building an inclusive practice. Although many of the suggested changes may take time to implement, the urgency to act is immediate.

References

Agaronnik, N., Campbell, E. G., Ressalam, J., & Iezzoni, L. I. (2019). Communicating with patients with disability: Perspectives of practicing physicians. *Journal of General Internal Medicine*, *34*, 1139–1145.

Beukelman, D., & Light, J. (2020). *Augmentative and alternative communication: Supporting children and adults with complex communication needs* (5th ed.). Baltimore, MD: Paul H. Brookes Publishing.

Brown, S. E. (2019). Self-reflection and bias awareness. *Journal of Counseling and Development, 97*(1), 13–21.

Brown, S. E. (2002). What is disability culture?. *Disability Studies Quarterly*, *22*(2), 34–50. https://doi.org/10.18061/dsq.v22i2.343

Charlton, J. I. (1998). *Nothing about us without us: Disability oppression and empowerment*. Berkeley: University of California Press.

Crenshaw, K. W. (1989). Demarginalizing the intersection of race and sex: A black feminist critique of antidiscrimination doctrine. *University of Chicago Legal Forum*, *1989*(1), 139–168.

Crenshaw, K. (1991). Stanford law review mapping the margins: Intersectionality, identity politics, and violence against women of source. *Stanford Law Review*, *43*(6), 1241–1299. https://doi.org/10.2307/1229039

Davis, L. J. (2011). Why is disability missing from the discourse on diversity? *The Chronicle of Higher Education*, *25*, 38–40.

Deroche, M. D., Herlihy, B., & Lyons, M. L. (2020). Counselor trainee self-perceived disability competence. *Counselor Education and Supervision, 59*(3), 187–199. https://doi.org/10.1002/ceas.12183

Emir Öksüz, E., & Brubaker, M. D. (2020). Deconstructing disability training in counseling: A critical examination and call to the profession. *Journal of Counselor Leadership and Advocacy*, *7*(2), 163–175. https://doi.org/10.1080/2326716X.2020.1820407

Feather, K. A., & Carlson, R. G. (2019). An initial investigation of individual instructors' self- perceived competence and incorporation of disability content into CACREP-accredited programs: Rethinking training in counselor education. *Journal of Multicultural Counseling and Development*, *47*(1), 19–36.

Friedman, C. (2023). Explicit and implicit: Ableism of disability professionals. *Disability and Health Journal*, *16*(4), 101482. https://doi.org/10.1016/j.dhjo.2023.101482

Goodley, D. (2016). *Disability studies: An interdisciplinary introduction*. Thousand Oaks, CA: Sage.

Hartley, M. T., & Saia, T. (2022). Rehabilitation counseling associations and the disability community: A return to social action. *Rehabilitation Counselors and Educators Journal*, *11*(2), 1–13. https://doi.org/10.52017/001c.38192

Heumann, J., & Joiner, K. (2021). *Being Heumann: An unrepentant memoir of a disability rights activist* (Young readers' edition). New York, NY: Beacon Press.

Ho, S., Mingus, M., & Wong, A. (n.d.). *Further readings & resources*. https://www.disabilityintersectionalitysummit.com/access-is-love/

Lewis, T. A. (2022, January 1). *Working definition of ableism—January 2022 update*. https://www.talilalewis.com/blog

Mace, R. (1985). Universal design: Barrier free environments for everyone. *Designers West*, *33*(1), 147–152.

McDonald, G., & Oxford, M. (1995). *History of independent living*. Dayton, OH: Access Center for Independent Living.

Mingus, M. (2011, February 11). *Changing the framework: Disability justice*. https://leavingevidence.wordpress.com/2011/02/12/changing-the-framework-disability-justice/

Miserandino, C. (2003, April 8). *The spoon theory*. But You Don't Look Sick. https://butyoudontlooksick.com/articles/written-by-christine/the-spoon-theory/

Purlang, A. (2021, March 21). *What disabled people are thinking and feeling about the pandemic, one year later*. Forbes. https://www.forbes.com/sites/andrewpulrang/2021/03/21/what-disabled-people-are-thinking-and-feeling-about-the-pandemic-one-year-later/?fbclid=IwAR3VIgfor-jqjc6LNyvvzq5BAmRUfN6zb-ecIohXv2nVeK3gCAxPmISxH4o&sh=df0e6193277c

Priester, P. E., Jones, J. E., Jackson-Bailey, C. M., Jana-Masri, A., Jordan, E. X., & Metz, A. J. (2008). An analysis of content and instructional strategies in multicultural counseling courses. *Journal of Multicultural Counseling and Development, 36*(1), 29–39. https://doi.org/10.1002/j.2161-1912.2008.tb00067.x

Purlang, A. (2022, Febuarary 21). *Ableism is more than a breach of etiquette — It has consequences*. Forbes. https://www.forbes.com/sites/andrewpulrang/2022/02/17/ableism-is-more-than-a-breach-of-etiquette---it-has-consequences/

Rivas, M. (2020). Disability in counselor education: Perspectives from the United States. *International Journal for the Advancement of Counselling*, 42, 1–16. https://doi.org/10.1007/s10447-020-09404-y

Rivas, M., & Hill, N. R. (2018). Counselor trainees' experiences counseling disability: A phenomenological study. *Counselor Education and Supervision, 57*(2), 116–131. https://doi.org/10.1002/ceas.12097

Ruiz-Grossman, S. (2021, May 7). *What your disabled friends want you to know about 'going back to normal' post-vaccine*. Huffington Post. https://www.huffpost.com/entry/disabled-post-vaccine-coronavirus-masks-safety_l_6091b424e4b05af50dc8c61e

Saia, T. (2023). Embracing disability culture in schools. *Language, Speech, and Hearing Services in Schools*, *54*(3), 794–798.

Saia, T., Nerlich, A. P., & Johnston, S. P. (2021). Why not the "new flexible"?: The argument for not returning to "normal" after COVID-19. *Rehabilitation Counselors and Educators Journal*, *11*(1), 1–7. https://doi.org/10.52017/001c.28332

Shakespeare, T. (2016). The social model of disability. In Davis, L. J. (Ed.), *The disability studies reader* (pp. 195–203). New York: Routlege.

Slesaransky-Poe, G., & García, A. M. (2014). The social construction of difference. In *Condition critical: Key principles for equitable and inclusive education* (pp. 66–85). New York: Teachers College Press.

Strike, D. L., Skovholt, T. M., & Hummel, T. J. (2004). Mental health professionals' disability competence. *Rehabilitation Psychology*, *49*(4), 321–327. https://doi.org/10.1037/0090-5550.49.4.321

Thomas, A. (2020, January 23). *Why access is love and there is no such thing as "barrier-free."* Akimbo. https://akimbo.ca/akimblog/why-access-is-love-and-there-is-no-such-thing-as-barrier-free/

Vash, C. L., & Crewe, N. M. (2003). *Psychology of disability*. New York: Springer Publishing Company.

Wehman, P. (2013). Transition from school to work: Where are we and where do we need to go?. *Career Development and Transition for Exceptional Individuals*, *36*(1), 58–66.

Wentz, B., Jaeger, P. T., & Lazar, J. (2011). Retrofitting accessibility: The legal inequality of after-the-fact online access for persons with disabilities in the United States. *First Monday*, *16*(11), 1–15. https://doi.org/10.5210/fm.v16i11.3666.

Woo, H., Goo, M., & Lee, M. (2016). A content analysis of research on disability. *Journal of Multicultural Counseling and Development, 44*(4), 228–244. https://doi.org/10.1002/jmcd.12051

Bibliography

Heumann, J., & Joiner, K. (2020). *Being Heumann: An unrepentant memoir of a disability rights activist.* Boston, MA: Beacon Press.

SECTION IV

Clinical Supervision and Program Development

PART IV

I am.

Pramod Shankar

Watching the rain,
I see a raindrop
that isn't quite one.
A half-raindrop.

The other half,
robbed by the sun
and the sleet.

I am that.

A leaf singed by the solstice.
A lake shrunk around the edges,
a horizon abandoned by the songbirds.

A river flowing over eroded pebbles,
a wind shredded by the woods it tries to embrace.

I am the cry of the crescent
that can never wax fully;
the dance of a hundred feet,
shod with broken ballerina shoes.

A gale with a tear,
a song at half-mast,
a brush with tangled bristles.

And yet, I am.

DOI: 10.4324/9781003362586-23

15

ADDRESSING THE MISSING PIECE

Developing Inclusive Programmatic Structures, Modules, and Coursework

Brittany A. Williams, Derek X. Seward, and Kahyen Shin

Introduction

Across mental health disciplines, a recognition of the pressing need to provide culturally responsive services that honor the diverse identities and realities of clients has surged. Accreditation bodies and professional codes of ethics mandate that students and professionals receive multicultural-competence training (CACREP, 2023; CSWE, 2022; APA, 2017; ACA, 2014). Despite these professional mandates, disability, a pivotal dimension of diversity, is persistently neglected in mental health training (Öksüz & Brubaker, 2020). This is concerning, since one in four adults in the United States lives with some form of disability (Center for Disease Control [CDC], 2023). Marriage and family therapists, counselors, and other mental health professionals are expected to assume pivotal roles in aiding disabled individuals. Yet, graduate-level training programs frequently falter in adequately preparing future therapists to cater to the distinctive requisites of this demographic (Kim & Sellmaier, 2020; Oksuz & Brubaker, 2020). This oversight curtails therapists' efficacy in serving disabled clients proficiently and perpetuates ableist prejudices prevalent in mental health care.

This chapter investigates the contemporary landscape of disability inclusion across graduate-level mental health training programs. After delving into the detrimental ramifications of inadequate disability training, an array of strategies will be presented to address this deficiency. The overarching objective is to prioritize disability as a foundational component interwoven throughout mental health curricula and training programs. This reform is imperative for upholding professional standards of multicultural competence, dismantling ableist attitudes and inaccessible practices, and ultimately enhancing affirmative, quality, mental health services for disabled clients.

 DOI: 10.4324/9781003362586-24

The Historical Marginalization and Medical Model Framing of Disability in Mental Health

The interaction between disability and mental health is intricate, influencing individuals' lived realities, sense of self, and ability to access appropriate clinical care. Despite this connectedness, disability often receives insufficient attention within mental health training programs, leading to a deficiency in therapists providing competent and inclusive care (Feather & Carlson, 2019; Deroche et al., 2020). The marginalization of disability in these training curricula mirrors broader patterns of historical oppression, exclusion, and the medicalization of disability within societal and healthcare contexts. Historically, disability has been predominantly viewed through a medical lens, portraying it as an individual flaw, functional limitation, or personal hardship necessitating medical intervention, rehabilitation, or cure (Olkin, 2022). This medical perspective frames disability as a problem to be remedied or conquered, rather than recognizing it as a multifaceted aspect of human diversity.

This medical model ideology has permeated mental health fields, shaping how disability is conceptualized and addressed in research, theory, and practice. Traditionally, mental health professions have attended to disability primarily from a stance of remedial intervention, aiming to reduce or manage client symptoms and functional limitations. Training has concentrated on diagnostic categories, assessing client deficits, and prescriptive treatment modalities – all of which are anchored through an individual, deficit model (Brinkman et al., 2023). Consequently, training has lacked emphasis on examining disability as an intersectional identity and culture, a valuable dimension of human diversity, and an issue of social justice.

The framing of disability through a deficit-oriented, medical lens reflects and reinforces deeply ingrained ableist assumptions, stigma, and discrimination that have systematically marginalized disabled individuals. Ableism is defined as a set of beliefs or practices that devalue and discriminate against people with physical, intellectual, or psychiatric impairments and often rests on the assumption that disabled people need to be "fixed" in one form or another (Center for Disability Rights, n.d.). The medical model's delineation of abnormal/pathological identities and bodies has been a driving force behind the ableist institutionalization, dehumanization, and denial of rights for disabled populations (Hogan, 2019). Contemporary mental health practices continue to grapple with the residual ableist biases sthat stem from this marginalization.

The Disability Rights Movement has challenged ableist medical model hegemonies and catalyzed a paradigm shift toward the social model of disability (Andrews et al., 2019). The social model conceptualizes disability as a socially constructed phenomenon where societal attitudes, environments, and a lack of accommodations are disabling, as opposed to individualized impairments (Oliver, 2013). Mental health training programs have been slow to integrate this affirmative and intersectional recognition of disability as a valued identity and culture into their curricula. This is concerning, as training rooted in an ableist medical model can leave therapists without essential awareness of critical disability concepts, including ableism, identity-first language, accessibility as a human right, and the principles of the disability justice movement (Brinkman et al., 2023).

In order to "produce" therapists who are capable of providing responsive, affirmative, clinical care, training programs must prioritize moving beyond ableist and deficit-based medical model frameworks. Incorporating disability studies perspectives can promote a nuanced exploration of how disability intersects with other marginalized identities, as well as the psycho-emotional effects of ableism and internalized oppression. It also highlights the importance of self-determination, culture, and community in shaping disability experiences (Joshi & Pappageorge, 2023). In addition to strengthening clinical competencies, this reconceptualization empowers therapists to serve as allies in dismantling social and systemic barriers that disable people and communities.

It is necessary for mental health training programs to explicitly confront the problematic, historical landscape of ableism. Training programs can disrupt persisting ableist biases and shift toward a holistic, affirmative understanding of disability that is grounded in human rights, intersectionality, and social justice. This ideological reform is essential for equipping future systemic therapists to work in partnership with the disability community toward the collective removal of disabling barriers and the pursuit of true equity.

Impacts of Insufficient Disability Training

The absence of adequate disability education within mental health programs yields adverse effects across various domains, including client treatment outcomes and satisfaction, therapist-client relationships, client engagement, overall client well-being, quality of care, systemic healthcare disparities, cultural competence, and inclusivity in mental health services (Conner et al., 2023). These effects include individual therapist biases and a diminished quality of clinical services and outcomes. At a broader level, they also contribute to barriers in care accessibility and reinforce systemic injustices that impact the disability community.

Clinician-Level Training

For the individual clinician, insufficient exposure to disability perspectives and affirmative paradigms, facilitates the perpetuation of unconscious, ableist biases and assumptions. Research indicates that more than 70% of doctoral students of clinical and counseling psychology receive minimal to no disability-specific training and hold implicit and explicit biases such as associating disability with being helpless, incompetent, and burdensome (Right, 2020). Counselors-in-training lack core disability competencies, such as ensuring accessible service-provision and accommodating needs (Smith, 2021). These ingrained biases shape therapists' attitudes and clinical judgments about disabled clients' presenting concerns, strengths, and capabilities. Feather and Carlson (2019) argue that counselor educators recognize a lack of sufficient attention to disability-related issues and guidelines in training programs, a gap that contributes to the persistence of ableist biases in clinical practice.

Clinical Services

Therapists with inadequate proficiency in disability issues contribute to the provision of insufficient, insensitive, and inaccessible interventions that affect the quality of service delivery. The Substance Abuse and Mental Health Services Administration (SAMHSA) advocates for therapists to alter interventions to meet the specific needs of disabled individuals. For instance, therapists should explicitly explore disability aspects with their clients rather than overlooking disability as a relevant cultural identity. Therapeutic outcomes are significantly compromised without such adaptations and attention to disability. One reason for the lack of appropriate interventions is a significantly limited body of research on culturally responsive treatment. Mental health providers frequently neglect to appropriately adapt evidence-based assessments and interventions to accommodate various disabilities (SAMHSA, 2021). Therapists tend to prioritize a deficit/rehabilitation model focused on "fixing" impairments, rather than an empowerment approach attentive to environmental barriers and human rights (Smart, 2016). This approach prioritizes individual pathology and rehabilitation needs, while frequently neglecting broader social factors that contribute to disability. Alternatively, the empowerment approach aligns with the social model of disability and emphasizes the importance of removing societal barriers and advocating for the human rights of disabled individuals (Smart, 2016). These disconnects undermine therapeutic rapport, heighten client dissatisfaction, and limit treatment engagement and positive outcomes.

Access and Systemic Barriers

Deficient disability education contributes to systemic barriers that hinder access for disabled individuals to essential mental health services. Over 50% of disabled individuals avoid seeking treatment due to previous encounters with discrimination, inaccessibility, and invalidation from providers lacking competence in disability studies (Hill & Delgado, 2023). These barriers exacerbate long-standing mental health disparities for disabled people who experience depression and anxiety at exponentially higher rates than non-disabled people (NIMH, 2022). The failure to confront these systemic barriers propagates unjust disparities in access to quality care.

Social Injustice and Oppression

Broadly, the insufficient emphasis on disability education in mental health curricula reflects and perpetuates systemic ableism, marginalization, and oppression of the disability community. The exclusion of disability from core training competencies signals that it is not considered a vital aspect of diversity and social justice (Brinkman et al., 2023). This omission upholds ableist norms that portray disability as an individual deficiency rather than a socio-political issue rooted in societal attitudes and environments (Joshi & Pappageorge, 2023). Ultimately, this oversight in education impedes future providers from meeting ethical mandates to advocate for positive social change across all populations. Inadequate disability education in mental health programs generates a cascade of negative effects from individuals to the community at large. These effects include hindering clinical competence and reinforcing unconscious biases, compromising the quality of services and outcomes for clients with disabilities. This perpetuates systemic barriers that impede equitable access to affirmative care, propagating oppressive ableist norms and the societal marginalization of the disability community (Feather & Carlson, 2019; Meidert et al., 2023; Yzaguirre et al., 2022). There is both an ethical imperative and practical urgency to comprehensively integrate disability education throughout mental health curricula and clinical training experiences.

Multi-Level Strategies for Inclusive Programmatic Structures

Addressing the significant lack of disability training requires a multi-level, systemic reform approach spanning individual course requirements, experiential learning standards, resource allocation, faculty development initiatives, and program evaluation practices. Mental health training programs have experienced the detrimental results of piecemeal efforts that have insufficiently addressed the substantive cultural shift required to centralize disability inclusion. Hence, recommended approaches for mental health training programs will be outlined. In the sections below, we will provide a framework to combat the challenges described above, making mental health training programs truly diversity-focused.

Curriculum Reform

At the core of what we propose is the revamping of curricula to ensure disability receives dedicated, mandatory coverage through requisite coursework. Programs can implement a semester-long "Disability Studies" course employing interdisciplinary perspectives from fields like Disability Studies, Disability Justice Theory, Disability Critical Race Theory, and Disability Bioethics (Annamma et al., 2013). This comprehensive overview would cover models of disability, disability history and culture, ableism and ableist oppression, disability laws and ethics, intersections with other marginalized identities, and affirmative clinical practices. Learners should become familiar with disability-related counseling competencies (Chapin et al., 2018). Existing required courses, including the multicultural counseling course, can be updated to thoroughly integrate disability perspectives across all content areas (Hill & Delgado, 2023). Educators and supervisors can use disability-focused case studies, assignment projects that explore disability identity, broach topics of disability, and ensure program policies and literature are not ableist (Deroche et al., 2024). Program activities (e.g., classes, orientation, and continuing education training) should be universally accessible in terms of digital and physical accessibility.

Experiential Learning

Beyond classroom learning, programs can infuse service learning or applied experiential requirements for developing skills in working alongside the disability community (Langellier et al., 2020). These service-learning activities could include interventions co-facilitated with local community leaders with self-identified disabilities. They may also involve rotating practicum placements at disability service organizations and consultation with Disabled Cultural Brokers (Balcazar & Suarez-Balcazar, 2016). Experiential learning can boost students' multicultural competence in working with disabled individuals (Feather & Carlson, 2019). These immersive experiences offer invaluable perspective and counter harmful societal narratives. Supervisors during practicum/internships should assess trainees' disability competencies using evaluations like the Disability Competence Assessment (Deroche et al., 2020).

Resource Allocation

Programs must invest resources toward supporting disability curriculum and community engagement. This includes dedicating a budget for compensating speakers, consultants, and interventionists with disabilities or expertise in disability studies. Funds should also cover accessible classroom technologies, textbooks foregrounding disability perspectives, and professional development for teaching this content. Disability services offices should expand to provide technical assistance for accommodation, implementation, and university-wide disability inclusion efforts.

Faculty Training and Scholarship

Initiatives are essential to invest in existing faculty's capacity for integrating disability throughout curricula. Professional development workshops, guest lectures, and learning communities can increase faculty members' knowledge of disability models, culture, and clinical skill sets (Keesler et al., 2023). Incentivizing disability-related research and scholarship through grants, course releases, and tenure/promotion criteria could further advance faculty expertise and leadership in this area. Additionally, programs can actively recruit disabled faculty members and students to foster disability identity representation.

Program Evaluation and Accountability

Graduate programs must develop systematic evaluation mechanisms to ensure accountability for disability training priorities. This includes assessing the quantity and quality of disability-focused curricula during regular program reviews from accrediting bodies like CACREP and COAMFTE. Student competencies in disability should be benchmarked, and programmatic data should be transparently reported. Town halls and surveys can solicit feedback from local disability communities about the adequacy of programs' inclusion efforts.

These proposed reforms require stakeholder investment from administrators, faculty, students, community partners, and accreditors. By implementing this comprehensive, multi-pronged approach, mental health programs can centralize disability within diversity frameworks and fulfill their ethical obligations. Therapists would then benefit from foundational training and feel more equipped to provide affirming, responsive services that eliminate attitudinal, institutional, and clinical service barriers for disabled clients. This systemic prioritization of disability training is vital for advancing justice, equity, and affirmative care for disabled communities.

Future Directions and Recommendations

Future efforts to enhance disability inclusion in mental health training should prioritize ongoing curriculum development, faculty support and development, student involvement, and collaboration with disability stakeholders. Several practical strategies to develop inclusive programmatic structures, modules, and coursework for disability inclusion in mental health training programs are outlined below to support the aforementioned multi-pronged approach.

Inclusive Programmatic Structures

1 Establish a Disability Studies specialization/concentration: Create a dedicated specialization track focused on disability studies within the broader mental health program. This ensures a comprehensive set of coursework and requirements centered on disability (Hill & Delgado, 2023).
2 Develop a disability resource center: Partner with the university's disability services office to create a disability resource center specific to the mental health program. This center can provide technical assistance, resource libraries, training for accessibility/accommodations, and connections to the local disability community (Keesler et al., 2023).
3 Prioritize representation in program leadership: Actively recruit and hire faculty, staff, and administrators with lived experience of disability to serve as leaders, instructors, supervisors, and role models within the program structure (Annamma et al., 2013).
4 Form disability advisory boards: Create advisory boards comprised of students, faculty, alumni, and local disability community members to provide ongoing guidance on programmatic inclusion efforts, curriculum development, policies/procedures, and quality improvement (Stuntzner & Hartley, 2014).

Inclusive Modules/Coursework

1. Implement a core Disability Studies course: Develop and require a foundational course solely focused on disability studies, covering models/theories, culture, identity, history, ethics, affirmative therapy approaches, and intersectionality (Olkin, 2022).
2. Integrate disability throughout existing courses: Systematically review and update all courses (e.g. theories, ethics, techniques, multicultural) to incorporate disability perspectives, literature, case examples, and experiential activities related to course content (Goodman-Scott et al., 2018).
3. Develop an intervention-focused disability course: Create a skills-based course on affirmative interventions, therapeutic modalities, assessments, and community approaches specifically tailored for clients with disabilities (Keesler et al., 2023).
4. Embed experiential learning components: Design applied learning experiences such as consultations with local disability organizations, interventions facilitated with disabled community members, practicum rotations focused on disability services, and accessibility audits or trainings (Balcazar & Suarez-Balcazar, 2016).

By embracing these future directions and recommendations, mental health training programs can advance the agenda of disability inclusion, promote social justice, and empower future therapists to provide compassionate, culturally competent, and person-centered care to disabled individuals.

Sample Course Description and Assignment

Disability-Affirming Practices in Mental Health Settings

This course will provide an overview of the history of disability, with an emphasis on inclusionary practices in mental health settings. The objective of the course is an in-depth exploration of affirmative, inclusive, and socially just approaches for mental health practice with disabled clients. Students will examine the implications of ableism, disability identity development, and intersectionality. The course will emphasize the shifting social and cultural constructions of disability through multiple modalities of instruction, such as small group discussions, individual projects, lectures, community immersion experiences, facilitated reflection, and simulated activities.

The course objectives include: exploring disability models and theories; critiquing ableist language and practices; examining cross-cultural understandings of disability, including the intersection of identities, accessibility, and accommodations; identifying social, emotional, intrapersonal, and motivational factors associated with the experiences of being labeled/identified as disabled; and discussing therapeutic practices by therapists with disabilities, family and community systems, utilizing disability-affirmative assessments, and evidence-based affirmative interventions and disability justice approaches. Students will develop the knowledge, skills, and awareness necessary for providing affirming, responsive, and socially just services to address the needs of disabled clients across mental health settings.

Sample Assignment: Cultural Conversations and Immersion Project

This assignment aims to deepen students' understanding of disability through interaction with disabled individuals. Each student is required to engage in ongoing dialogue with a disabled individual. Ideally, this person will be different from the student in multiple ways beyond ability status (e.g., race, social class, sexual orientation, gender, religion, country of origin, etc.). Students should prepare to interview this individual at least three times over a minimum of a six-week time interval. The interviews should consist of a discussion of the interviewee's family background and heritage, personal cultural identities and identity development-with specific attention to their identity as a disabled person-cultural attitudes, values, beliefs, understandings, and acculturative experiences. Additionally, students should inquire about any important cultural or historical events, multigenerational trauma, and current issues impacting the interviewee and/or members of their cultural communities, as well as coping behaviors and help-seeking behaviors from individual, interpersonal, community, and societal levels. Students should expect each interview to last at least one hour, and notes should be taken. Students will benefit from having questions prepared to make the most out of these interviews. In addition to the interviews, students are required to attend an activity or event with this individual that represents the cultural values of that group.

Finally, in order to help facilitate student personal development and knowledge of cultural groups, students will write a 7–10-page double-spaced paper that summarizes the content of the interviews, personal experiences (e.g., thoughts, feelings, behaviors) from the cultural activity/event, knowledge gained about cultural groups as reflected by the interviewee, and perceptions of the learning process. In other words, how did these experiences change or shape the way you view yourself, the world, and your role as a future counselor? Students are required to submit the paper as a PDF document. Prior to submission, students must ensure their paper can be accessed by an individual using assistive technology such as a screen reader or enlarger.

Conclusion

To effectively tackle the deficiency in disability inclusion within graduate-level mental health training, a comprehensive strategy is necessary, spanning various dimensions such as curriculum enhancements, faculty-training, experiential learning, and community engagement. Through the adoption of specific strategies and the cultivation of an environment that embraces disability inclusion, mental health training programs can equip aspiring professionals with the skills and mindset needed to deliver affirming, proficient, and accommodating services to disabled clients.

References

American Counseling Association. (2014). ACA code of ethics. *2014 ACA code of ethics*. Alexandria, VA: Author. Retrieved from https://www.counseling.org/docs/default-source/ethics/2014-aca-code-of-ethics.pdf

American Psychological Association. (2017). Multicultural guidelines: An ecological approach to context, identity, and intersectionality. https://www.apa.org/about/policy/multicultural-guidelines.pdf

Andrews, E. E., Forber-Pratt, A. J., Mona, L. R., Lund, E. M., Pilarski, C. R., & Balter, R. (2019). #SaytheWord: A disability culture commentary on the erasure of "disability." *Rehabilitation Psychology*, *64*(2), 111–118. https://doi.org/10.1037/rep0000258

Annamma, S. A., Connor, D., & Ferri, B. (2013). Dis/ability critical race studies (DisCrit): Theorizing at the intersections of race and dis/ability. *Race Ethnicity and Education*, *16*(1), 1–31, https://doi.org/10.1080/13613324.2012.730511

Balcazar, F. E., & Suarez-Balcazar, Y. (2016). Promoting empowerment among individuals with disabilities. In M. A. Bond, C. B. Keys, & I. Serrano-García (Eds.), *APA handbook of community psychology* (Vol. 2). American Psychological Association.

Brinkman, A. H., Rea-Sandin, G., Lund, E. M., Fitzpatrick, O. M., Gusman, M. S., Boness, C. L., & Scholars for Elevating Equity and Diversity (SEED). (2023). Shifting the discourse on disability: Moving to an inclusive, intersectional focus. *American Journal of Orthopsychiatry, 93*(1), 50–62. https://doi.org/10.1037/ort0000653

Center for Disability Rights. (n.d.). Ableism. https://cdrnys.org/blog/uncategorized/ableism/

Centers for Disease Control and Prevention. (2025, April 11). *Prevalence of disabilities and health care access by disability status and type among adults.* U.S. Department of Health and Human Services. Retrieved from https://www.cdc.gov/disability-and-health/articles-documents/disabilities-health-care-access.html

Chapin, M., McCarthy, H., Shaw, L., Bradham-Cousar, M., Chapman, R., Nosek, M., Peterson, S., Yilmaz, Z., & Ysasi, N. (2018). *Disability-related counseling competencies*. American Rehabilitation Counseling Association, a Division of ACA.

Conner, K. J., Acosta, V. M., Nouri, R., Tyler von Wrangel, M., Gramillo, E., & Conner, A. (2023). Psychotherapy experiences of U.S. adults with physical disabilities: Recommendations for affirmative practice. *The Counseling Psychologist*, *51*(7), 970–1004. https://doi.org/10.1177/00110000231186824.

Council for Accreditation of Counseling and Related Educational Programs. (2023). 2024 CACREP standards. https://www.cacrep.org/news/2024-cacrep-standards/

Council on Social Work Education. (2022). *Educational policy and accreditation standards* (EPAS). Alexandria, VA: Council on Social Work Education. Retrieved from https://www.cswe.org/getmedia/bb5d8afe-7680-42dc-a332-a6e6103f4998/2022-Educational-Policy-and-Accreditation-Standards-(EPAS).pdf

Deroche, M. D., Herlihy, B., & Lyons, M. L. (2020). Counselor trainee self-perceived disability competence: Implications for training. *Counselor Education and Supervision, 59*(3), 187–199. https://doi.org/10.1002/ceas.12183

Deroche, M. D., Ong, L. Z., & Cook, J. M. (2024). Ableist microaggressions, disability characteristics, and nondominant identities. *The Professional Counselor*, *13*, 404–417.

Feather, K. A., & Carlson, R. G. (2019). An initial investigation of individual instructor's self-perceived competence and incorporation of disability content into CACREP-accredited programs: Rethinking training in counselor education. *Journal of Multicultural Counseling and Development*, *47*, 19–36. https://doi.org/10.1002/jmcd.12118

Goodman-Scott, E., Bobzien, J., & Milsom, A. (2018). Preparing preservice school counselors to serve students with disabilities: A case study. *Professional School Counseling*, *22*(1) , 1–10. https://doi.org/10.1177/2156759X19867338

Hill, J. C., & Delgado, H. (2023). Incorporating disability knowledge and content into the counselor education curriculum. *ACES Teaching Practice Briefs*, Issue 2. Retrieved from: https://acesonline.net/wp-content/uploads/2023/10/TPB-iss2-Incorporating-Disability-Knowledge-and-Content-into-the-Counselor-Education-Curriculum.pdf

Hogan, A. J. (2019). Moving away from the "medical model": The development and revision of the World Health Organization's classification of disability. *Bulletin of the History of Medicine*, *93*(2), 241–269. https://doi.org/10.1353/bhm.2019.0028

Joshi, P., & Pappageorge, J. (2023). Reimagining disability: A call to action. *Developmental Disabilities Network Journal*, *3*(2), 88–97.

Keesler, J. M., Purcell, A., & Thomas-Giyer, J. (2023). Advancing trauma-informed care in intellectual and developmental disability services: A pilot study of a digital training with direct service providers. *Journal of Applied Research in Intellectual Disabilities*, *36*(3), 615–628. https://doi.org/10.1111/jar.13085

Kim, J., & Sellmaier, C. (2020). Making disability visible in social work education. *Journal of Social Work Education, 56*, 496–507.

Langellier, K. A., Astramovich, R. L., & Doughty Horn, E. A. (2020). Infusing service learning into the counselor education curriculum. *Professional Counselor, 10(2)*, 194–203.

Meidert, U., Dönnges, G., Bucher, T., Wieber, F., & Gerber-Grote, A. (2023). Unconscious bias among health professionals: A scoping review. *International Journal of Environmental Research and Public Health*, *20*(16), 6569. https://doi.org/10.3390/ijerph20166569

National Institute of Mental Health. (2022). Mental health disparities: People with disabilities experience depression and anxiety at higher rates than people without disabilities. https://www.nimh.nih.gov/research/priority-research-areas/mental-health-disparities-research

Oliver, M. (2013). The social model of disability: Thirty years on. *Disability & Society*, *28*(7), 1024–1026. https://doi.org/10.1080/09687599.2013.818773

Öksüz, E. E., & Brubaker, M. D. (2020). Deconstructing disability training in counseling: A critical examination and call to the profession. *Journal of Counselor Leadership and Advocacy*, *7*(2), 163–175. https://doi.org/10.1080/2326716X.2020.1820407

Olkin, R. (2022). *Disability studies: An interdisciplinary introduction* (4th ed.). Sage Publications.

Right, A. (2020). Explicit and implicit attitudes towards people with disabilities. *Psychology Research Methods Journals*, *1*(22), 199–219.

SAMHSA. (2021). Evidence-based practices resource center. Retrieved from https://store.samhsa.gov/sites/default/files/pep21-05-02-001.pdf

Smart, J. (2016). *Disability, society, and the individual* (3rd ed.). PRO-ED, Inc.

Smith, T. J. (2021). Multicultural ethics in rehabilitation services. *Journal of Vocational Rehabilitation, 54*(3), 295–304.

Stuntzner, S., & Hartley, M. (2014). Disability and the counseling relationship: What counselors need to know. *Vistas Online* (9), 1–12. Alexandria, VA: American Counseling Association. Retrieved from https://scholarworks.utrgv.edu/coun_fac/26/

Yzaguirre, M. M., PettyJohn, M. E., Tseng, C.-F., Asiimwe, R., Fang, M., & Blow, A. J. (2022). Marriage and family therapy master's students' diversity course experiences. *Journal of Feminist Family Therapy*, *34*(1–2), 15–37. https://doi.org/10.1080/08952833.2022.2052534.

Bibliography

Baglieri, S., & Shapiro, A. (2012). *Disability studies and the inclusive classroom: Critical practices for creating least restrictive attitudes*. Routledge.

Centers for Disease Control and Prevention. (2018). Disability impacts all of us. National Center on Birth Defects and Developmental Disabilities. Retrieved from https://www.cdc.gov/disability-and-health/media/pdfs/disability-impacts-all-of-us-infographic.pdf

Freedman, J., Applebaum, A., Woodfield, C., & Ashby, C. (2019). Integrating disability studies pedagogy in teacher education. *Journal of Teaching Disability Studies*, *1*(1), 1–40.

National Parks Service, U.S. Department of the Interior. (n.d.). *Disability history: The disability rights movement*. https://www.nps.gov/articles/disabilityhistoryrightsmovement.htm

Olkin, R. (2017). *Disability-affirmative therapy: A case formulation template for clients with disabilities*. Oxford University Press.

Siebers, T. (2011). *Disability theory*. University of Michigan Press.

16

MULTI-DISCIPLINARY COLLABORATION, REPRESENTATION, AND ETHICAL RESEARCH OF DISABILITY EXPERIENCES[1]

Lydia Qualls, Lyndon Frommer, and Ashley Shew

Introduction

Why is a chapter on research important to include in a handbook of clinical practice? Anyone who has been in a graduate program or continuing education (so likely everyone reading this book) knows the emphasis placed on "evidence-based practice" (Patterson, Miller, Carnes, & Wilson, 2004). However, evidence-based practice is only as good as the research base for clinical practice. For disability-focused research, this literature base often ignores, misinterprets, and misrepresents the interests of disabled people and the disability community. Therefore, to create a comprehensive handbook for disability-affirmative therapy, there needs to be a discussion of disability-affirmative research. Multi-disciplinary collaboration, the hallmark of any effective research in the 21st century, often includes different interest groups, researchers, and experts with similar interests or concerns to work together to develop solutions to complex problems. Indeed, it is almost impossible to obtain any funding, from a departmental position to an NIH grant without listing several collaborators across different fields. While it is true that multi-disciplinary collaboration is an effective tool that leads to important breakthroughs, in disability research the most important collaborators are often left out – disabled individuals themselves.

Disability rights leaders and self-advocates have used the rallying cry of "Nothing about us, without us" for decades when it comes to research, legislation, and

 DOI: 10.4324/9781003362586-25

policies involving disabled people. The position that disabled people should be involved at all levels of investigation and policy-making on issues that concern them is a cornerstone in the disability rights movement. However, to date, research has an especially poor track record of involving disabled people in the conception, execution, and application of disability research. Disability justice advocates add concerns about intersectional disabled approaches as well, where the beneficiaries of disability rights have often been otherwise-privileged disabled people (those who are financially more secure, often white, or who have disabilities that are more "palatable" or relatable to the public; see The Principles of Disability Justice; Sins Invalid, 2015).

Research about disability often features biases and tropes that influence researchers (Ymous et al., 2019; Botha & Cage, 2022; Williams, 2019), including their research questions (what researchers take as a problem), their methods (what avenues of inquiry and setups they see as yielding data), their interpretations of data (what they infer from observations), and the conclusions they draw. Ymous and Colleagues (2019) discuss how technology for disabled people is developed by not (yet) disabled researchers, who often dismiss, put down, and invalidate the perspectives and lived experiences offered by disabled researchers.

A mixed-methods study by Botha and Cage (2022) examined views of Autism researchers toward Autistic people and found that those researchers who constructed Autism in a medical narrative were more likely to endorse ableist cues. The authors also found that objectification was pivotal in considering a person's value to society, with Autistic people that have normal to above average intellectual ability and capacity for greater independence being perceived as more valuable. Language use was also important, as talking about eliminating "Autism" as a concept is more palatable than talking about eliminating Autistic people. Alarmingly, these authors found Autism researchers used language that was quite stigmatizing, including one participant and researcher who described Autistic people as, "shut down from the outside world; rigid; emotional; fat" (Botha & Cage, 2022, p. 8). These words are not neutral in a context of evaluation where autistic people seeking help are dehumanized and othered by researchers. Some of their language also echoes misunderstandings and scientific ignorance stemming from outdated autism theories that describes autistic people as "empty fortresses" (in the work of Bruno Bettleheim; there is important critique of these theories and their perpetuation in Human-Computer Research approaches to autism therapies in Williams, 2021). Research about researchers' biases also shows what can counter some of this ableist bias: greater inclusion of Autistic people in the research, which was found to indicate a lower likelihood of ableist cues (Botha & Cage, 2022).

Another way to conceptualize the view of disability-as-deficit in medicine and mental health is through pathologization. Pathologization is the process by which a person's difference is seen as disordered, deviant, or abnormal and needing correction (Liebert, 2014). Moreover, this deviance is often defined in medical or clinical terms because the definition of this difference remains in the medical and corrective sphere (Liebert, 2014). Disability is often pathologized in medicine and mental health, which is problematic for both fields because it neglects a disabled person's personhood and reduces them to their disability (Eickers, 2023). Additionally, it neglects the fact that a person's disability does not necessarily need to be cured but rather that it is other social and systemic issues that create real challenges for disabled people (Baár, 2017). Pathologizing a disabled person also does not lead to better care for disabled people in clinical settings because it focuses on normalizing disabled people rather than focusing on the mental health care that fits their needs that may or may not be related to their disability and even if it is related to their disability it does not mean that the disability needs correcting (Baár, 2017). By adopting some of the critical and reflexive research explored in this chapter, we hope that research can help de-pathologize disabled people by recognizing their autonomy and perspectives in research done about them, reestablishing their personhood.

There are many mismatches between researcher ideas and disability community interests in therapies and assistive technologies. Labeled as #DisabilityDongles, some devices like exoskeletons and sign-language gloves are roundly criticized by people in the disability community as a "well intended, elegant, yet useless solution to a problem we never knew we had" (Jackson, Haagaard, & Williams, 2022, para. 2). Sometimes people imagine what it would be like to be disabled and project what they would want from there; this practice, often aligning with disability simulation approaches (which have been themselves the subject of disabled criticism and produce different outcomes for the participants than what is intended, see Silverman, 2015, 2017; Nario-Redmond et al., 2017), often "gets the story wrong" when it comes to disabled people's experiences (Shew, 2022). Recent work on technoableism highlights the many ways in which negative and biased perceptions of disability undermine disabled testimony and voices about actual lived experience. These perceptions put nondisabled people as the experts regarding disabled people's lives and desires, and shape therapist and social opinions about what it is disabled people want or need (Shew, 2023; Mauldin, 2016; Virdi, 2020). Oftentimes, we see a failure of imagination and of proper listening and understanding where people imagine what it is disabled people want and need (and of course internalized ableism can play a role in what disabled people ask for too).

Given the importance of disabled expertise on anything pertaining to disability, the remainder of this chapter will explore some concerns about conducting research with disabled people and how to conduct disability-focused research. To begin this discussion, this chapter will first explore the ways that disability is often defined in research, as well as how these definitions reduce disabled people's identities and neglect to identify some members of the disability community accurately. Section "Defining 'Fair Research': Principles and Practices for Ethical Inquiry" discusses fairness and inclusion of disabled people in research and how disabled people are often excluded unnecessarily from research either due to ability exclusion criteria or non-inclusive research recruitment and methodologies.

This section concludes with suggestions for creating fair research. From there, the conversation turns to suggestions on ways to include disabled people's voices in research, inviting researchers to confront and change their ableist mentalities and suggesting participatory research (PR) methods such as advisory boards with multiple disabled adults or participatory evaluation. This chapter concludes with a list of questions researchers can use to evaluate whether their or others' work includes disabled people.

Defining Disability in Research

Disability-focused Questionnaires

Creating a diverse sample in research typically focuses on racial/ethnic identities and gender, although there has been more focus recently in including sexual orientation as an aspect of diversity. However, unless the focus of the study is explicitly examining disability, this important identity characteristic is rarely described. Furthermore, various ways of characterizing disability can under-identify disabled people. The most commonly used measures of disability in federal surveys in the United States are the American Community Survey six-question measure (ACS-6) and the Washington Group Short Set (WG-SS). The questions in the ACS-6 ask yes-no questions about disabilities in six categories: hearing difficulty, vision difficulty, cognitive difficulty, ambulatory difficulty, self-care difficulty, and independent living difficulty (Census.gov, accessed 12–20–2023). The WG-SS questions measure a continuum of difficulty performing activities of daily living from "no difficulty" to "cannot do at all" in the areas of seeing, hearing, mobility, cognition, self-care, and communication (https://www.washingtongroup-disability.com/, accessed 12–20–2023) and are preferred when doing international research due to producing data on disabilities that can be compared internationally (Miller et al., 2011).

Standardization among questions is helpful for looking at categories over time, but these categories do not account for many other factors and are often inaccurate in identifying those with disabilities. Landes et al. (2025) found that these two most commonly used measures of disabilities failed to detect a large percentage of respondents (ACS-6, 20% and WG-SS, 43%) who reported disabilities in response to other questions on the National Survey on Health and Disability (NSHD). These measures most often excluded respondents with psychiatric or chronic health disabilities (Landes et al., 2025). The NSHD used open-ended function-based and condition-based questions to have respondents describe their disabilities and had respondents self-select one of seven major disability categories (intellectual or cognitive, mental illness or psychiatric, physical or mobility, chronic illness or disease, sensory, developmental, and neurological) to describe their most disabling condition (Institute for Health and Disability Policy Studies, 2022). This method was also more accurate at identifying those who had short-term rather than long-term disabilities, a population often overlooked in many discussions of disabilities (Hall et al., 2022). One potential drawback to this approach is that many disabled people have multiple disabilities, and it is often difficult to choose which one is "primary," especially with conditions that wax and wane over time or that vary based on circumstance.

A key reason why disabled respondents may not have been identified as disabled by the ACS-6 and WG-SS is that disabled people who have access to appropriate accommodations and supports may not have difficulty with the task or activity in question and therefore may be missed by both of these measures. As Hall and Colleagues (2022) note, both sets of questions ask if participants have "difficulty" with a particular task or activity, which ignores respondents who may only have difficulty without accommodations, or only had difficulty temporarily, or only sometimes (in the case of many chronic illnesses where level of disability fluctuates). They also note that the ACS-6 and WG-SS have many fewer categories of functioning than defined by the International Classification of Functioning, Disability and Health, which may be part of the reason these measures underestimated people with psychiatric and chronic health disabilities. In their recommendations, the authors recommend three additional questions to include in measuring disability (Hall et al., 2022). The first, if the survey respondent "has a mental or physical condition, impairment, or disability that affects daily activities or requires use of equipment or technology" (Hall et al., 2022, p. 1440). This question captures disabled people who have assistive devices (like prosthetic limbs for amputees and glucose monitors for those with diabetes), although it may still exclude individuals who rely on other people and systems for support rather than equipment or technology. The authors also recommend asking respondents the age of onset or expected duration of the condition, and to name or self-categorize their condition(s) and describe which one is their primary condition (Hall et al., 2022). While it is important for disabled people to have autonomy in naming and describing their conditions, it may be difficult for disabled people to choose one primary condition, as the relative impact of each condition may vary from situation to situation.

Recruiting Disabled Participants

In addition to intentionally and inclusively selecting the questions that measure disability, information about the goals of the survey, how participants were recruited, and other demographic characteristics of the sample besides disability can all define how representative the sample is of larger groups of disabled people (Hermans, 2023). For example, if the investigated disabled population in a study is primarily white, but a researcher wants to apply the findings to disabled people in their area, which has a large Latino population, the findings may not translate as accurately. Another example is the American Community Survey, which historically does not collect information on people living in institutions, such as adult and juvenile correction facilities, as well as nursing facilities (Popkin et al., 2022; Oneto, Farrell, and Popkin, 2022; United States Census Bureau, 2017). This would exclude a large percentage of the disabled population who are incarcerated, including those that are incarcerated for reasons associated with their disability and those that acquire health conditions, mental and physical, from their incarceration. Due to its size, the prison system is the largest system to house disabled people in the United States. A survey by the Bureau of Justice Statistics estimates that disabled people make up as much as 40% of those incarcerated, and for women in state prisons that estimate rises to 50% of the total population (Maruschack, Bronson, & Alper, 2021). The findings from studies that exclude institutionalized disabled people may not be beneficial or applicable to the large population of disabled people in the prison system.

Case Vignette

B takes medication for both ADHD and anxiety. In the absence of medication, B often has difficulty concentrating at work and doing household chores. Because of her anxiety about public hostility due to her gender presentation as a transgender woman, B often avoids doing errands outside of the house, such as grocery shopping and picking up medication. On the ACS-6, B may deny having "serious" difficulty concentrating, remembering, or making decisions, because she is helped with medication or reminders from her partner for most tasks. Similarly, on the WG-SS, she might mark "some difficulty" with remembering or concentrating, again because of the help of medication and care from those around her. Additionally, she sees her difficulty running errands as being related to her gender presentation, and not a "physical, mental, or emotional condition" on the ACS-6. Therefore, both the ACS-6 and WG-SS could fail to identify B as disabled.

Defining "Fair Research": Principles and Practices for Ethical Inquiry

Avoiding Unnecessary Exclusion

Even if disabled people are able to be accurately identified as disabled by researchers, they are often excluded from research because of their disability. Most research, including that on therapy interventions, is considered "more robust" if it has a "well defined" sample, meaning participants with no other diagnoses other than the one under investigation. This means that disabled people, due to their "diagnosed" disability, will oftentimes be excluded from a study. This brings the effectiveness of an intervention into question, as mental health comorbidity is the rule rather than the norm (McGrath et al., 2020) and disabled people are more likely than non-disabled people to have a mental health diagnosis (Cree et al., 2020). Unfounded exclusions such as these can lead to cases such as using risperidone in children and adults for behavioral management for several years before it was found to be clinically ineffective in this population (Singh et al., 2005).

Van Spall, Toren, Kiss, and Fowler (2007) note that instead of running separate trials for first examining efficacy with a more exclusive patient population, and then examining effectiveness with a more representative population, many medical researchers merely complete the first set of trials and then recommend doctors "proceed with caution" when using the treatment on any individuals outside the population. These authors examined a selection of randomized control trials (RCTs) found in high-impact medical journals from 1994 to 2006 and found 84% of trials contained at least one "poorly justified" exclusion criteria, many of which excluded disabled people. The exclusion was considered to be "poorly justified" if it did not affect the person's ability to provide informed consent or if the intervention would be harmful, ineffective, or the effects of which would be difficult to determine. Of these overly-exclusive criteria, 11% of trials excluded participants due to physical or functional disabilities, 8% excluded participants because of cognitive disabilities, 81% excluded people due to an additional medical condition, and 11% excluded participants due to language and communication barriers (Van Spall et al., 2007).

Feldman, Battin, Shaw, and Luckasson (2013) specifically examined the exclusion of children with disabilities from child development research and found that one-third of studies explicitly excluded disabled children from their research and this number rose to 90% when including studies that did not even mention disabled children, noting that no mention of disabled participants likely indicated exclusion. In almost three quarters of the studies, no justification for exclusion was provided. When justification was provided, they often included reasons that could potentially be accommodated (e.g., "unable to complete surveys and questionnaires independently") or were vague and subjective (e.g., "incapable of meaningful participation," excluded to "minimize disruptions to the study"; Feldman et al., 2013, p. 1002) The authors also noted that of the studies that did not mention or that explicitly excluded children with disabilities, one-half could have included disabled children *even without accommodations* according to the study's methodology, for at least one of three categories of disabilities the authors used in their review (sensory, physical/health, developmental/learning; Feldman et al., 2013). For many researchers, it appears the exclusion of disabled participants is based more on assumptions about the capabilities of disabled people rather than "evidence-based."

Unfortunately, it appears that exclusion of disabled people from clinical research has persisted since the review conducted above. Plosky and Colleagues (2022) reviewed 97 registered clinical trials across the areas of depression, dementia, diabetes, and lung cancer and found that rates of exclusion ranged from 3% (speech and communication disabilities) to 93% ("other chronic conditions"). Other excluded disability-related conditions included being in long-term care (6%), mobility (9%), hearing (10%), visual (34%), cognitive and intellectual (42%), HIV or hepatitis (53%), substance use (62%), and psychiatric disabilities (68%). Only 18% of studies explicitly permitting disabled people to use forms of support (e.g., supported decision making, assisted devices) to complete the study, and up to 85% of protocols allowed for exclusion at the investigator's discretion. This was most commonly diabetes research and dementia research (100% and 93% respectively) but was also present in depression (67%) and lung cancer research (76%). This discretion was often phrased broadly, such as "any disorder which in the investigator's opinion might jeopardize subject's safety or compliance with the protocol" (Posky et al., 2022, Study Results, para. 1). This makes it easier for investigators to exclude individuals with any "inconvenient" disabilities as opposed to accommodating them. The authors also found a wide variance between what disabilities were excluded for what studies, such that depression research more often excluded those with cognitive disability (83% of studies) and less often excluded visual disability (29%), whereas the opposite was true of diabetes research (only 6% excluded cognitive disability, while 50% excluded visual disability[2]). Justification for exclusion criteria was often not present, ill-defined and subjective, or for reasons that could be overcome with typical accommodations. All studies were in Phase III of research, the period in which broader efficacy outside of a strictly defined group is studied in order to inform the product label (Posky et al., 2022).

Accessing Research Participation

Even when disabled people are not intentionally excluded from research, other aspects of recruitment and research design may limit their participation. In a 2000 research study, Meyers and Andresen noted that methods commonly used in research and research recruitment at the time often excluded disabled people. For example, random digit dialing often excluded telephone devices for the deaf (TDDs) and self-administered surveys created barriers for blind people or those with low-vision, fine motor difficulties, traumatic brain injury, and other common disabling conditions (Meyers & Andresen, 2000). Although assistive devices and multiple methods of recruitment are now common, many foundational research studies were performed at a time when research was more exclusionary to disabled people, and these studies have likely not been replicated with a more inclusive sample. Additionally, researchers who want to do better are not always allowed to do so: institutional review boards (IRBs) sometimes still push back against researchers who want to allow multiple modes of feedback, interviewing, and participant response, especially in the context of people who use things like alternative and augmentative communication (AAC) devices with an ableist assumption being that AAC users cannot properly give believable testimony or feedback, or report back in meaningful ways (Personal Communication). Furthermore, as Posky and Colleagues (2022) found, many IRBs and therefore researchers insist that participants must be able to read and sign informed consent documents themselves, despite any difficulties with this being readily accommodatable (e.g., having a recording available for visually disabled people, allowing for recording of a person's verbal assent, or clicking a button or making a mark to indicate consent).

Williams and Moore (2011), writing in the field of biomedical research, introduced the concept of Universal Design of Research (UDR), suggesting researchers follow "a few simple rules" to include as many disabled people as possible: (1) plan to include any participants who meet inclusion criteria regardless of disability status, (2) do not use exclusion criteria without strong scientific justification (access Posky et al., 2022 for examples of what this can look like in including individuals with multiple types of disabilities), (3) use multisensory options for recruitment, research instruments (e.g., questionnaires), measurements, and responses from participants, and (4) when the researcher themselves does not know how to include a particular disability or category of disabilities, consult someone who does (Williams & Moore, 2011).

Rios, Magasi, Novak, and Harniss (2016) also include UDR in their suggestions on how to include disabled people in public health, epidemiological, and outcomes studies, as well as additional suggestions for how to provide accommodations and modifications of research protocol to include those with disabilities. Their suggestions for accommodations include examining the physical setting, mode of presentation of instructions, mode of response, and schedule or timing of tasks to tailor the research participation of a particular person to that person's needs, without altering the primary construct being measured. Modifications are an additional way to make the task accessible to some disabled people, although these may involve changes that affect the measurement of the primary construct. While modifications come with internal validity concerns, further studies can aid in establishing measurement equivalence (Rios et al., 2016).

Fair and Inclusive Research Questions

Research questions themselves can also be presumptive about expectations of disabled people. Often, disabled participants are judged against "normal" standards. This can be a problem where healthy norms for a disability group may be different than for nondisabled people. A great example of this is in critiques of autism research. Maxfield Sparrow, an autistic writer, points to the ways in which researchers observe compliance as a success, often in highly problematic ways:

> We autistic people need researchers to develop better criteria for success than our symptoms, compliance, and manageability. I'm more compliant when I have a fever, more compliant when I'm too depressed to care anymore, more compliant when dissociating from a trauma response. Not all reduction of symptoms is a success. Symptoms are just what other people see; they aren't what we are experiencing inside.
>
> (Sparrow, 2023)

Because so much Autism research involves observed behavior, a lot of the research diverges from the self-reports of Autistic people. An Autistic person may be more compliant, but at the expense of long-term mental health. This is often a critique of Applied Behavioral Analysis (ABA) therapy for Autistic individuals, which often has poor long-term outcomes in terms of health and safety, even though it's often called the "gold standard" in terms of approaches by its well-funded proponents (see critiques of ABA by the Autistic Self-Advocacy Network, 2024). This emphasis also extends to other forms of Autism research, which often presumes that Autistic groups should be like (or should be trying to be like) non-Autistic ones. Maxfield Sparrow particularly talks about the importance of screentime to Autistic children, and its role supporting Autistic children in socializing, understanding, and participating in ways that are unlike non-Autistic children. iPads and other tools can be essential technologies for Autistic people, and Sparrow calls for us to change our expectations:

> Research is beginning to catch up with what we've been telling the world for decades: it takes a lot of energy to try to be "indistinguishable from our peers." Not all of us are able to perform neurotypicality. Some of us literally kill ourselves trying to maintain the act. For those of us who go on to be social or who work at school and jobs, letting us have unstructured screen time as children, whether in addition to structured screen time or on its own, will pave the way for more connection with the world in the future, whatever that connection ends up looking like… everyone deserves access to the tools that allow them to connect with the world in the ways that foster their well-being.
>
> (Sparrow, 2023)

We should not expect that all technologies operate in the same way in different people's lives or malign a technology based on expectations of normalcy. In this case, more technology use might be better, but the filter of neurotypical norms often restricts dialogue about technology presumed to be predominantly negative.

Ethics at the Community Level

Even when "fair" research practices are followed for individuals, most of the ethical analysis of costs and benefits of the research is done at the level of the individual, rather than the community. Herington, Li, and Pisani (2024) argue that "research projects should not only respect individual participant autonomy but should also ensure a just allocation of the benefits and burdens of research for all community members" (Herington, Li, & Pisani, 2024, p. 131). They note that this is especially important to consider in contexts such as secondary research with "de-identified" electronic data, since the original research participants are unable to consent to their data being used for this specific research purpose. The authors note that because communities can "reasonably disagree with each other" (Herington, Li, & Pisani, 2024, p. 131), it is important to consider the Belmont Principles of beneficence, autonomy, and justice (National Commission for the Protection of Human Subjects of Biomedical & Behavioral Research, 1979) at the community level rather than only at the individual level. This necessitates an equitable distribution of burdens and benefits across a population of people who each have different values, abilities, and interests (Herington, Li, & Pisani, 2024).

An example of considering the impact of research to a broad community of disabled people can be seen in the Autistic community's response to the Spectrum 10k study. This study was launched in August of 2021 by Simon Baron-Cohen, director of the Autism Research Centre at the University of Cambridge and was designed to collect both questionnaire data and DNA samples from Autistic participants for genomic and environmental factors contributing to autism. Autistic people and family members, allies, and professionals who work with autistic people pushed back over concerns around research transparency, data storage, and uncertainty of aims of the study led for recruitment for the study to be paused a month later (Ellis & Asbury, 2023). An autistic-lead research study conducted by Ellis and Asbury (2023) used interviews to qualitatively explore opinions of late-diagnosed Autistic adults residing in the UK on this project specifically. Concerns raised by these participants included how this research would influence the negative rhetoric surrounding Autism in public opinion; lack of transparency of research aims, procedures, and data storage; the focus on genetics over other priorities of the Autistic community; and the exclusion of marginalized voices within the Autism community in the decision-making process (Ellis & Asbury, 2023). The study was resumed after Spectrum 10K internally evaluated itself, but many detractors remain steadfast in opposing this research project because of its potential harms in terms of genetic diagnostics and elimination of autistic people, and of distrust for the research team running the study (many of whom are seen to have engaged in ableist work about autistic people in the past).

Case Vignette

Researchers want to solicit feedback from disabled participants about the use of robot dogs for various applications and usability. Researcher A recruits disabled people with only mobility-related disabilities, broadly construed, for individual feedback through survey methods where participants have to be able to read and click to respond. Researcher B does one-on-one verbal interviews with disabled participants after they play with the device, which requires two hands to operate (so some participants are excluded). Researcher C recruits participants for both in-person and online observation; participants can either play with the device or watch others play with the device or watch a series of videos about the device (for people who do not want to be in-person or are afraid of the device) and provide feedback through a variety of formats, including short live interview, written documents, or recorded response.

Strategies for Ethical and Inclusive Research and Therapy Practices

Background on Participatory Research

A way to include disabled people in research is to explore methods of PR. PR is broadly defined as the practice of including members of the community in research that will directly impact them (Vaughn & Jacquez, 2020). PR developed out of two categories of traditions of emancipatory theories: the "northern" and "southern" traditions (Macaulay, 2017). The participatory science which developed out of the "northern" tradition in the 1940s emphasized the "continuous inquiry, action and evaluation" of research and that this process should be done with rather than for/on a community (Macaulay, 2017, p. 256). However, out of this tradition, some groups started to adopt it for organizational efficiency. In contrast, the "southern" traditions developed in the 1970s out of the work of the *Pedagogy of the Oppressed* by Paulo Freire which questioned traditional values in science and emphasized the capacity of lay people to participate in inquiry. For both traditions, researchers in the academic community saw the development of participatory science as less rigorous than other forms of inquiry (Macaulay, 2017).

The perceived validity of participatory science began to shift in the 1980s when public health organizations such as the CDC and PRC started to recommend PR methodologies. Some of the first adopters of these methods started to develop in the 1990s with primary care practitioners in Indigenous communities, while the full shape of PR methods started to form in the late 1990s into the 2000s with the development of PR guidelines and evaluations. More publications and testimonials to the efficacy of PR methods emerged through the 2000s to the point that it was more widely seen in the scientific literature as an effective and sometimes more effective research method compared with more traditional modes of research (Macaulay, 2017).

PR seeks to be inclusive research that comes in different forms, settings, and populations. Inclusion of members of the community can range from enlisting people to help collect data, such as in citizen science, to people being involved in the early stages of planning and helping to formulate research questions used in Participatory Action Research, to having community-based advisory boards for the project (Vaughn & Jacquez, 2020). Skorburg, O'Doherty, and Friesen (2024) provide an overview of both epistemic and ethical considerations for PR, particularly in light of the growing inclusion of artificial intelligence and machine learning in mental health research.

Some examples of beginning to explore PR in research include community science, patient-centered outcomes research, and user-centered design research. Community Science, a method used in community psychology, focuses "on building strong communities through partnered prevention, treatment, education, and health promotion efforts" (Vaughn & Jacquez, 2020). This method recognizes the importance of a strong community to build lasting improved outcomes for the target populations, emphasizing the individual, institutions, and the community as "active and responsible" contributors (Wandersman, 2003). Patient-centered outcomes research focuses on the outcomes participants are most interested in and theorizes that higher quality clinical research comes from end-users' input (Vaughn & Jacquez, 2020). Similarly, user-centered design research describes an iterative design process with the end user to develop a product or service that is intended for them (Vaughn & Jacquez, 2020). All three of these methods focus on including the community or end-users most impacted by the research and either emphasize a holistic perspective on well-being or the importance of relevant research rather than prescriptive.

Application of Participatory Research

The assortment of PR methods has been used with a whole host of different communities, including adolescents, refugees, immigrants, native populations, and other marginalized populations that have historically been excluded from research (Vaughn & Jacquez, 2020; Ozer, 2017; Kia-Keating & Juang, 2022; Hearod et al., 2019; Macaulay, 2017). Some Indigenous nations, which have historically been discriminated against and abused by researchers, have developed an intertribal IRB board which not only reviews research being done about or with their community but also sets the requirement that this research must contribute to the wellbeing of the community. This often necessitates PR as a central part of research development when working with the intertribal IRB by prioritizing the needs of the community over specific research questions (Kelley, 2013). Kelley (2013) outlines different criteria for determining how and when to establish an intertribal IRB. These include:

1. Identify the context in which research involving Tribal members or communities is regulated
2. Determine whether the level of regulation is adequate for the potential risks involved
3. Assess the views of Tribal leaders, community members, and researchers on research regulation
4. Create a working group under the direction of Tribal leaders to assess areas of need relating to the development of formal research regulations, policies, or an IRB
5. Review the existing policies and practices of the Indian Health Service area IRB, Tribal consortia, and the local Tribal IRB
6. Encourage community-level protections and formal research review processes as appropriate (based on steps 1–5).

Multiple methods of PR are available, and Hodges and Colleagues (2024) review how these methods collectively can give researchers the best chance at truly upholding the core ethical principles of the Belmont Report – respect for persons, beneficence, and justice (National Commission for the Protection of Human Subjects of Biomedical & Behavioral Research, 1979) when working with participants from historically excluded and underserved communities (Hodges et al., 2024). The first, community-based participatory research (CBPR) involves investigating research questions the community deems to be priorities, collective identification of ecological resources, building long-term relationships in the community, information gathering through focus groups and interviews, and relying on "cultural brokers," individuals who are both part of the research team and the community who can liaise between the two groups and promote active and equitable collaboration (Hodges et al., 2024). An additional approach, Transdisciplinary Team Science (TDTS) composes a team with a variety of educational and cultural backgrounds united by digital communication, drawing models from diverse perspectives and creating new solutions to multi-faceted problems (Ferguson et al., 2019). This method combines effective forward-thinking leadership with collaborative decision making to engender both the flexibility and stability to make real-time decisions and changes to the research protocol to adapt to community needs as they arise (Hodges et al., 2024).

Another collaborative research design is representational ethics (Haarlammert et al., 2017), which uses knowledge of both "insiders" and "outsiders" to reduce bias and provide ecological context for research findings. Research performed solely by "insiders" has the strength of providing a community viewpoint through which to interpret findings in contextualized and nuanced ways, while being vulnerable to biased conclusions based on the salience of the individual researcher's lived experiences. In contrast, research performed only by "outsiders" can provide "objective detachment" but may not always center community needs in selecting research questions and can perpetuate dominant cultural biases in interpreting outcomes. A combination approach instructs researchers to consider their individual and combined positionality and the effect these positions have on the research (Haarlammert et al., 2017). This approach can also work in conjunction with Cross-Cultural Psychology (CCP), which can be used methodologically to distinguish between culture specifics from cultural universality (Van De Vijver, 2009). This approach can benefit historically excluded groups by highlighting and rejecting the myth that there is a singular "best" way to be across the range of human diversity. This method promotes situating research findings contextually by advocating for interpreting structural findings (e.g., invariance) in addition to construct level (e.g., mean differences; Van De Vijver, 2009).

There are instances where PR has been used with different members of the disability community, such as McDonald and Stack (2016) in which the authors evaluated the effectiveness of CBPR with developmentally disabled people. The CBPR projects McDonald and Stack reviewed sought to explore violence, victimization, and the health of people with developmental disabilities. To gauge the effectiveness, they conducted interviews that asked whether the participants had felt heard, respected, and valued during the research process and compared that to the effectiveness of the findings that researchers developed. This study found that

CBPR is an effective method to respect disabled people and produce significant findings at the same time (McDonald & Stack, 2016).

In our own work, we are cultivating a research consulting group as part of a larger project on community building. The research facet of our "DisCoTec Center" – Disability Community Technology Center – provides cross-disabled recruiting and consulting feedback on scientific and technological research (including on projects that are not centered on disability). The consulting process is founded on PR principles to inform where and how disabled people's voices should be heard during the research process, and our project is led by a predominantly disabled group of investigators. The consulting process involves the recruiting of disabled community members who wish to provide their expertise and experience to STEM research to give feedback about devices and research that will positively impact disabled people rather than the assumed needs or interests placed upon disabled people by nondisabled researchers. We prioritize mutiply-disabled people on our teams, and our work is on-going.

Earlier we discussed the tendency of researchers to reduce people to one singular disability, which can lead to the exclusion of people with multiple disabilities and a narrowing of the experience of being a disabled person. The multiplicity in the experience of members of the community is incredibly important because the experience of different disabilities (and other demographic factors) can lead to a variety of experiences and perspectives. We also find that disabled people are better listened to when we are not the only one in the room: where we can amplify each other's concerns and discuss together. If we want to accurately gauge how different disabled people experience the world and maximize who can be included in research, it is crucial to have a wealth of experiences within the disability community. No one member of the community can speak to the experience of the whole of the community.

Case Vignette

Dr. A is interested in doing research using wearable technology to track biomarkers of Autistic participants that can be sent to their healthcare providers in real time. As Dr. A is not Autistic, they gather a research board of community members to review their research proposal. Some Autistic adults on the research board are worried that Dr. A's plan is not aligned with their privacy interests as Autistic adults, while parents of Autistic children (some parents are Autistic themselves and some are not) are in favor of knowing more about their children's health, but worried about the comfort of the wearable device for their children. Dr. A listens to input from the Autistic adults about how they would prefer the information from the wearables be used, given directly to them as participants rather than sent to their doctor's office. That way, they have control over their own data. Study protocol is developed so that there are a number of ways the Autistic children can wear the devices, and the Autistic children are asked for assent in the way most accessible to them, are provided with options for how their data can be used at a developmentally-appropriate level, and are informed that they can ask for the study to be stopped at any time.

Evaluating Research for Use in Practice

Transitioning from the decades- and centuries-long view of disability-as-deficit that has shaped medical and therapeutic research to one that values the lives, expertise, and contributions of disabled people is a process that we hope is underway, but it is not happening overnight. While we might not discount all helpful research when it does not focus on or include those with disabilities, it is our responsibility as consumers of research to consider what effects using the results of such research with our disabled clients, students, participants, and so forth may be. For researchers, it is important to be *as inclusive as possible* (not as inclusive as is convenient) in including disabled people, and those from other traditionally excluded groups as well, in research, and to check our own biases for presumptions we may have about disabled people and disability research. The following questions are ones that researchers and research consumers can ask themselves to gauge whether or not the work is accessible and inclusive of disabled people.

1 Does the article have a position statement that describes how the author(s)' identities influenced the research? Many journals currently require or encourage such statements to allow authors to name their identities for reasons such as "nothing about us, without us." However, it is still difficult for academics in many environments to be "out" as disabled (see Price, Salzer, O'Shea, & Kerschbaum, 2017). Disabled researchers who do not want to center their disabled identities can do the same things as non-disabled researchers in collaborating with those who can take on the role of being the "out" disabled person, centering these people's experiences, and paying them for their contributions.
2 If there is not a position statement, how do the authors describe centering disabled people in their research? Are disabled people involved from the beginning or are they used as a "sounding board" for ideas the authors had already developed? This does not mean research done this way is bad, but it is a point to keep in mind that the therapy or practice being described may not always serve the interests of that particular disabled community.
3 If the evidence-based practice being used is for a broader population than just disabled people, do any researchers include disabled people in their research samples? If adapting general research to disabled clients, learn about the experiences of disabled people to see if any of the therapy practices are contraindicated (e.g., a focus on mindful breathing may not always be the best for those on ventilators or respiratory disorders). One of our authors has had two lung surgeries due to cancer, and being asked to take in and hold her breath makes her think about where two little chunks of her lungs were taken out!

4 How is disability described and measured? Is it through a deficit-based model, strengths-based/social model, or integrated model (which recognizes that while some disabilities have inherent impairment, much of what is disabling is society's attitude toward disabilities)? Is there a possibility the questions asked about disability may exclude (or alienate) some disabled people? How does this study account for those with multiple disabilities? How does the sample of disabled people in your study compare to the demographics of disabled people in the United States?
5 Is the method described as being accessible to people with a variety of disabilities? Are online surveys screen-reader accessible? Are videos captioned?
6 Can you find what the specific disability community being served says about this particular practice? The Autistic community in particular is very vocal about some "evidence-based practices" that can actually be harmful to Autistic people, such as behavioral approaches that do not address the issues underlying behavior, take into account sensory experiences, or even recognize what autistic distress looks like in its research subjects.

This list is not exhaustive, and no list or book chapter can cover all the possible considerations for conducting and reviewing research that focuses on disabled people. The needs and priorities of the disability community may also change depending on the political climate, built infrastructure, disasters, and world events. The best way to continue to work in the interests of disabled people in research is to immerse oneself in disability culture, through reading books (*Disability Visibility* edited by Alice Wong (2020) and *Care Work* by Lakshmi Piepzna-Samarasinha (2018) are two good ones), following disability activists on social media (Sins Invalid is an excellent place to start), and connecting with your local disability community. Above all, listen to disabled clients, and don't presume to know their experiences. Listen to disabled activists and researchers about research priorities and listen to your own disabled clients about their treatment priorities and what modalities are and are not accessible to them. Remember that there are no truly non-disabled people, only people who have not been disabled yet, and by listening to and supporting the disabled community, you are supporting your own inclusion in the future.

Notes

1 **Authors' Note**: As a team of disabled researchers, sometimes we refer to disabled people as "them" and at other times as "us."
2 The exclusion of visual disability from research on diabetes is especially strange and will lead to an unrepresentative sample because blindness and changes to vision are one outcome and potential long-term condition from diabetes! Diabetic people are more likely to be blind, and more likely to be amputees. Excluding people with mobility and visual disabilities from diabetic research suggests that researchers are not adequately familiar with what they are studying. The same is true for autistic researchers who

are unfamiliar with the high incidences of postural orthostatic tachycardia syndrome (POTS), Ehlers-Danlos syndrome (EDS), mast cell activation syndrome (MCAS), and other conditions that often co-occur with autism.

References

Autistic Self-Advocacy Network. (2024). *What We Believe*. https://autisticadvocacy.org/about-asan/what-we-believe/

Baár, M. K. (2017). De-pathologizing Disability: Politics, Culture and Identity. *Neue Politische Literatur, 62*(2), 281–304. https://doi.org/10.3726/NPL2017-2_281

Botha, M., & Cage, C. (2022). "Autism Research Is in Crisis": A Mixed Method Study of Researcher's Constructions of Autistic People and Autism Research. *Frontiers in Psychology, 13*. https://doi.org/10.3389/fpsyg.2022.1050897

Cree, R. A., Okoro, C. A., Zack, M. M., & Carbone, E. (2020). *Frequent Mental Distress among Adults by Disability Status, Disability Type, and Selected Characteristics – United States 2018*. Morbidity and Mortality Weekly Report (MMWR).

Eickers, Gen (2023). Pathologizing Disabled and Trans Identities: How Emotions Become Marginalized. In Shelley Lynn Tremain (Ed.), *The Bloomsbury Guide to Philosophy of Disability* (pp. 360–379). Bloomsbury Academic.

Ellis, R., & Asbury, K. (2023). An Investigation of Autistic Opinions about Autism-related Genomic Research. https://doi.org/10.31234/osf.io/7x8cw

Feldman, M. A., Battin, S. M., Shaw, O. A., & Luckasson, R. (2013). Inclusion of Children with Disabilities in Mainstream Child Development Research. *Disability & Society, 28*(7), 997–1011. https://doi.org/10.1080/09687599.2012.748647

Ferguson, G. M., Fiese, B. H., Nelson, M. R., & Meeks Gardner, J. M. (2019). Transdisciplinary Team Science for Global Health: Case Study of the JUS Media? Programme. *The American Psychologist, 74*(6), 725–739. https://doi.org/10.1037/amp0000383

Haarlammert, M., Birman, D., Oberoi, A., & Moore, W. J. (2017). Inside-Out: Representational Ethics and Diverse Communities. *American Journal of Community Psychology, 60*(3–4), 414–423. https://doi.org/10.1002/ajcp.12188

Hearod, J. B., Wetherill, M. S., Salvatore, A. L., & Jernigan, V. B. B. (2019). Community-Based Participatory Intervention Research with American Indian Communities: What Is the State of the Science? *Current Developments in Nutrition, 3*(2), 39–52. https://doi.org/10.1093/cdn/nzz008

Herington, J., Li, K., & Pisani, A. R. (2024). Expanding the Role of Justice in Secondary Research Using Digital Psychological Data. *American Psychologist, 79*(1), 123–136. https://doi.org/10.1037/amp0001190

Hermans, A. (2023, January 3). *How Can Research Better Represent People with Disabilities?* Urban Institute. https://www.urban.org/urban-wire/how-can-research-better-represent-people-disabilities.

Hodges, H. R., Gillespie, S., Cherubini, F. D. S., Ibrahim, S. A., Gibson, H., Ali Daad, A. M., Davis, S. L., Abdi, S. M., Senesathith, V., Food Culture and Health Study Data Collection Team, & Ferguson, G. M. (2024). Ethical Applications of Digital Community-based Research with Black Immigrant and Refugee Youth and Families. *American Psychologist, 79*(1), 9–23. https://doi.org/10.1037/amp0001191.

Institute for Health & Disability Policy Studies. (2022). *NSHD Background and Overview.* Lawrence, KS: University of Kansas. Retrieved from https://ihdps.ku.edu/nshd-background-and-overview

Jackson, L., Haagaard, A., & Williams, R. (2022, April 19). *Disability Dongle*. Platypus: The CASTAC Blog. https://blog.castac.org/2022/04/disability-dongle/.

Kelley, A., Belcourt-Dittloff, A., Belcourt, C., & Belcourt, G. (2013). Research Ethics and INDIGENOUS COMMUNITIES. *American Journal of Public Health, 103*(12), 2146–2152. https://doi.org/10.2105/AJPH.2013.301522.

Kia-Keating, M., & Juang, L. P. (2022). Participatory Science as a Decolonizing Methodology: Leveraging Collective Knowledge from Partnerships with Refugee and Immigrant Communities. *Cultural Diversity and Ethnic Minority Psychology, 28*(3), 299–305. https://doi.org/10.1037/cdp0000514

Lakshmi Piepzna-Samarasinha, L. (2018). *Care Work: Dreaming Disability Justice.* Arsenal Pulp Press.

Landes, S. D., Hall, J. P., Swenor, B. K., & Vaitsiakhovich, N. (2025). *Comparative Performance of Disability Measures. PLOS ONE, 20*(1), Article e0318745 (*Public Library of Science*). https://doi.org/10.1371/journal.pone.0318745

Liebert, R. (2014). Pathologization. In T. Teo (Ed.). *Encyclopedia of Critical Psychology.* Springer. https://doi.org/10.1007/978-1-4614-5583-7_572

Macaulay, A. C. (2017). Participatory Research: What Is the History? Has the Purpose Changed? *Family Practice, 34*(3), 256–258. https://doi.org/10.1093/fampra/cmw117

Maruschack, L. M., Bronson, J., & Alper, M. (2021). *Medical Problems Reported by Prisoners: Survey of Prison Inmates, 2016.* (Report No. 252644). Bureau of Justice Statistics.

Mauldin, L. (2016). *Made to Hear: Cochlear Implants and Raising Deaf Children.* Minneapolis, MN: University of Minnesota Press.

McDonald, K. E., & Stack, E. (2016). You Say You Want a Revolution: An Empirical Study of Community-based Participatory Research with People with Developmental Disabilities. *Disability and Health Journal, 9*(2), 201–207.

McGrath, J. J., Lim, C. C. W., Plana-Ripoll, O., Holtz, Y., Agerbo, E., Momen, N. C., Mortensen, P. B., Pedersen, C. B., Abdulmalik, J., Aguilar-Gaxiola, S., Al-Hamzawi, A., Alonso, J., Bromet, E. J., Bruffaerts, R., Bunting, B., de Almeida, J. M. C., de Girolamo, G., De Vries, Y. A., Florescu, S., Gureje, O., … de Jonge, P. (2020). Comorbidity Within Mental Disorders: A Comprehensive Analysis Based on 145 990 Survey Respondents from 27 Countries. *Epidemiology and Psychiatric Sciences, 29*, e153. https://doi.org/10.1017/S2045796020000633

Meyers, A. R., & Andresen, E. M. (2000). Enabling Our Instruments: Accommodation, Universal Design, and Access to Participation in Research. *Archives of Physical Medicine and Rehabilitation, 81*(2), S5–S9. https://doi.org/10.1053/apmr.2000.20618

Miller, K., Mont, D., Maitland, A., Altman, B., & Madans, J. (2011). Results of a Cross-national Structured Cognitive Interviewing Protocol to Test Measures of Disability. *Quality and Quantity, 45*, 801–815.

National Commission for the Protection of Human Subjects of Biomedical & Behavioral Research. (1979). *The Belmont Report.* Department of Health, Education, and Welfare. https://www.hhs.gov/ohrp/regulations-and-policy/belmont-report/read-the-belmont-report/index.html

Nario-Redmond, M. R., Gospodinov, D., & Cobb, A. (2017). Crip for a Day: The Unintended Negative Consequences of Disability Simulations. *Rehabilitation Psychology, 62*(2), 190–203. https://doi.org/10.1037/rep0000127

Ozer, E. J. (2017). Youth-Led Participatory Action Research: Overview and Potential for Enhancing Adolescent Development. *Child Development Perspectives, 11*, 173–177. https://doi.org/10.1111/cdep.12228

Patterson, J. E., Miller, R. B., Carnes, S., & Wilson, S. (2004). Evidence-based practice for marriage and family therapists. *Journal of Marital and Family Therapy, 30*(2), 183–195. https://doi.org/10.1111/j.1752-0606.2004.tb01233.x

Plosky, D. W., Ne'eman, A., Silverman, B. C., Strauss, D. H., Francis, L. P., & Bierer, B. E. (2022). Excluding People with Disabilities from Clinical Research: Eligibility

Criteria Lack Clarity and Justification. *Health Affairs, 41*(10), 1423–1432. https://doi.org/10.1377/hlthaff.2022.00520

Popkin, S. J., Hermans, A. D., Oneto, A. D., Farrell, L., Connery, M., & Cannington, A. (2022, October). *People with Disabilities Living in the US Face Urgent Barriers to Housing* (Fact sheet). Washington, DC: Urban Institute & The Kelsey. Retrieved from https://www.urban.org/sites/default/files/2022-10/People%20with%20Disabilities%20Living%20in%20the%20US%20Face%20Urgent%20Barriers%20to%20Housing.pdf

Price, M., Salzer, M. S., O'Shea, A., & Kerschbaum, S. L. (2017). Disclosure of Mental Disability by College and University Faculty: The Negotiation of Accommodations, Supports, and Barriers. *Disabilities Studies Quarterly, 37*(2), 1–16. https://doi.org/10.18061/dsq.v37i2.5487

Rios, D., Magasi, S., Novak, C., & Harniss, M. (2016). Conducting Accessible Research: Including People with Disabilities in Public Health, Epidemiological, and Outcomes Studies. *American Journal of Public Health, 106*(12), 2137–2144. https://doi.org/10.2105/AJPH.2016.303448

Shew, A. (2022). How to Get a Story Wrong: Technoableism, Simulation, and Cyborg Resistance. *Including Disability, 1*(1), 13–36. https://doi.org/10.51357/id.vi1.169

Shew, A. (2023). Against Technoableism: *Rethinking Who Needs Improvement.* New York, NY: W. W. Norton & Company.

Silverman, A. M., Gwinn, J. D., & Van Boven, L. (2015). Stumbling in their Shoes: Disability Simulations Reduce Judged Capabilities of Disabled People. *Social Psychological and Personality Science, 6*, 464–471. https://doi.org/10.1177/1948550614559650

Silverman, A. M., Pitonyak, J. S., Nelson, I. K., Matsuda, P. N., Kartin, D., & Molton, I. R. (2017). Instilling Positive Beliefs about Disabilities: Pilot Testing a Novel Experiential Learning Activity for Rehabilitation Students. *Disability and Rehabilitation, 40*(9), 1108–1113. https://doi.org/10.1080/09638288.2017.1292321

Singh, A. N., Matson, J. L., Cooper, C. L., Dixon, D., & Sturmey, P. (2005). The Use of Risperidone among Individuals with Mental Retardation: Clinically Supported or Not? *Research in Developmental Disabilities*, *26*(3), 203–218. https://doi.org/10.1016/j.ridd.2004.07.001

Sins Invalid. (2015, September 17). *10 Principles of Disability Justice.* Sins Invalid. https://www.sinsinvalid.org/blog/10-principles-of-disability-justice

Skorburg, J. A., O'Doherty, K., & Friesen, P. (2024). Persons or Data Points? Ethics, Artificial Intelligence, and the Participatory Turn in Mental Health Research. *American Psychologist, 79*(1), 137–149. https://doi.org/10.1037/amp0001168

Sparrow, M. (2023, September 26). "We autistic people need researchers to develop better criteria for success than our symptoms…" *Autistic Screen Time: Swipe Left on Stigma.* Petrie-Flom Center. https://petrieflom.law.harvard.edu/2023/09/26/autistic-screen-time-swipe-left-on-stigma/

United States Census Bureau. (2017). *American Community Survey Information Guide.* https://www.census.gov/content/dam/Census/programs-surveys/acs/about/ACS_Information_Guide.pdf

Van De Vijver, F. J. (2009). Types of Comparative Studies in Cross-Cultural Psychology. *Online Readings in Psychology and Culture*, *2*(2). https://doi.org/10.9707/2307-0919.1017

Van Spall, H. G. C., Toren, A., Kiss, A., & Fowler, R. A. (2007). Eligibility Criteria of Randomized Controlled Trials Published in High-impact General Medical Journals: A Systematic Sampling Review. *JAMA, 2297*(11), 1233–1240. https://doi.org/10.1001/jama.297.11.1233

Vaughn, L. M., & Jacquez, F. (2020). Participatory Research Methods – Choice Points in the Research Process. *Journal of Participatory Research Methods, 1*(1), 1–13. https://doi.org/10.35844/001c.13244

Virdi, J. (2020). *Hearing Happiness: Deafness Cures in History*. Chicago, IL: University of Chicago Press.

Wandersman, A. (2003). Community Science: Bridging the Gap Between Science and Practice with Community-Centered Models. *American Journal of Community Psychology, 31*, 227–242. https://doi.org/10.1023/A:1023954503247

Williams, R. M. (2019). Metaeugenics and Metaresistance: From Manufacturing the 'Includeable Body' to Walking Away from the Broom Closet. *The Canadian Journal of Children's Rights Revue Canadienne Des Droits Des Enfants, 6*(1), 60–77. https://doi.org/10.22215/cjcr.v6i1.1976

Williams, R. M. (2021). I, Misfit: Empty Fortresses, Social Robots, and Peculiar Relations in Autism Research. *Techné, 25*(2), 451–478. https://doi.org/10.5840/techne20211019147

Williams, A. S., & Moore, S. M. (2011). Universal Design of Research: Inclusion of Persons with Disabilities in Mainstream Biomedical Studies. *Science Translational Medicine, 3*, 82. https://doi.org/10.1126/scitranslmed.3002133

Wong, A. (Ed.). (2020). *Disability Visibility: First-person Stories from the Twenty-first Century.* Vintage Books.

Ymous, A., Spiel, K., Keyes, O., Williams, R. M., Good, J., Hornecker, E., & Bennett, C. L. (2019). "I am just terrified of my future" - Epistemic Violence in Disability Related Technology Research. In *Extended Abstracts of the 2020 CHI Conference on Human Factors in Computing Systems (CHI EA '20)*. Association for Computing Machinery, New York, 1–16. https://doi.org/10.1145/3334480.3381828

Bibliography

Washington Group on Disability Statistics (2020). *An Introduction to the Washington Group on Disability Statistics Question Sets*. https://www.washingtongroup-disability.com/fileadmin/uploads/wg/Documents/Primer.pdf

17

CLINICAL SUPERVISION OF DISABILITY-SPECIFIC CASES

Shakeela Gray, Brittany A. Williams, and Briana Gaines

Introduction

Clinical supervision is a critical component of counselor development (Barnett & Molzon, 2014) and is one of the primary methods for training new clinicians (Cummings et al., 2015). Supervision provides a structured framework to enhance clinical skills, ensure ethical practice, and promote professional growth (Corey et al., 2021). It supports counselors-in-training in developing their clinical and professional skills in meaningful ways (Corey et al., 2021; Bernard & Goodyear, 2018; Bernard, 1979). Supervision becomes even more nuanced when working with disability-specific cases, especially since most clinicians are not trained in working with disabled people (Olkin, 2017). To effectively supervise disability-specific cases, counselors must navigate complex client needs, advocate for social justice, and address stigmas surrounding disability.

Despite the advancements within the counseling field regarding multiculturalism, there remains a deficit of comprehensive resources dedicated to clinical supervision of disability-specific cases. There is a significant lack of research within the counseling field, and the available research is mostly from the discipline of Rehabilitation Psychology (Olkin, 2017). Since there is limited attention to disability overall within counselor education and clinical training, it is not surprising that supervisors are unprepared to address the unique needs of supervisees who work with disabled clients.

This chapter will aim to bridge that gap by offering guidance on how supervisors can support supervisees with disability-specific cases holistically. It explores supervision models, techniques, methods of supervision, therapist considerations, challenges, and resources relevant to disability-specific cases. The primary objectives of this chapter are to: (1) identify the gaps in knowledge and skills

DOI: 10.4324/9781003362586-26

that supervisors and supervisees encounter when working with disability-specific cases; (2) understand the importance of integrating social justice principles into the supervisory relationship as they relate to disability-specific cases; and (3) apply appropriate supervision models and techniques to work effectively with these cases. By meeting these objectives, this chapter encourages therapists to enhance their supervision practices in the context of disability-specific cases, ultimately improving outcomes for both supervisees and their clients.

The target reader of this chapter includes graduate students, trainees, and supervising professionals in counseling and related fields who are seeking to improve their competence and skills in supervising disability-specific cases. Regardless of their level of clinical experience, readers will find valuable insights and tools to enhance their supervision skills, address clinical challenges, manage ethical issues, and contribute to inclusive counseling practices for disabled individuals. Through this chapter, readers will better understand the unique supervisory dynamics involved in working with disability-specific cases, along with practical methods for fostering growth and development for supervisees within clinical supervision. The authors aim to contribute to creating a more inclusive and effective counseling profession, where disabled individuals receive high-quality care, supported by competent clinical supervision.

Models of Supervision

Corey et al. (2021) define clinical supervision as "a process whereby consistent observation and evaluation of the counseling process is provided by a trained and experienced professional who is competent in the unique body of knowledge and skills required for professional development" (p. 3). According to the Council for Accreditation of Counseling and Related Educational Programs (CACREP), clinical supervision is a required component of counselor training during practicum and internship experiences (CACREP, 2024). Although all graduate counseling students participate in supervision (Corey et al., 2021), the methods and approaches supervisors employ can vary significantly. Regardless of the chosen supervision model, personalizing the process to meet the developmental needs of each counselor-in-training or supervisee is essential for effective supervision (Barnett & Molzon, 2014).

Theoretical models of supervision offer structured frameworks to help supervisors organize, evaluate, and guide the developmental process of supervisees (Rubel & Okech, 2006). These models define the nature of supervision and explain how supervisees' learning and professional identity evolve over time (Corey et al., 2021). Numerous models exist (Crunk & Barden, 2017; Walsh et al., 2017), typically classified into four categories: developmental models, psychotherapy-based models, process models, and second-generation models (Corey et al., 2021). However, current research offers little empirical support for the superiority of any single model (Crunk & Barden, 2017). In practice, many supervisors draw from multiple approaches. This chapter highlights two models particularly relevant to disability-specific supervision: Bernard's Discrimination Model (DM) and the Person-of-the-Therapist Training (POTT) Model.

Bernard's Discrimination Model

A developmental supervision model recognizes that supervision is an evolving process of growth and refinement (Bernard, 1979; Bernard & Goodyear, 2018; Corey et al., 2021).

The DM, developed by Janine Bernard, is one such model and is considered one of the most accessible approaches to clinical supervision (Bernard & Goodyear, 2018; Crunk & Barden, 2017). It is empirically supported and adaptable in complexity (Crunk & Barden, 2017), making it suitable for a wide range of clinical issues that may arise in supervision.

In her seminal work, "Supervisor Training: A Discrimination Model" (1979), Bernard emphasized the importance of including supervision skills in counseling literature to better support supervisors guiding counselors-in-training. The development of the DM aimed to systematically align supervision practices with the evolving needs of supervisees. Addressing this gap resulted in what is arguably one of the most influential models of clinical supervision. The DM is grounded in its central aim of developing competent counselors (Bernard, 1979). It is called the DM because the supervisor's approach is not one-size-fits-all; rather, it is shaped by the specific developmental needs of each supervisee (Corey et al., 2021).

The model revolves around the supervisor taking on one of three roles: teacher, counselor, or consultant (Bernard, 1979; Corey et al., 2021; Tümlü, 2022). Within these roles, the supervisor may focus on three key processes: intervention (formerly known as process), conceptualization, and personalization (Bernard, 1979; Bernard, 2018). This structured yet flexible approach allows the supervisor to meet supervisees where they are developmentally. To determine the most appropriate supervisory role for a given case, the supervisor must assess the supervisee's skill set (Bernard, 2018) and developmental level (Corey et al., 2021). This ensures a personalized supervisory approach aligned with the supervisee's learning needs. The model's flexibility – its ability to shift fluidly between teacher, counselor, and consultant roles – makes it particularly effective for supervision in disability-specific cases, enabling supervisors to tailor their methods to both the supervisee and their client population.

The Teacher

The supervisor assumes the role of the "teacher" when the supervisee needs more information, instruction, modeling, or feedback (Bernard, 2018; Tümlü, 2022). For example, a supervisee working with a client with autism spectrum disorder (ASD) might want to implement social skills training but may lack clinical experience with this population. In this scenario, the supervisor adopts the teacher's role and guides the supervisee in techniques to develop social skills, such as role-playing or using visual aids to support client engagement.

Similarly, if a supervisee struggles to understand how a client's physical disability shapes their self-concept and interpersonal relationships, the supervisor can provide guidance to enhance the supervisee's conceptualization of how the impairment affects the client's lived experiences. In such cases, the supervisor may observe a live session or review a session recording to help the supervisee identify patterns or themes related to the client's experiences of stigmatization or challenges with self-concept. Lastly, if a supervisee finds it difficult to discuss how a client's disability influences their career goals, the supervisor takes on the teacher role by helping the supervisee examine their own biases and discomfort, while also offering strategies to effectively address disability-related challenges in the workplace and advocate for the client.

The Counselor

When the supervisor takes on the role of a "counselor," they help the supervisee enhance self-reflectivity (Bernard & Goodyear, 2018). Examining this role from the personalization perspective, the supervisor may engage in the counselor role if they notice the supervisee is struggling with countertransference. For instance, if a counselor is in a session with a client who uses a wheelchair, the supervisee may feel excessive sympathy for the client, which, in turn, can impact the therapeutic process. The supervisor would benefit from taking a personalized approach to explore this challenge in a safe and supportive supervisory context.

Additionally, if the supervisee has difficulty conceptualizing a client's problems – such as understanding the impacts of lupus on a client's daily functioning and personal relationships – the supervisor can provide support to enhance their clinical reasoning. Lastly, if the supervisee struggles to process emotional reactions from a session with a client with a developmental disability, the supervisor might encourage them to reflect on their feelings, biases, and beliefs. This reflective process can deepen the supervisee's self-awareness.

Of course, within the counselor role, clear communication of professional boundaries is essential for effective supervision. Though the role is labeled "counselor," supervisors are not engaging in therapeutic work with their supervisees. This distinction must be explicitly stated at the outset of supervision, and referrals should be made when appropriate to ensure supervisees receive appropriate support beyond the scope of supervision.

The Consultant

As the "consultant," Bernard and Goodyear (2018) explain that the supervisor adopts more of a collegial role. For example, the supervisor would act as a consultant when the supervisee expresses interest in using mindfulness techniques to support a client with chronic pain from fibromyalgia. In this role, the supervisor provides feedback based on their expertise and may offer additional resources for mindfulness practices tailored to clients with chronic pain.

Another scenario where the supervisor acts as a consultant is when the supervisee explores strategies to support a client with Down syndrome who has challenges with verbal communication. The supervisor would then discuss various communication techniques and aids, such as augmentative and alternative communication systems, and how to integrate them into therapy sessions.

Lastly, if a supervisee shares discomfort in working with a client with a visual impairment, the consultant role allows the supervisor to engage in a personalized discussion around these developmental concerns and offer guidance on effectively navigating the challenge while supporting the client.

By assessing the supervisee's abilities and functioning level, supervisors can tailor their approach using the roles of teacher, counselor, and/or consultant (Bernard, 1979). Each role provides a unique opportunity to strengthen the supervisee's intervention, conceptualization, and personalization skills when working with disability-specific cases.

Person of the Therapist

The POTT Model, developed by Harry Aponte, posits that therapists can benefit from actively utilizing their personal struggles, wounds, and life experiences in their therapeutic work, rather than attempting to maintain complete neutrality. This model emphasizes the integration of the therapist's personal self into their professional work (Aponte & Kissil, 2016). In disability-specific supervision, this framework becomes particularly relevant as it creates space for personal-professional integration and positions signature themes as potential therapeutic tools rather than limitations. Supervisees are encouraged to explore how their own experiences with disability-whether personal or through family or friends-influence their clinical work (Reeve, 2014). They are also encouraged to identify recurring patterns in their responses to disabled clients. According to Aponte and Kissil (2016), this model validates the importance of lived experiences while maintaining professional boundaries.

Strength and Limitations

The POTT Model represents a profound paradigm shift in understanding clinical supervision, particularly within the complex landscape of disability-informed practice. The strengths of this model lie in its ability to enhance the authenticity of the therapeutic process, deepen understanding, and build confidence in professional development. The core of this model lies in challenging the traditional notion of professional detachment, instead recognizing personal experience as a powerful clinical instrument that can be carefully and intentionally leveraged to enhance therapeutic effectiveness.

Authenticity emerges as the fundamental strength of this approach. In disability-specific contexts, where lived experience carries unique depth and nuance, therapists are no longer required to maintain an artificial separation between their personal and professional selves. Instead, they are invited to view their own disability-related experiences as a rich, complex source of clinical wisdom (Aponte & Kissil, 2016). This approach validates the intricate ways personal understanding can inform professional practice, transforming what might have been seen as potential bias into a sophisticated form of empathetic attunement.

Traditional supervision models might encourage suppressing or compartmentalizing personal experiences. In contrast, POTT emphasizes the therapist's personal integration of disability-related experiences, which often carry complex emotional landscapes-stories of adaptation, resilience, medical navigation, and identity reconstruction-as a powerful mechanism for professional development. This model provides a structured, supportive framework for exploring how these personal narratives can be carefully and ethically woven into clinical understanding (Aponte & Kissil, 2016). As a straightforward example, a supervisor may help a therapist with a hearing impairment explore how their experience of communication challenges informs their work with hearing-impaired clients. The goal is not to project personal experience onto the client, but to develop a deeper, more nuanced understanding of potential therapeutic dynamics.

POTT also addresses a critical gap in traditional supervision approaches: the emotional and psychological impact of disability on professional identity. Many disabled therapists have historically been encouraged to minimize or hide their personal experiences, creating unnecessary psychological fragmentation. The POTT Model offers a healing alternative, creating institutional and professional space for disabled therapists to integrate their full, complex selves into their clinical work (Aponte & Kissil, 2016). By encouraging disabled therapists to explore their own disability narratives, the model inherently promotes a more sophisticated, nuanced understanding of disability. It moves beyond medical or deficit-based models, instead embracing disability as a complex intersection of personal, social, and systemic experiences.

Ultimately, the POTT Model's greatest strength lies in its radical reimagining of the meaning of professional expertise. It suggests that the most powerful clinical tools are not found in detached objectivity, but in the careful, intentional integration of personal experience. Professional confidence subsequently emerges as another significant strength of this model. By transforming potential vulnerability into professional strength, it encourages disabled therapists to see their personal experiences as professional assets rather than potential limitations. The supervisory relationship becomes a critical site of this transformation. Skilled supervisors using the POTT Model create a safe environment where therapists can explore the intricate connections between personal experience and professional practice. For therapists working in disability-informed practice, this means embracing a more holistic, authentic approach to professional development.

Despite its transformational potential, the POTT Model is not without significant challenges, particularly when applied to disability-specific supervision. The limitations emerge from the complex intersections of personal experience, professional boundary challenges, and supervision complexity due to the inherent vulnerabilities of both disabled therapists and clients navigating disability-related experiences. Additional examples to further concretize these model gaps are provided in the following section. The invitation to integrate personal experience creates a delicate tightrope walk between meaningful self-disclosure and inappropriate professional intimacy. This boundary management represents the most persistent challenge in implementing the POTT Model. Disabled therapists may find themselves susceptible to over-identification, unconsciously projecting their own disability narratives onto clients' experiences. This risk is amplified in contexts where shared lived experiences can create powerful, potentially destabilizing emotional resonances (Aponte & Kissil, 2016).

Supervision becomes exponentially more complex when personal experiences are brought to the forefront, and supervisors lack the nuanced skills required to navigate the intricate terrain of disability-related personal narratives. Many traditional supervision models don't possess the sophisticated framework needed to help disabled therapists process their personal experiences without allowing those experiences to become overwhelming or inappropriately centralized in the therapeutic work. The result can be a supervision process that inadvertently becomes more therapeutic than educational, blurring critical professional boundaries.

The model's approach reveals significant gaps in addressing the intersectionality of disability experiences (Aponte & Kissil, 2016). Similar to many cultural identities, disability is never a monolithic experience, and therapists may find themselves struggling to recognize the unique nuances of clients' experiences that differ from their own. For instance, a therapist with a congenital disability may find it challenging to fully comprehend the emotional landscape of someone acquiring a disability later in life. While well-intentioned, the POTT Model can potentially create limited awareness that reinforces rather than challenges narrow understandings of the disability experience. The emotional labor required to enact the POTT Model cannot be understated. Disabled therapists are asked to repeatedly revisit potentially traumatic personal experiences, transforming them into clinical insights. This process demands extraordinary emotional resilience and can lead to significant compassion fatigue or burnout if not carefully managed.

Societal dimensions and systemic aspects of disability often receive insufficient attention within the POTT framework (Reeves, 2014). Personal experience, while powerful, can sometimes lead to an overly individualized understanding of disability, creating a biased approach to treatment. This approach runs the risk of over-pathologizing disability as a personal challenge instead of recognizing it as a complex social construct. Training becomes a critical challenge in implementing the POTT Model effectively, specifically related to disability. Supervisors need extensive training in disability studies, intersectionality, and advanced relational skills to guide therapists through complex terrain. Most clinical training programs currently remain ill-equipped to teach the advanced skills requisite for integrating personal experiences into professional practice.

These limitations don't negate the model's potential; instead, they call for a more nuanced, critically reflexive approach to its implementation. It necessitates a commitment to ongoing critical reflection, robust supervision frameworks, and a willingness to continually challenge our understanding of personal experiences in professional contexts (Reeves, 2014). The future of the POTT Model lies not in avoiding these limitations but in developing increasingly mature ways to navigate them. This is an approach that is simultaneously deeply personal and rigorously professional, which demands a delicate balance that challenges traditional notions of therapeutic expertise and opens new possibilities for genuine, transformative clinical practice.

In summary, the POTT Model offers a valuable framework for disability-specific supervision, particularly in its validation of personal experience as a therapeutic tool. Yet, successful implementation requires careful attention to boundaries, thorough supervisor training, and ongoing evaluation of its effectiveness. Future development of this model could include more specific guidance for disability-related situations and consideration of intersectional identities.

Techniques and Methods of Supervision

Supervision in counseling involves various techniques and methods administered by the supervisor to help develop the supervisee's skills and competencies. Just as a counselor may incorporate techniques from different theoretical orientations that are not their primary framework but suit a particular situation, clinical supervisors can also draw from multiple supervision models (Barnett & Molzon, 2014). This flexibility enables supervisors to tailor their approach to best support the needs of their supervisees. While various supervision techniques and methods exist, the following interventions are particularly useful when working with both novice and experienced supervisees on disability-specific cases.

Case Consultation

The case consultation method involves discussing the supervisee's cases and is the most frequently used supervision strategy (Corey et al., 2021). In the case of a supervisee working with a client who has a speech impediment, the supervisor would conduct a detailed review of the case. This process would include examining the clinical diagnosis, the purpose of counseling, therapeutic goals, interventions, challenges, and overall progress. During the review, the supervisor might also address the speech impediment directly, guiding the supervisee on how to navigate situations where understanding the client's speech may be difficult. Through case consultation, the supervisor can gain insight into how the supervisee navigates communication with the client. This includes acknowledging and addressing any challenges that may arise in understanding a client with a speech impediment, rather than overlooking or avoiding them. This is important because if there are barriers, they can be addressed and corrected-not neglected-to ensure that the client's welfare is prioritized through a clear understanding of their concerns. A limitation of case consultation is that its effectiveness depends on the supervisee's accurate self-report, and the retelling of the case during supervision may not always be precise (Corey et al., 2021).

Self-Reflection

Self-reflection is an intellectual and affective process through which a supervisee examines their experiences and thoughts to evaluate their clinical understanding and practice. It can also be described as a neutral, non-judgmental focus on the condition of the supervisee's emotions (Prasko et al., 2021). For instance, this technique can be implemented for a novice supervisee who does not have experience working with a client who has a mobility impairment. During supervision, the supervisor can instruct the supervisee to reflect on emotional responses, thoughts, and interactions during the counseling session. The supervisee may think about any conscious or unconscious biases they might have had about the client's abilities and limitations. They may reflect on their ability to continue with sessions or whether they felt unequipped due to a lack of experience working with someone with a mobility impairment. The supervisee's self-reflective insights serve as a learning tool to help them grow in their clinical skills with the supervisor's support while navigating unfamiliar territory.

Cognitive Restructuring

Cognitive restructuring is a therapeutic technique derived from Cognitive Behavioral Therapy (Beck, 1979). Ezawa and Hollon (2023) explain that cognitive restructuring is a collection of therapeutic techniques used to identify, evaluate, and correct inaccurate beliefs and underlying schemas. It is instantiated through a thought record, correcting negative thoughts and considering alternative positive narratives. This technique can be applied to a supervisee working with an adult client who is blind and wants to move out of their parent's home to live independently. In supervision, the supervisee expresses concerns that the client may not have the capability to live independently due to the risks associated with the client's visual impairment. Using cognitive restructuring, the supervisor would help the supervisee assess these assumptions by identifying and evaluating their concerns and supporting them in challenging limiting beliefs and negative thoughts. The supervisor may then guide the supervisee toward developing a more inclusive, strengths-based view of the client's independence and support the supervisee in helping the client work toward that goal.

Homework

Homework involves assigning the supervisee a task that contributes to their professional development and clinical skill-building. It can be a collaborative process, and the supervisee comes to supervision prepared to review the assignment (Corey et al., 2021; Bernard & Goodyear, 2018). For instance, if the supervisee wants to learn more about the barriers and microaggressions that disabled clients experience, homework could include reading articles or watching videos that depict the firsthand experiences of disabled individuals. In the following supervision session, there would be a discussion of what was learned and how it can inform the supervisee's understanding and practice with disabled clients.

Role Play

Role play is an enactment of what can or has occurred in a session between the therapist and client. It can be an effective technique that allows the supervisee to practice a new clinical skill or refine existing ones. It enables the supervisor to observe the supervisee's abilities in session and provide feedback (Prasko, 2023; Corey et al., 2021).

In summary, implementing a variety of techniques and interventions in supervision provides supervisees with opportunities to refine their skills while receiving meaningful support. As previously noted, several techniques used in clinical supervision have not been covered in this chapter. Due to the limited research available on working with disabled clients in a counseling setting, existing methods, techniques, and interventions must be critically adapted and thoughtfully applied. This approach supports supervisees handling disability-specific cases and helps them navigate the complexities of counseling this population while continually working to enhance their development as inclusive clinicians.

Additional Clinical Supervision Considerations

Therapy involves interacting with clients and supervisees with diverse identities, including race, ethnicity, gender, nationality, sexuality, abilities, language, and religion, among other factors. Given these differences, therapists bring their lived experiences, beliefs, and values into relationships. These varying perspectives may include stereotypes, biases, and assumptions, which can impact how people interact. Therapists must cultivate self-awareness to ensure their engagement with clients is respectful and non-judgmental. Without such awareness, there is an increased likelihood that microaggressions, biases, and assumptions may negatively affect relationships.

While the ACA Code of Ethics (2014) outlines principles related to multiculturalism, equitable practice, and client welfare, not all counselors immediately possess the level of competence needed to integrate these principles into their practice. Therefore, the incorporation of social justice principles must be intentional. This holds true for the clinical supervision process as well, especially when working with a minoritized identity such as disability. The section below will explore how supervisors can support supervisees in identifying and addressing their biases when working with disabled clients, to prevent perpetuating stigma and ensure equitable practice.

Every day, disabled people are subjected to prejudice, discrimination, stigma, and microaggressions (Olkin, 2017). The supervisee must self-reflect and explore how their experiences, beliefs, and exposure to disability may influence their engagement and clinical approach-and ensure they do not perpetuate the stigma faced by disabled clients. A supervisee who is able-bodied and has limited experience working with disabled clients may bring their biases and assumptions into sessions, potentially jeopardizing the therapeutic relationship. For example, an able-bodied therapist might unintentionally assume that a client with a mobility impairment cannot live independently. This bias may stem from the supervisee's limited knowledge of accessibility accommodations or lack of exposure to people with mobility impairments who live independently.

During supervision, the supervisor may facilitate strategies of self-reflection and guide supervisees to explore personal experiences that have contributed to bias. For example, a supervisee working with an adult client with Down syndrome who expresses a desire to have sex with her boyfriend might raise concerns in supervision about the client's cognitive ability to make such a decision. In this instance, the supervisee may believe the client should not be engaging in sexual activity, which could be stigmatizing. This assumption – that the client, due to her disability, is incapable of making autonomous, adult decisions about intimacy – highlights the importance of addressing biases in supervision to ensure ethical practice.

Issues in Supervision

As previously noted, clinical supervision is an essential part of supervisees' skill-building and professional development. While the supervision process must be flexible and fluid, it does not come without challenges. Issues in clinical supervision vary depending on several factors, including ethical concerns, legal considerations, power dynamics, and issues related to multiculturalism.

Ethical issues are often tied to balancing the rights of clients, the rights and responsibilities of supervisees, and the responsibilities of the supervisor (Corey et al., 2021). Legal challenges pertain to state and federal regulations, as well as ethical violations that may escalate into legal matters (Bernard & Goodyear, 2018). Power dynamics are a concern in supervision because the process involves persons with deeply marginalized and oppressed identities, which can make establishing a collaborative, non-hierarchical relationship difficult (De Stefano et al., 2017). Multiculturalism can also present challenges in supervision, as both the supervisor and the supervisee must demonstrate cultural competence. According to the ACA

Code of Ethics (2014), standard F.2.d., "counseling supervisors are aware of and address the role of multiculturalism/diversity in the supervisory relationship."

Ethical Issues

Disability-specific ethical and legal issues add to the existing complexities within counseling. Clinical supervisors must work intentionally with their supervisees to understand legal obligations and ethics through a disability lens.

Informed Consent

The informed consent process and format may demand adaptation and flexibility when working with disabled clients, such as those with cognitive or communication impairments. This may also include obtaining consent from a legal guardian, where applicable. Some related codes of ethics of the counseling profession are detailed below.

ACA CODE OF ETHICS (2014)

A.2.a. Informed Consent: Clients have the freedom to choose whether to enter into or remain in a counseling relationship and need adequate information about the counseling process and the counselor. Counselors have an obligation to review in writing and verbally with clients, the rights and responsibilities of both counselors and clients. Informed consent is an ongoing part of the counseling process, and counselors appropriately document discussions of informed consent throughout the counseling relationship.

A.2.d. Inability to Give Consent: When counseling minors, incapacitated adults, or other persons who are unable to give voluntary consent, counselors still seek the assent of clients to services and include them in decision-making as appropriate. Counselors recognize the need to balance the ethical rights of clients to make choices, their capacity to give consent or assent to receive services, and parental or familial legal rights and responsibilities to protect these clients and make decisions on their behalf.

F.1.c. Informed Consent and Client Rights: Supervisors make supervisees aware of client rights, including the protection of client privacy and confidentiality in the counseling relationship. Supervisees provide clients with professional disclosure information and inform them of how the supervision process influences the limits of confidentiality. Supervisees make clients aware of who will have access to records of the counseling relationship and how these records will be stored, transmitted, or otherwise reviewed.

Confidentiality

Issues of confidentiality may arise with disability-specific cases. Disabled individuals often receive support from multiple organizations, as well as from family members and caregivers. A supervisee may need to coordinate with various sources while still maintaining confidentiality, including ensuring a release of information is on file where relevant.

ACA CODE OF ETHICS (2014)

B.1.a. Multicultural/Diversity Considerations: Counselors maintain awareness and sensitivity regarding cultural meanings of confidentiality and privacy.

B.1.c. Respect for Confidentiality: Counselors protect the confidential information of prospective and current clients.

Legal Obligations: Counselors cannot offer legal advice, but it is important to inform clients of their rights (Olkin, 2017). Counselors should be aware of two important laws: the Americans with Disabilities Act (ADA) and the Individuals with Disabilities Education Act (IDEA). In clinical supervision, a supervisor may need to provide support and guidance to supervisees in understanding these laws so that they can best support and advocate for their clients.

ACA CODE OF ETHICS (2014)

I.1.a. Knowledge: Counselors know and understand the ACA Code of Ethics and other applicable ethics codes from professional organizations or certification and licensure bodies of which they are members. Lack of knowledge or misunderstanding of an ethical responsibility is not a defense against a charge of unethical conduct.

Competence in Disability

Disability competence involves having foundational knowledge of disabilities and an awareness of the challenges that disabled individuals experience and the resources available in their communities. While there is no expectation for a supervisor or supervisee to know everything about all disabilities, both parties are expected to do their due diligence in increasing competence in areas such as understanding common disabilities, distinguishing between impairments, recognizing apparent vs. non-apparent disabilities, and using appropriate language such as person-first vs. identify-first preferences. If an uncharted area arises in supervision, it should be openly discussed and explored to ensure the client receives the best care possible

Resources and Tools for Supervision

To help guide supervisees in disability-specific cases, it is best practice for supervisors to have educational and community resources readily available. Disabled people often experience gaps or delays in support, such as long waitlists for federally or state-funded services, limited access to accommodations, reliance on others for assistance, or lack of a strong support system. Being prepared in advance with appropriate resources and tools supports the supervisee's development and ensures better clinical outcomes for the client.

Community Resources

1. Local non-profit organizations
2. Local county government programs and funds for disabled people

Federal/State-Funded Resources

1. Medical Assistance (income-based health insurance or eligibility-based disability programs)
2. Supplemental Security Income (SSI): Monthly income for individuals who meet the disability criteria
3. Social Security Disability Insurance (SSDI)
4. State-funded community integration programs supporting social inclusion, residential services, and employment for people with disabilities
5. ABLE Accounts (Achieving a Better Life Experience): Tax-advantaged savings accounts for individuals with disabilities, allowing them to save and invest for qualified disability expenses without jeopardizing eligibility for public benefits like Medicaid or SSI
6. Veterans Benefits: https://www.va.gov/disability/

References

American Counseling Association. (2014). *ACA code of ethics.* Retrieved from https://www.counseling.org/docs/default-source/ethics/2014-aca-code-of-ethics.pdf

Aponte, H. J., & Kissil, K. (2016). *The person of the therapist training model: Mastering the use of self.* Routledge. https://doi.org/10.4324/9781315676685

Barnett, J. E., & Molzon, C. H. (2014). Clinical supervision of psychotherapy: Essential ethics issues for Supervisors and supervisees. *Journal of Clinical Psychology, 70*(11), 1051–1061. https://doi.org/10.1002/jclp.22126

Beck, A. T. (1979). *Cognitive therapy and the emotional disorders.* Penguin.

Bernard, J. M. (1979). Supervisor training: A discrimination model. *Counselor Education and Supervision, 19*(1), 60–68. https://doi.org/10.1002/j.1556-6978.1979.tb00906.x

Bernard, J. M., & Goodyear, R. K. (2018). *Fundamentals of clinical supervision* (6th ed.). Pearson.

Council for Accreditation of Counseling and Related Educational Programs. (2024). *2024 CACREP Standards.* https://www.cacrep.org/wp-content/uploads/2024/04/2024-Standards-Combined-Version-4.11.2024.pdf

Corey, G., Haynes, R., Moulton, P., & Muratori, M. (2021). *Clinical supervision in the helping professions: A Practical Guide* (3rd ed.). American Counseling Association.

Crunk, A. E., & Barden, S. M. (2017). The common factors discrimination model: An integrated approach to counselor supervision. *The Professional Counselor, 7*(1), 62–75. https://doi.org/10.15241/aec.7.1.62

Cummings, J. A., Ballantyne, E. C., & Scallion, L. M. (2015). Essential processes for cognitive behavioral clinical supervision: Agenda setting, problem-solving, and formative feedback. *Behavior Therapy*, *46*(4), 510–520. https://doi.org/10.1016/j.beth.2015.05.004

De Stefano, J., Hutman, H., & Gazzola, N. (2017). Putting on the face: A qualitative study of power dynamics in clinical supervision. *The Clinical Supervisor*, *36*(2), 223–240. https://doi.org/10.1080/07325223.2017.1295893

Ezawa, I. D., & Hollon, S. D. (2023). Cognitive restructuring and psychotherapy outcome: A meta-analytic review. *Psychotherapy*, *60*(3), 396–406. https://doi.org/10.1037/pst0000474

Olkin, R. (2017). *Disability-affirmative therapy: A case formulation template for clients with disabilities*. Oxford University Press.

Prasko, J., Abeltina, M., Vanek, J., Dicevicius, D., Ociskova, M., Krone, I., Kantor, K., Burkauskas, J., Juskiene, A., Slepecky, M., & Bagdonaviciene, L. (2021). How to use self-reflection in cognitive behavioral supervision. *Activitas Nervosa Superior Rediviva, 63*, 68–83.

Prasko, J., Vanek, J., Ociskova, M., Krone, I., Slepecky, M., Abeltina, M., Burkauskas, J., Grambal, A., & Bagdonaviciene, L. (2023). Role-playing in cognitive behavioral supervision. *Neuroendocrinology Letters, 44*(2), 74–85. https://www.nel.edu/userfiles/articlesnew/1685917501_44_2_prasko_74-pdf.pdf

Reeve, D. (2014). Counselling and disabled people: Help or hindrance? In J. Swain, S. French, C. Barnes, & C. Thomas (Eds.), *Disabling barriers - enabling environments* (3rd ed., pp. 255–261). Sage Publications.

Rubel, D., & Okech, J. E. A. (2006). The supervision of group work model: Adapting the discrimination model for supervision of group workers. *The Journal for Specialists in Group Work, 31*(2), 113–134. https://doi.org/10.1080/01933920500493597

Tümlü, G. Ü. (2022). The effect of discrimination model-based group supervision on counseling self-efficacy and insights of novice supervisees. *International Journal of Psychology and Educational Studies*, *9*(4), 1270–1285. https://doi.org/10.52380/ijpes.2022.9.4.905

Walsh, R., Bambacus, E., & Gibson, D. (2017). An approach to supervision for doctoral and entry-level group counseling students. *The Journal for Specialists in Group Work*, *42*(4), 338–363. https://doi.org/10.1080/01933922.2017.1350231

Bibliography

Bernard, J. M., & Goodyear, R. K. (2014). *Fundamentals of clinical supervision* (5th ed.). Pearson Education.

Corey, G. (2023). *Theory and practice of counseling and psychotherapy*. Mindtap Course List.

Sahu, A., Bell, A.-S., Ridley, C. R., & Tran, V. (2024). Multicultural counseling skills evaluation form: A tool for clinical supervision. *The Counseling Psychologist*, *52*(6), 842–873. https://doi.org/10.1177/00110000241248099

Timm, M. (2015). Creating a preferred counselor identity in supervision: A new application of Bernard's discrimination model. *The Clinical Supervisor*, *34*(1), 115–125. https://doi.org/10.1186/1472-6963-14-99

Wilcox, M. M., Farra, A., Black, S. W., Pollard, E., Drinane, J. M., Tao, K. W., DeBlaere, C., Hook, J. N., Davis, D. E., Watkins, C. E., & Owen, J. (2024). Cultural humility and racial microaggressions in cross-racial clinical supervision: A moderated mediation model. *Journal of Counseling Psychology*, *71*(4), 304–314. https://doi.org/10.1037/cou0000732

18

DISABILITY JUSTICE AND THE PERSON-OF-THE-THERAPIST FRAMEWORK

James Tillett, Jody Russon, and Shalini Srinivasan

Introduction

Therapy offers opportunities for genuine person-to-person encounters-moments in which clients experience being deeply understood by another human being. For those who have been disabled by the social systems in which they live, these moments are especially vital. Indeed, many disabled clients have few spaces where they are not only accepted but actively celebrated for their uniqueness. In cultivating these experiences of being understood, therapists can offer disabled clients a new way of relating to themselves. Achieving this, however, requires the therapist to remain fully connected and responsive to the client's emotional world and worldview. Sustaining this kind of presence in therapeutic practice demands skill and intentionality and can be difficult to operationalize within traditional therapy training programs. Fortunately, the Person-of-the-Therapist Training (POTT; Aponte & Kissil, 2016) framework offers sequenced guidelines to support therapists in cultivating such presence. POTT aims to build therapists' capacity to selectively and purposefully use their personal selves to enhance therapeutic effectiveness, including in work with clients whose life experiences may differ significantly from their own.

Becoming a Wounded Healer: Recognizing Our Connections with Disablement

POTT is centered on helping therapists systematically find points of connection between themselves and their clients in order to foster authentic understanding and empathy. The POTT training framework draws on Nouwen's (1972) concept of the "wounded healer." In this role, therapists learn to recognize their personal

 DOI: 10.4324/9781003362586-27

vulnerabilities and how these are shaped by the interplay between internal discourses (e.g., self-talk and inner voice) and external discourses (e.g., dominant cultural narratives about disability). Once recognized, these vulnerabilities can be reframed as clinical assets and used intentionally in service of others. Therapists who engage this process are better able to recognize shared human experiences and, in turn, connect with the existential and emotional struggles of their clients. For therapists seeking to understand their disabled clients in ways that challenge the internalization of ableism, they must first examine the processes of disablement embedded within society-and how these external forces shape their own internal discourses. To begin this work, it is essential to critically reconceptualize the language therapists use to describe both their clients and the lived experiences of disablement.

Using "Disability" as a Verb

When using the word "disabled," most people strictly understand it either as an adjective or a noun. In other words, they might refer to "disabled people" as those they associate with being in wheelchairs, having formal accommodations in school and work environments, using braille, and so on. In this way, "disabled" merely serves as a description of an individual person or some aspect of their being (i.e., being Deaf, autistic). We are inviting therapists to shift toward understanding and using the word "disabled" as a verb (Union of the Physically Impaired Against Segregation & The Disability Alliance, 1976), reconceptualizing "disabled" as something one *experiences* rather than something one *is*, akin to theories of gender performativity (i.e., being a woman is something one is socialized and/or elects to *do* rather than something one *is*, per say; Butler, 1990). This shift is important for therapists, as wounded healers, because it moves us away from simply thinking of "the disabled" as people who experience neurobiological impairments (that many of their counterparts do not) toward understanding how external discourses about disability shape clients' experiences. The former line of thinking locates all the responsibility (and often blame) for a person's disable*ment* within their individual "bodymind," a term referring to the inseparable combination of their mind and body (Dychtwald, 1986). Instead, therapists can better connect with their clients through recognizing the *process* of disable*ment* as something enacted on specific bodyminds, which then become "dis*abled*." In other words, clients who experience certain neurobiological impairments are "dis*abled*" by social contexts which both passively neglect to facilitate their fuller participation within society and actively facilitate their disconnection from society (Wolf-Meyer, 2020). This way of thinking shifts the onus onto society to change its systemic practices of ableism, rather than problematizing disabled bodyminds and trying to "fix" them without attending to the core issue of their social oppression.

Whether we realize it or not, as therapists, our recognition of disablement as a process has world-changing consequences for our clients. For instance, from the traditional medical model perspective of disability (consistent with using the word "disabled" as a noun/adjective), clients in wheelchairs are expected to wait indefinitely for medical advances that "cure" their bodies of ambulation impairments (Oliver, 1990). Instead, from the social model perspective of disability (consistent with using the word "disabled" as a verb), clients in wheelchairs are ideally met with ramps, elevators, automatic doors, wheelchair-accessible public transport and bathrooms, and other infrastructure needed to facilitate their full participation in society *as they already are*. Not only is the social model more realistic about what is medically and scientifically possible (and affordable) at this sociocultural moment, but it does not demand a person's bodymind (e.g., how they move through the world, how they perceive and exist through specific experiences, and the unique wheelchair-using and disabled cultures they belong to) fundamentally change to enable their full participation in society. In other words, viewing our clients as dis*abled* by their societies, rather than simply sick and/or deficient, does more than hold societies responsible for changing their relationships to these individuals; it protects their ways of being from cultural and literal genocide via eugenics. Indeed, arguments about whether certain impairments should be "corrected" or not, amounts to deciding what lives are worth living versus which are not. It is not an accident that the fascist regime of Nazi Germany condemned disabled children as "life unworthy of life" before murdering them through what they called "euthanasia," often by administering them barbiturates to induce fatal pneumonia (Sheffer, 2018). As people, we often assume that ways of being which are pathologized by external discourses are not worthwhile or are lesser than in some capacity. As therapists, we must be very careful that we do not allow such assumptions to insidiously sneak into our work and harm our disabled and otherwise socially marginalized clients.

Finally, acknowledging the process of disablement enables therapists to meet the inevitable neurobiological diversity of clients, as opposed to (1) problematizing and pathologizing this inherent variety only in people deemed "abnormal," (2) setting an arbitrary standard of what is relatively "normal" via diagnosis and assessments, (3) coercing conformity to "normal" through medical "cures" and mental health "treatments," and (4) blaming these clients for being too difficult when such "treatments" fail, and even harm them (Walker, 2021). It is difficult to write this to an audience of therapists knowing that, in reading this, they must face the painful realization that most psychotherapies readily play into and even *constitute* these injustices; that eugenics has been woven into the very premise of our work as mental "health" professionals. We – along with medical professionals – are the ones who are given the power to decide who is too "disordered" to be fixed, who is too "sick" to be healed, and ultimately, who is unworthy of life in this world. Perhaps most dauntingly, in taking up the mantle of the "expert" role by deciding which clients are worth holding out hope for and worth supporting, our verdicts are lethal. Effectively shifting toward an anti-ableist (and disability-just) future means that our ways of thinking about disability must undergo an earth-shaking transformation. It is a harrowing journey to embark on, but – just as our disabled clients must fight to stay alive in a world that is actively hostile to their ways of being – we must learn to "stay with the trouble" of an inherently troubled world (Haraway, 2016). Our clients need us to stay with them through their troubles, rather than locating the trouble within them (and within our points of relation with them). Accordingly, using the word "disability" as a verb provides an avenue of empathy for therapists – who may or may not have explicit experiences of disablement themselves – to personally connect with the impact of being misunderstood, pathologized, or "othered" by the external processes discussed here. Constant engagement with this avenue allows for therapists to embrace their own vulnerabilities as wounded healers.

Both/And: Unraveling the Disabled vs. Non-Disabled Binaries

With new language to better understand experiences of disablement, we now offer another avenue to explore how external processes shape internal discourses for ourselves and our clients. This section focuses on helping therapists unravel their own ableist assumptions by inviting them to discover their *own* relationships to the process of disable*ment*. Exploring one's relationship to the social phenomenon of disability is a challenging process, as it asks us to discover ways in which we can make our thinking more complex. Specifically, we must reflect on the tendency to think in "binary opposition" (Saussure, 2005; Latour, 1993), which means "either/or" thinking rather than "both/and" thinking. In other words, we tend to think that things must be *either* one way *or* another, and that they cannot be *both at once*. Systemic therapists are taught to be mindful of binary thinking in our work with relational cases, because it derails our ability to exercise multidirected partiality (Boszormenyi-Nagy, 1966), and other techniques essential for attuning to multiple client perspectives within the same case.

On a societal scale, people are also taught to think about sociocultural identities in binaries. For instance, most people are raised with the understanding that they can only be (and must only be) *either* a boy *or* a girl, and eventually, *either* a man *or* a woman. Yet, even within the same social context, men vary widely in their definition of what "manhood" means to them, as do women of "womanhood," and there are expansive and non-binary ways of expressing gender in reference to its constant cultural evolutions (Stryker, 2017). Furthermore, a gender binary is argued based on a sex binary of male *or* female, which is also inaccurate to the full complexity of how human sex characteristics tend to vary within different people (e.g., there is a wide variety of hormone compositions spread across assigned female at birth people and assigned male at birth people, intersex people exist, and people may change their sex characteristics with hormones and procedures). In other words, everyone's way of doing "man" or "woman" (and "male" or "female") would look very different and overlap greatly with one another, no matter the degree to which one might identify with these labels and separate them mentally.

We are asking therapists to apply a similar paradigm shift to their understanding of disability as a lived experience. In this case, the imposed binary in question is understanding people as *either* disabled *or* non-disabled (a.k.a. able-bodied). Additionally, given that psychiatric and cognitive disabilities fall under the umbrella of disability (hence, the term "bodymind"), the binaries of *either* "mentally ill" *or* "healthy," and *either* neurotypical *or* neurodivergent, must be questioned as well. Indeed, in teaching an introduction to disability studies course at a university many times, I (James) have found that most students who came into the course identifying as non-disabled were surprised to learn that they technically met the criteria for being disabled; depression and anxiety are common disabled experiences. This is not to suggest that those who experience, say, low vision and full blindness are not uniquely disabled by a world that prioritizes the seeing. Nor is it to encourage those who are – for all intents and purposes – 'not blind' to unfairly equate their experiences with that of those who 'are blind,' dismissing their lived expertise. However, it is to question why we simply think of people as *either* blind (and low vision) *or* seeing, when many people use some type of glasses or contacts to support their seeing. Moreover, sight – like any other neurobiological possibility for human beings – represents a wide range of "abilities," such as exterior-world seeing, phantasia (visual seeing in the "mind's eye"), seeing certain colors, and seeing certain letters/numbers as more or less distinct when reading. How can we fully separate ourselves from the experience of neurobiological impairment when, given the countless neurobiological possibilities that exist, we are all surely impaired in some way or another? Again, this is not to draw false equivalences of marginalization across all embodied experiences of impairment and subsequent disablement, but it is to argue that we all *do* experience impairment, whether we recognize and identify with these aspects of our experience or not.

One might ask: Does this mean that we all experience disablement too? The short answer is that anyone *could be* disabled, in varying ways and degrees of salience, based on our own unique combination of experiences. For instance, it is not generally taboo nor socially marginalized to obtain and use a common glasses prescription in the United States (although some people are teased for theirs). Yet, up-to-date prescription glasses are an additional, expensive cost for those who need them, and can be inaccessible on that basis alone. In this way, *the cost of being impaired is put on the individual,* and some can afford the costs of enabling themselves while some cannot. In the case of the current example, if one does not get glasses for one's visual impairment, one *will be* disabled (i.e., receiving poor grades in school or poor performance evaluations at work for not being able to read easily/quickly). Furthermore, researchers estimate that approximately 2.5 billion people in the world cannot afford the eye care they need, which is primarily prescription glasses (Vision Impact Institute, 2012). However, some social environments may not require a person to use glasses to meet their daily needs (i.e., if they need reading glasses but do not have to read in their daily life). Thus, whether this type of visual impairment incurs the process of disablement depends on a person's context as well as their location and social mobility within it. Finally – and this is very important – even if an individual is not currently disabled in a salient way, they are much more likely to become disabled as they age and their bodymind acquires new impairments (Brault, 2008). Rather than thinking of being disabled as something we *either* "are" *or* "are not," it's more accurate to think of disablement as a phenomenon we all have varying experiences of, which are prone to changing over time.

In our work with psychiatrically disabled therapy clients, the dismantling of the disabled vs. non-disabled (mentally ill vs. healthy) binary is equally, if not more vital. In general, social scientists are prone to "chicken vs. egg" binaries when explaining psychiatric disability, most evident in classical debates about how much *nature* (i.e., genetics, inborn temperament) shapes individual bodyminds, versus *nurture* (i.e., how we were parented, our cultural milieu growing up). Contemporary professionals trained within the social sciences typically agree that *both* nature *and* nurture are important factors in shaping a person, but many do not honor just how inseparable these two concepts are in practice. Specifically, with increasing research and understandings of epigenetics (how DNA is shaped by environmental experiences, which then shapes genetic lineages) and socialization (how people are raised to think about their contexts and respond, which also deeply shapes what their "personalities" look like and reinforces which social contexts they tend to seek out), it is perplexing that nature and nurture continue to be treated as divisible phenomena at all. Moreover, the continued naming and separation of these two concepts has serious consequences for clients in a world that seeks to find *causes* – and thereby *cures* – of psychiatric "disorders." As Yergeau (2018) explains in their foundational work on neurological queerness (italics added for emphasis):

> Research on autistic people's so-called homosexual behaviors in sex-segregated institutional settings likewise interweaves the rhetorical, the gendered, and the sexual. Researchers routinely lock themselves into polar arguments around queer causation, reverting to the all-too-common innateness versus choice debate about what causes the Gay or the Trans. *The hidden premise, of course, is that possessing causal knowledge will provide mechanisms for eradicating both disability and queerness.* With regard to autism, the social/biology dichotomy often takes shape as follows: are institutionalized autistics behaving queerly because they lack biorhetorical concepts of gender and social propriety, or are they behaving queerly because they do not have access to opposite-sex partners? In other words, sexuality, gender identity, neurobiological development, and rhetoricity are interconnected constructs in clinical theory and practice, and their shared trajectory often takes form, rhetorically, as *quests for causes and cures*.
>
> (pp. 185–186)

Thus, even if psychiatric causes *could* be separated from effects, questions about causes are slippery slopes into eugenicist "solutions" for "problems" with the bodyminds of *certain* people.

This brings us back to the very beginning of the foundation of the systemic therapy field, which started as a movement of psychotherapists to de-pathologize the individual person, and a fervent insistence that everything is situated in the relational and contextual (Brodkin, 1980). The beliefs of these revolutionary therapists were wildly different from the medicalized views of psychiatry today. Some of these foundational figures believed that the collective phenomena called schizophrenia were *entirely* family dynamic-caused, taking the opposite extreme in this nature vs. nurture binary. Yet, we suggest that there is a nugget of wisdom held in this history of our field, wherein the nurture/social experiences of individuals are not dismissed in lieu of nature/neurobiology. Additionally, we do not deny that individual neurobiology plays part in – for example – experiencing perceptive phenomena that other individuals do not (i.e., hallucinations and hearing voices). Yet, we maintain that social experiences *strongly* shape (1) which voices one hears, (2) whether hearing voices is even considered a problem, and ultimately, (3) how disconnected one's perspective becomes from that of others when their perceptive experiences are culturally treated as cause to dismiss their knowledge entirely. In this sense, "mental illness" is *a world of experience*, and both nature and nurture are inseparable elements of that experience.

In light of these reflections, we sincerely ask the following question: How is the binary of mental disorder vs. health serving our clients whom we consider psychiatrically dis*abled* (e.g., by minority stressors, systemic ableism), how is it harming them, and is the result worth it? Additionally, how can we know which parts of our clients *are* them – versus which parts are "disordered" and might be externalized or cured – when clients *are* the result of their own experiences? Yergeau (2018) offers more on this point (italics added for emphasis):

> When one is schizophrenic, for example, her rhetorical actions are rendered less as symbolic actions and more as *biological motions*: schizophrenia causes the person to act. The schizophrenic person, in these constructions, *has no volition* – or whatever volition she has is tempered by the schizophrenia. In this regard, it's important to note that whatever the placeholder – whether schizophrenia, autism, depression, cerebral palsy, ADHD, bipolar – mental disability signals a kind of rhetorical *involuntariness*. Mental disability wields more agency than mentally disabled people… Involuntarity is a project of *dehumanization*.
>
> (p. 10)

To avoid playing into this style of dehumanization, we maintain that people do the best they can with what they have, whether their unique patterns of "doing" are labeled mentally disordered or not. Furthermore, we argue that the binary distinction between mental illness and health serves no one. A disability-informed iteration of psychotherapy must venture into uncharted territories, moving beyond the oversimplified dichotomy of sanity versus insanity, which has historically been used to create and exploit positions of power over psychotherapy clients. Thus, being curious and compassionate about the most vulnerable parts of *our own* bodyminds and internal discourses (rather than hiding or denying them under the guise of professionalism) is another avenue to dismantle the oppressive power of the traditional therapist-expert role. Indeed, it is likely that every client could find a therapist whose sense of reality was so different from theirs, they thought them insane and vice versa. As our field previously sought to do, we must champion a social/relational understanding of what our clients – who may or may not be labeled with disability and/or disorder – experience, and what to do about it. Given that we are *part of* the therapeutic relationship, this change starts with the internal work of unraveling these binaries *within ourselves* and exploring our relationships to the phenomena of impairment, disablement, and mental pathologization. In the following sections, we will introduce readers to the POTT framework and then offer an example how it may be utilized to facilitate this self-exploration toward a more disability-just therapy practice.

Person-of-the-Therapist Applications

Once therapists begin to recognize how processes of disablement impact themselves and their clients, they can more fully engage in the POTT applications that further support becoming a wounded healer for their clients who have been disabled. Aponte and Kissil's (2016) POTT guide focuses on three applications that enhance moment-by-moment engagement. *Self-knowledge* (having insight into one's own experiences), *self-access* (being in touch with one's experiences when conducting therapy), and *self-management* (using one's experiences to actively relate, assess, and respond with clients) are essential for facilitating effective use of self. In the paragraphs below, these applications are described in light of the concepts discussed earlier in this chapter. Finally, a case study illustrates each of these applications in action.

The building of self-knowledge is not a passive process. The POTT approach requires therapists to examine their intergenerational histories, family of origin experiences, and sociocultural positionalities *while* attending to the reactions that occur during this process. These reactions are then excavated for the purposes of understanding how we, influenced by our current social systems, are conditioned to hide our vulnerabilities as weaknesses. The idea that the pain, failings, and struggles that shape our personal experiences strengthen our therapeutic practices challenges the tendency to hide these matters from ourselves and others. The POTT model suggests that it is through examining and sharing ourselves that we learn the importance of our vulnerability. In turn, we can let go of the psychic energy required to contain our personal issues so that they cannot interfere with our work. Instead, therapists become free to examine personal vulnerabilities as an asset to guide our own process of relating to another person. This way of gaining self-knowledge parallels the aim of disability-just practice. Indeed, just as POTT asks therapists to reframe vulnerabilities as critical assets, clients can be asked to consider how the aspects of them that have been pathologized by society may be assets to themselves and others in their lives. In doing so, the therapist demonstrates a deep and fundamental respect for social diversity, as well as the importance of self-compassion for navigating spaces where differences are problematized. As recommended in sections above, if therapists can move toward embracing all aspects of their personhoods for the purposes of connecting with their clients, there is space for clients to do the same for the purposes of connecting with themselves and others.

Self-access requires that therapists not only know the aspects of themselves that can help them relate to their clients, but also draw on those aspects when relevant to therapy. In doing so, therapists must practice the internal process of connecting with their experiences while maintaining focus on the client and their presenting problems. This requires therapists to find ways of being selective and thoughtful about what experiences they access and when they access them in the context of therapy. When working with clients who have experiences of being disabled by society, it is important for therapists to consider how they, themselves, have sacrificed aspects of their personhoods to conform to standards or expectations that do not fit for them. That is, we have felt the push to "be normal" or "fit" to avoid isolation, judgement, and condemnation and, in doing so, have struggled to embrace our own imperfectness. It is these instances that can be accessed when the therapist aims to provide their clients with a unique experience that counters ableist values. When we, as therapists, can connect to the burden of having to fit ourselves into the binary structures existing in our social norms, we are pushed to create spaces where we welcome our clients by letting them be all of who they are with us.

Self-management allows for aspects of the therapist's personal experience to guide their practice with clients. It is through connecting that we can expand the ways in which we relate to our clients and understand their unique experiences. To embrace a disability-just stance, self-management can be used to cultivate humility and honesty on behalf of the therapist. We must ask if we are allowing ourselves to grow and change in response to our clients. Are we considering who they need in the therapy room today? Do we draw on the parts of ourselves that can offer them a refuge from normative performance (i.e., performing able-bodiedness, neurotypicality, and wellness) in our broader society? As therapists who are providing an environment where our clients can be themselves, a stance of humility is required. For example, what does a Deaf person notice that I, as a hearing therapist, may not? With an explicit stance of humility, therapists are managing themselves so that their clients have space to connect that is authentic to them. In sum, self-management is a stance that is maintained by the therapist for the purposes of countering experiences where clients are devalued instead of respected and appreciated for who they are.

Case Study

The following case study illustrates POTT applications within a Disability Justice framework. The clinical information for this case study was based on our (the authors') experiences working with clients who have been impacted by processes of disablement. As such, the case study is not reflective of one single client and, instead, is representative of themes that emerged across many cases. In organizing the material for this case study, we made certain that no identifying information was retained in the narrative below.

Eliseo (a 38-year-old, White-passing Hispanic American, straight, cisgender man) and Jane (a 37-year-old, White American, queer, cis woman) have been partnered for three years, and have lived together for two years. Eliseo reports no disabilities, and Jane is a wheelchair user and autistic. Eliseo works a full-time office job and is responsible for physical household labor, and Jane is paid a monthly disability check. Jane is often very vocal about her appreciation and gratitude for everything Eliseo does for their household. They experience conflict when Eliseo is tired from a long workday and wants some quiet, down time. In these moments, Jane expects them to spend some quality time together. Most of Jane's friends are online, so Eliseo is her only in-person close relationship. Eliseo has remarked that sometimes it can be overwhelming to "be on" all the time in the relationship. They said they have been arguing more frequently, which leaves them feeling hurt and helpless.

The therapist, Ali (a 30-year-old, South Asian-American, queer, cis man), sees this couple virtually. Ali has not considered himself disabled before, but often resonates with the experiences of autistic and ADHD friends and has sometimes wondered if these labels fit him too. In the first session, he finds himself readily identifying with Jane's experiences of being autistic (and queer) and wanting to learn more. He also readily connects with Eliseo's accounts of being a second-generation immigrant in the United States, and often feeling like an outsider in one's home country. Moreover, Ali notices how Jane feels shame for being disabled, and relies on Eliseo for love and social connection. He also recognizes how Eliseo both appreciates Jane for who she is and reassures her of this, while also struggling to empathize with her experience of disablement. Going into the second session, Ali is prepared to explore Jane's experience of being disabled within the relationship. The following is an excerpt from his second session with Jane and Eliseo.

Ali: How have things been this week?

Jane: *[Twirls her hair repeatedly] I'm exhausted after the day we had. Eliseo, would you be willing to tell him what happened?*

Eliseo: *[Nods] Sure. Jane has been trying to get a wheelchair through her disability insurance, and they have taken almost a year to accept it, even when she was eligible for a new one. The insurance is supposed to cover the wheelchair cost, but we ended up paying 50% of the price. And we just found out that they are not going to reimburse us.*

Ali: That's really awful news. How are you both feeling about it?

Jane: *They make it so hard to live in this country. How am I supposed to cover the wheelchair cost when they know I rely on my disability check? [Tears up] Eliseo has been covering the difference and it's not fair.*

Eliseo: *I don't mind doing that, Jane [moves closer to Jane and holds her hand]. I'm glad I can help, especially dealing with the insurance company.*

Jane: *I just feel like I'm broken – like I'm a burden. I know it's hard to live with me, and I'm afraid Eliseo will find someone better and leave [cries and covers her face with her hands]. I'm also not attractive enough and don't think I can please Eliseo sexually. It just seems like he is taking pity on me and will eventually get tired of it.*

Eliseo: *[Frowns and looks worried] Jane… I love you; I only want to be with you.*

Ali: *[Leans in and speaks softly] Jane, what makes you believe that you are a burden and hard to live with?*

Jane: *[Pauses] I was unwanted my whole life… My parents did not know how to care for me, and I had to mask my autism a lot to pretend that I was normal enough. Even then, no one wanted to be my friend. My parents didn't want to have people over because they were worried they'd be judged about me. In my previous relationships, partners did not want much to do with me besides having sex occasionally. I feel hurt all the time – I'm scared all the time. And nothing good seems to last in my life.*

During this session, Ali feels himself doubt whether he has the knowledge or ability to "fix" Jane's problem of social disablement without trying to fix *her*. In particular, he worries that no therapy training has prepared him to embrace that Jane is autistic without trying to "treat" it. For instance, he recalls that other therapists have often talked about teaching autistic clients "social skills," which mostly seem to aim at helping them pass as neurotypical from the perspective of others. Yet, Ali knows if that if a client was presenting with any other minoritized and stigmatizing way of being – much like, for himself, being a person of color in the United States and a queer person – he would not be trying to "change" those things about them but help them externalize their associated stigmas. Finally, Ali is unsure of how to help Jane feel better when the systemic disablement of her mobility impairment and neurological proclivities *is* devastating, and ableism *has been* pervasive throughout her life. He begins to blame himself for not knowing or learning more about these issues before working with this case.

In his POTT training, Ali is asked to lean into this feeling of inadequacy when working with a disabled client and explore what it means for him (self-knowledge). Ali remembers that when he was growing up, authority figures repeatedly told him that he had the potential to do better, and he was compared to others who were considered more "normal" or "successful" than him. These experiences instilled the message that he was not intrinsically worthy of love, and that he needed to push himself harder to meet the expectations of people around him. Ali begins to recognize that this feeling of unworthiness serves as a connection to Jane's experience of being disabled by society. He also begins to access his own assertive anger, wondering to himself: "Why have I internalized that something is wrong with me because I don't feel good about changing my client?" He holds these personal reflections consciously when going into the next session with Eliseo and Jane, preparing to rely on this self-knowledge to use "empathic conjecture" with Jane (Goldman et al., 2021). In other words, Ali begins drawing from his inner experience of feeling unworthy of love (self-access) to guess how Jane is feeling, and to help her access this part of herself in turn.

Ali: *Jane, during our last session you mentioned feeling like you are a burden in your relationship, and Eliseo responded by telling you that he loves you. I'm wondering – do you doubt that you're worthy of Eliseo's love as you already are?*

Jane: *Yes, I think so. It's hard to believe that anyone can love me, being this way. Everyone talks about having a partner who cooks them dinner when they come home from work, going out and buying them things, or just helping them do laundry or whatever. There are so many things I can't do on my own, let alone for Eliseo. [Looking downward] And I know he says he doesn't care, but I just can't believe him. Who wouldn't get tired of this life with me?*

Ali: *[Blocking Eliseo from reassuring Jane again] Eliseo, I love your instinct to reassure Jane that she's loved, but before you do, I have another question for her. [Turns toward Jane again] Jane, I want you to imagine I was your friend who was also in a wheelchair and autistic, coming to you with the same worry about being lovable. What would you say to me?*

Jane: *[Laughs] Well, I guess I'd say, "screw anyone who's made you feel unlovable for that in the past." And maybe I'd reassure them I love them too. But I guess it's different when it's me.*

Ali: Yeah? What's different about you?

Jane: *[Pauses] Maybe it feels like I should still be trying harder, I guess. Like even within the limits of what I* can *do, I'm still never doing enough. Like* I'm *not enough.*

Here, Ali remembers his own feeling that he did not know or learn enough about disability – that he wasn't a capable or good enough therapist – before working with Jane and Eliseo and observes the connection with what Jane just shared. He also remembers that, for him, what helped was having compassion for himself *in* the past and present, and understanding that he has internalized a lot of pressure from others to be more or different. From here, he helps Jane explore what happens when she feels like she's not enough, and to recognize that she is shaming herself for not working harder to be what she thinks other people want or expect from her. He also helps her attune to her younger self and notice her assertive anger that comes up on her own behalf, as well as the compassion she feels for that younger version of herself. To help Eliseo empathize more deeply with Jane, Ali asks him about his own experiences of being "not enough" for the people or world around him. Eliseo begins to share some of his personal history learning English as a second language during elementary school and being bullied by English-speaking peers for a time. Jane and Eliseo then begin to connect over their past experiences of feeling like they were not good enough and needing to be "fixed" or to do "better" in life.

After several months of therapy, and Jane increasingly embracing herself as a disabled person, she comes into session one day sharing her own personal success: she made a local friend (Carly) who is also a wheelchair user. Unlike Jane's experiences of being autistic, Ali does not have much experiential overlap with being in a wheelchair. Therefore, he suddenly recognizes at this moment that there may be things about Jane's new friendship that he cannot fully understand, nor connect with as easily. With this realization, he feels an insecurity and self-doubt creep up again, worrying that he might continue to miss things about Jane's experience because he is not in a wheelchair. He brings this up in his POTT training and is asked how other people are able to make him feel appreciated for what is *different* about him from them, rather than what is similar. Ali reflects on this and shares that he feels appreciated when other people listen, are curious about, and intrinsically value what is different about him, *because* it is different or new to them. He eventually identifies this as taking a stance of humility and curiosity when encountering difference from oneself within others. In the next session, Ali arrives ready to take up this stance (self-management) in response to Jane and her new friend's shared experiences.

Eliseo: *[Smiling and looking at Jane] Jane hung out with Carly again this week.*

Ali: *That's exciting news. How's that going for you, Jane?*

Jane: *It's still really fun! [Plays with her stim toy excitedly] We went around the neighborhood together this time. I've been nervous to go around outside without a buddy, so it's nice to have someone to do it with. And it's nice to do it with another wheelchair user.*

Ali: *[Smiling] How so?*

Jane: *Well, before I worried I was either holding people back and they were secretly mad at me for not going faster, or that they felt like they were there to babysit me. Eliseo doesn't make it a problem, but it is nice to not be "the person in the wheelchair" all the time, you know? Like, we're just two friends going down the street together and talking, who both happen to be disabled.*

Ali: *It sounds like you really feel like you belong when you're with her.*

Jane: *Yeah…I'm still getting used to that feeling. There was even this funny moment when a neighbor Eliseo and I are friendly with stopped us to say hi, and I realized that he was the only one standing in the interaction. Like,* he *looked like the odd one out. And I couldn't help but laugh to myself in that moment and be like, "is this what the normies feel like?" [Laughs] You* should have seen the look on his face when Carly did a wheelie spin. He did not expect it at all!

Conclusion

The case example of Ali, Jane, and Eliseo demonstrates how a POTT framework – particularly using one's vulnerabilities as a wounded healer when connecting with clients – can be especially powerful when working with disabled clients, who are often made to feel extremely vulnerable and that their vulnerabilities are "too much" for this world. Indeed, the more that we lean into our own vulnerabilities, make space for, and accept them (self-compassion), the more that we make space for our clients to do the same in our presences. While the whole world would benefit from this self-compassion, disabled people – who generally have less control over how much their efforts and energies are valued in our world – are among those who may benefit the most. However, we cannot ask our clients to take the risk of being self-compassionate in the face of a conditionally loving world without taking this risk on ourselves as therapists. Disability-just systemic therapy starts with defiantly choosing to unconditionally love *ourselves*, even as we hold ourselves accountable to transform and grow. Ali's work with Jane and Eliseo shows what beginning this inner POTT journey looks like on a singular case level. On a larger isomorphic scale, our willingness to take the risk of embracing our vulnerabilities across our careers and lives will create more space in the world for others to do the same, therein truly changing it inside out.

References

Aponte, H. J., & Kissil, K. (Eds.). (2016). *The person of the therapist training model: Mastering the use of self.*

Boszormenyi-Nagy, I. (1966). From family therapy to a psychology of relationships: Fictions of the individual and fictions of the family. *Comprehensive Psychiatry*, *7*(5), 408–423. https://doi.org/10.1016/S0010-440X(66)80070-6

Brault, M. W. (2008). *Americans with disabilities: 2005*. U.S. Department of Commerce. https://www2.census.gov/library/publications/2008/demo/p70-117.pdf

Brodkin, A. M. (1980). Family therapy: The making of a mental health movement. *American Journal of Orthopsychiatry*, *50*(1), 4–17. https://doi.org/10.1111/j.1939-0025.1980.tb03258.x

Butler, J. (1990). *Gender trouble: Feminism and the subversion of identity*. Routledge.

Dychtwald, K. (1986). *Bodymind*. J.P. Tarcher; Distributed by St. Martin's Press.

Goldman, R. N., Vaz, A., & Rousmaniere, T. (2021). Empathic conjectures. In *Deliberate practice in emotion-focused therapy* (pp. 93–101). American Psychological Association. https://www.jstor.org/stable/j.ctv1npx3pz.14

Haraway, D. J. (2016). *Staying with the trouble: Making kin in the Chthulucene*. Duke University Press.

Latour, B. (1993). *We have never been modern* (3. print.). Harvard University Press.

Oliver, M. (1990, July 23). *The individual and social models of disability*. Joint Workshop of the Living Options Group and the Research Unit of the Royal College of Physicians.

Saussure, F. (2005). *Course in general linguistics* (C. Bally, Ed.; Nachdr.). McGraw-Hill.

Sheffer, E. (2018). *Asperger's children: The origins of autism in Nazi Vienna* (First edition). W.W. Norton & Company.

Stryker, S. (2017). *Transgender history: The roots of today's revolution* (Second edition). Seal Press.

Union of the Physically Impaired Against Segregation & The Disability Alliance. (1976). *Fundamental principles of disability* (M. Priestley, Ed.). https://disability-studies.leeds.ac.uk/wp-content/uploads/sites/40/library/UPIAS-fundamental-principles.pdf

Vision Impact Institute. (2012). *The social and economic impact of poor vision* [White paper]. Vision Impact Institute.

Walker, N. (2021). *Neuroqueer heresies: Notes on the neurodiversity paradigm, autistic empowerment, and postnormal possibilities*. Autonomous Press.

Wolf-Meyer, M. J. (2020). *Unraveling: Remaking personhood in a neurodiverse age*. University of Minnesota Press.

Yergeau, M. (2018). *Authoring autism: On rhetoric and neurological queerness*. Duke University Press.

RESOURCES FOR EDUCATORS, CLINICIANS, AND ADVOCATES

In this section, you'll find a curated list of resources to support and strengthen disability-affirmative care. These materials have been contributed or vetted by disabled community members and the contributors of this handbook. This compilation also draws from the National Council on Disability (NCD), an independent federal agency that advises the president, congress, and executive branch agencies on disability policy. Please note that this is not an exhaustive list, and readers are encouraged to visit each source directly to ensure they are accessing the most current and updated versions, as many of these resources are revised regularly.

Civil Rights

1 *A Guide to Disability Rights Laws* (https://www.ada.gov/resources/disability-rights-guide/).

- This guide, a publication of the U.S. Department of Justice, provides summaries of all major disability rights laws and appropriate federal contact information for more information.

2 *Americans with Disabilities Act (ADA)* (https://www.ada.gov/index.html).

- This U.S. Department of Justice website contains valuable information regarding ADA standards, technical assistance, new or proposed regulations, an ADA Help Line, a toolkit for state and local governments, and other valuable information.
- ADA Information Line (800) 514-0301 (Voice) (800) 514-0383 (TTY)

3 *Employment Resource Hub* (https://adata.org/employment-resource-hub)
4 *Architectural Barriers Act* (https://www.access-board.gov/aba/)

5. *Civil Rights of Institutionalized Persons* (https://www.justice.gov/crt/civil-rights-institutionalized-persons)
6. *Rehabilitation Act* (https://www.dol.gov/agencies/oasam/centers-offices/civil-rights-center/statutes/section-504-rehabilitation-act-of-1973)
7. *Voting and Poll Place Accessibility* (https://www.ada.gov/topics/voting/)
8. *ADA Standards for Accessible Design* (https://www.ada.gov/law-and-regs/design-standards/)

    - The ADA mandates that buildings, including therapy facilities, must be accessible to disabled people. This includes providing equal access to services, making reasonable modifications to policies and procedures, and ensuring effective communication.

Pedagogical and Training Resources

1. *Implicit Association Test* (IAT) (https://implicit.harvard.edu/implicit/takeatest.html)

    - The IAT, developed by Harvard University measures unconscious associations between concepts, including those related to disability.

2. A disability-centered, sample curriculum can be found in Chapter 15 of this book, authored by Dr. Brittany A. Williams, Dr. Derek, X. Seward, & Kahyen Shin
3. *Working with Disability across the Counseling Professions* (British Association for Counseling and Psychotherapy) (https://www.bacp.co.uk/media/10780/bacp-working-with-disability-gpacp007-feb-21.pdf)
4. *Compliance Training Group* (https://compliancetraininggroup.com/2021/12/01/disability-bias-training/)

    - This organization provides training programs aimed at reducing disability bias in employment settings, such as graduate programs.

5. *Spokz People* (https://spokzpeople.org.uk/)

    - Cofounded by Mel Halacre, this UK-based social enterprise offers live online training and coaching to individuals, businesses, and universities on disability-affirmative mental health care. They also offer therapist-led forums, and live group consultations.

6. The Anti-Discrimination Focus (#TADF) (https://www.tadf.uk/)

    - A UK-based organization that offers numerous online courses for therapists and students working with disability.

7. *Teaching Disability: Practical Activities for In-Class and Homework*, Olkin, 2021.

    - An essential resource for educators seeking to move beyond superficial inclusion of disability in their syllabi.

8 "Providing Culturally Competent Supervision to Trainees with Disabilities in Rehabilitation Settings", Andrews et al., 2013.
9 *The Social Psychology of Disability*, Dunn, 2014.

- An essential text to use in undergraduate and graduate training programs that help understand the communication and psychological patterns between disabled and non-disabled individuals.

10 *Can you Hold the Door for Me: Including Disability in Diversity*, Olkin, 2002.

- An article intended to train graduate students on accessibility supporting disabled students.

11 *The Student voice: Recommendations for Supporting the Success of Graduate Students with Disabilities in Online Courses*, Anderson et al., 2022.
12 *10 Tips for Creating Accessible Course Content*, University of North Georgia (https://ung.edu/student-accessibility-services/resources-and-links/faculty-information/10-tips-for-creating-accessible-course-content.php)
13 *Creating an Accessible Course*, Cornell University (https://sds.cornell.edu/resources/faculty-staff/universal-design-instruction)
14 *Supervising Trainees with Disabilities*, American Psychological Association (https://www.apa.org/pi/disability/resources/supervising-trainees)
15 Various organizations provide regular training sessions, such as the Job Accommodation Network (JAN), the Association of University Centers on Disabilities (AUCD), and Coursera (https://www.coursera.org/learn/disability-inclusion-education)

Clinical Resources

1 *What psychotherapists Should Know about Disability*, Olkin, 1999.
2 *APA Guidelines for Assessment and Intervention with Persons with Disabilities* (2014) https://www.apa.org/about/policy/guidelines-assessment-intervention-disabilities.`pdf
3 *Disability Justice: An Audit Tool* (Leah Lakshmi Piepzna-Samarasinha wrote this tool, envisioned by Stacey Park Milbern to help organizations assess their commitment to disability justice, and strengthen as necessary)
4 Creating Accessible Therapy Offices: https://www.adapacific.org/healthcare-provider-responsibilities-under-the-ada/
5 *Creating Accessible Environments for People with Disabilities*, Pierce, 2020, https://cdn.ymaws.com/www.csinet.org/resource/resmgr/counselors_corner/Accessible_Environments.pdf
6 "*Resilience, Coping, & Disability: The Development of a Resilience Intervention*", Stuntzner & Hartley, 2024.

7 Preliminary Therapy Considerations for:

- **ADHD:** "Smart but Scattered: The Revolutionary 'Executive Skills' Approach to Helping Kids Reach Their Potential", Dawson & Guare, 2009; "Taking Charge of Adult ADHD", Barkley, 2010; "Cognitive-Behavioral Therapy for Adult ADHD: An Integrative Psychosocial and Medical Approach", Ramsay & Rostain, 2015.
- **Autism:** *The Gold Standard Fallacy of ABA: A Reference Guide for Therapists, Educators, & Parents*, Roberts, 2024; *Autism and Independence: Assessments and Interventions to Prepare Teens for Adult Life*, Marston, 2019; *Adapting Psychological Therapies for Autism - Therapist Experience, Skills and Confidence*, Cooper et al., 2018.
- **Blind/Low-Vision Clients:** A Guide to Counselling the Blind, Taylor, 2020.
- **Deaf/Hard-of-Hearing Clients** : *Treatment of Deaf Clients: Ethical Considerations for Professionals in Psychology*, Bones, 2015; *Culturally Affirmative Psychotherapy with Deaf Persons*, Glickman & Harvey, 1996.
- Therapy for Deaf Clients: *National Deaf Therapy*, https://nationaldeaftherapy.com/
- **ASLInterpretersforTherapists:**https://inclusiveasl.com/industries/mental-health-accessibility-services/; https://jeenie.com
- **Clients impacted by Mobility-Orthopedic impairments** *Psychotherapy Experiences of U.S. Adults with Physical Disabilities: Recommendations for Affirmative Practice*, Conner et al., 2023.
- **Traumatic Brain Injury** *Psychotherapy after Brain Injury: Principles and Techniques*, Klonoff, 2010; *Women Living with Traumatic Brain Injury: Social Isolation, Emotional Functioning and Implications for Psychotherapy*, Mukherjee et al., 2014.
- **Chronic Illness and Pain:** *Psychosocial Adaptation to Chronic Illness and Disability: A Primer for Counselors*, Livneh & Antonak, 2005.

Language, Terminology, and Etiquette

1 *What Psychotherapists Should Know about Disability*, Olkin, 1999.

- In Chapter 14, titled *Etiquette with Clients with Disabilities*, Dr. Olkin outlines ten general rules and provides practical guidance for clinicians interacting with disabled clients.

2 APA Style guide when writing about disability: apastyle.apa.org/style-grammar-guidelines/bias-free-language/disability

3 APA Inclusive Language Guide: https://www.apa.org/about/apa/equity-diversity-inclusion/language-guidelines

4 Standford University's Disability Language Guide: https://disability.stanford.edu/sites/g/files/sbiybj26391/files/media/file/disability-language-guide-stanford_1.pdf

Disability Justice, Lived Experiences, and Memoirs

1 *Nothing About Us Without Us*, James I. Charlton, 1998
2 Skin, Tooth, and Bone: The Basis of Movement is Our People, Sins Invalid, 2019
3 *Disability Visibility*, Alice Wong, 2020
4 *Demystifying Disability*, Emily Ladau, 2021
5 *The Anti-Ableist Manifesto*, Tiffany Yu, 2020
6 *Being Heumann*, Judith Heumann, Kristen Joiner, 2020
7 *Sitting Pretty*, Rebekah Taussig, 2020
8 *Leaving Evidence*, An ongoing blog by renowned advocate Mia Mingus, since 2006
9 *TourettesHero*, An ongoing blog by Jess Thom, since 2010

INDEX

Note: **Bold** page numbers refer to tables and *italic* page numbers refer to figures.

www.ingramcontent.com/pod-product-compliance
Ingram Content Group UK Ltd.
Pitfield, Milton Keynes, MK11 3LW, UK
UKHW022348190926
475702UK00015B/2170
9781032423869